BLUEPRINTS
CARDIOLOGY

Second Edition

For every step of your medical career,
look for all the books in the *Blueprints* series

Perfect for clerkship and board review!

Blueprints Cardiology, 2nd edition

Blueprints Emergency Medicine, 2nd edition

Blueprints Family Medicine, 2nd edition

Blueprints Medicine, 3rd edition

Blueprints Neurology, 2nd edition

Blueprints Obstetrics & Gynecology, 3rd edition

Blueprints Pediatrics, 3rd edition

Blueprints Psychiatry, 3rd edition

Blueprints Radiology, 2nd edition

Blueprints Surgery, 3rd edition

Visit www.blackwellmedstudent.com to see all the great
Blueprints:

Blueprints Notes & Cases

Blueprints Clinical Cases

Blueprints Pockets

Blueprints Step 2 Q&A

Blueprints USMLE Step 2 CS

Blueprints Step 3 Q&A

Blueprints Computer-Based Case Simulation Review:
USMLE Step 3

Blueprints Clinical Procedures

BLUEPRINTS
CARDIOLOGY

Second Edition

Editor

Eric H. Awtry, MD, FACC
Director of Education, Cardiology
Boston Medical Center
Assistant Professor of Medicine
Boston University School of Medicine
Boston, Massachusetts

Authors

Cathy Jeon, MD
Teaching Fellow in Medicine
Boston University School of Medicine
Fellow in Cardiology
Boston Medical Center
Boston, Massachusetts

Molly G. Ware, MD
Teaching Fellow in Medicine
Boston University School of Medicine
Fellow in Cardiology
Boston Medical Center
Boston, Massachusetts

Faculty Advisor

Joseph Loscalzo, MD, PhD
Wade Professor and Chair
Department of Medicine
Director, Whitaker Cardiovascular Institute
Boston University School of Medicine
Boston, Massachusetts

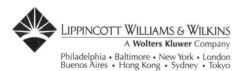
LIPPINCOTT WILLIAMS & WILKINS
A **Wolters Kluwer** Company
Philadelphia • Baltimore • New York • London
Buenos Aires • Hong Kong • Sydney • Tokyo

Copyright © 2006 by Eric H. Awtry, MD

351 West Camden Street
Baltimore, Maryland 21201-2436 USA

530 Walnut Street
Philadelphia, Pennsylvania 19106-3621 USA

ISBN-13: 978-1-4051-0464-7
ISBN-10: 1-4051-0464-3

Library of Congress Cataloging-in-Publication Data

Blueprints cardiology / editor, Eric H. Awtry; authors, Cathy Jeon, Molly G. Ware.—2nd ed.
 p. ; cm.
Rev. ed. of: Blueprints in cardiology / editor, Eric H. Awtry ; authors, Arjun V. Gururaj . . . [et al.]. c2003.
Includes index.
ISBN-13: 978-1-4051-0464-7 (pbk. : alk. paper)
ISBN-10: 1-4051-0464-3 (pbk. : alk. paper) 1. Heart—Diseases—Outlines, syllabi, etc. 2. Cardiology—Outlines, syllabi, etc. I. Awtry, Eric. II. Jeon, Cathy. III. Ware, Molly G. V. Blueprints in cardiology. IV. Title: Cardiology.
[DNLM: 1. Heart Diseases—Handbooks. 2. Cardiology—Handbooks. WG 39 B658 2006]
RC682.B558   2006
616.1´2—dc22

                                              2005011428

A catalogue record for this title is available from the British Library

Editor: Donna Balado
Managing Editor: Kathleen Scogna
Marketing Manager: Emilie Linkins

To purchase additional copies of this book call our customer service department at (800) 638-3030 or fax orders to (301) 824-7390. International customers should call (301) 714-2324.

Visit *Lippincott Williams & Wilkins on the Internet: http://www.lww.com*. Lippincott Williams & Wilkins customer service representatives are available from 8:30 am to 6:00 pm, EST, Monday through Friday, for telephone access.

                                                        07 08
                                          3 4 5 6 7 8 9 10

Dedication

To the students of Boston University School of Medicine and the residents and staff of the Department of Medicine at Boston Medical Center whose commitment, enthusiasm, and collegiality have created a superb learning environment.

C. J.
M. W
E. A.
J. L.

Contents

Contributors to the first edition ix
Reviewers x
Preface xiii
Acknowledgments xiv
Abbreviations xv

PART ONE: HISTORY & PHYSICAL EXAMINATION 1

1   History 2
2   Physical Examination of the Cardiovascular System 9

PART TWO: DIAGNOSTIC MODALITIES 15

3   The Electrocardiogram 16
4   Stress Testing 21
5   Echocardiography 26
6   Cardiac Catheterization 29
7   Diagnostic Modalities for Arrhythmias 34
8   Other Imaging Modalities 37

PART THREE: CORONARY ARTERY DISEASE 41

9   Coronary Artery Disease—Pathophysiology 42
10   Dyslipidemia 46
11   Chronic Stable Angina 51
12   Unstable Angina and Non-ST-Elevation Myocardial Infarction 55
13   ST-Elevation Myocardial Infarction 59
14   Complications of Myocardial Infarction 64

PART FOUR: HEART FAILURE 69

15   Cardiovascular Hemodynamics 70
16   Mechanisms of Heart Failure 73
17   Clinical Manifestations and Treatment of Heart Failure 76
18   Myocarditis 83
19   The Cardiomyopathies 85

PART FIVE: ARRHYTHMIAS 89

20 Mechanisms of Arrhythmogenesis 90

21 Tachyarrhythmias 93

22 Bradyarrhythmias (Bradycardia and Heart Block) 99

23 Syncope 103

24 Sudden Cardiac Death 107

25 Pacemakers and Implantable Cardioverter-Defibrillators 110

PART SIX: VALVULAR HEART DISEASE 113

26 Rheumatic Fever 114

27 Disorders of the Aortic Valve 117

28 Disorders of the Mitral Valve 121

29 Infective Endocarditis 125

30 Prosthetic Heart Valves 130

PART SEVEN: PERICARDIAL DISEASES 135

31 Pericarditis 136

32 Cardiac Tamponade 139

33 Constrictive Pericarditis 142

PART EIGHT: VASCULAR DISEASES 145

34 Hypertension 146

35 Peripheral Arterial Disorders 150

36 Diseases of the Aorta 154

37 Carotid Arterial Disease 160

38 Deep Venous Thrombosis and Pulmonary Embolic Disease 163

39 Pulmonary Hypertension 167

PART NINE: OTHER IMPORTANT CARDIAC CONDITIONS 171

40 Preoperative Cardiac Evaluation 172

41 Congenital Heart Disease 176

42 Pregnancy and Cardiovascular Disease 181

43 Traumatic Heart Disease 184

44 Cardiac Tumors 187

Questions 189

Answers 205

Appendix A: Evidence-Based Resources 219

Appendix B: Electrocardiograms 224

Appendix C: Commonly Used Cardiovascular Medications 244

Index 247

Contributors to the first edition

Arjun V. Gururaj, MD
Teaching Fellow in Internal Medicine
Boston University School of Medicine
Fellow in Electrophysiology
Division of Cardiology
Boston Medical Center
Boston, Massachusetts

Melanie Maytin, MD
Teaching Fellow in Medicine
Boston University School of Medicine
Fellow, Section of Cardiology
Boston Medical Center
Boston, Massachusetts

Michael W. Tsang, MD
Teaching Fellow in Medicine
Boston University School of Medicine
Fellow, Section of Cardiology
Boston Medical Center
Boston, Massachusetts

Benoy J. Zachariah, MD, MRCP
Teaching Fellow in Medicine
Boston University School of Medicine
Clinical Fellow in Interventional Cardiology
Boston Medical Center
Boston, Massachusetts

Reviewers

Jaime Aagaard, MD
Class of 2004
University of New Mexico
Albuquerque, New Mexico

Siddharth Agarwal, MD
Class of 2004
Boston University School of Medicine
Boston, Massachusetts

Jaspal Singh Ahluwalia
Class of 2006
Ohio State University
Columbus, Ohio

Jessica Brooks Anderson, MD
Class of 2004
Resident, Internal Medicine and Pediatrics
University of Texas Medical Branch, Galveston
Galveston, Texas

Alexander L. Ayzengart, MD
Resident in General Surgery
University of California San Francisco
San Francisco, California

Simin Bahrami
Class of 2005
David Geffen School of Medicine, UCLA
Los Angeles, California

Kara M. Barnett
Class of 2005
Washington University School of Medicine
St. Louis, Missouri

Kenneth Bryant, MD
Intern
University of Alabama Hospital
Birmingham, Alabama

Christian Clark, MD
PGY-2, Internal Medicine
Medical University of South Carolina
Charleston, South Carolina

Alexis Dang, MD
Orthopaedic Surgery Resident, University of California, San Francisco
Class of 2004, University of California, San Francisco
San Francisco, California

Sarah Davis
Class of 2005
Drexel University College of Medicine
Philadelphia, Pennsylvania

David Brian Feig, MD
Resident Physician
Department of Family Medicine
University of Michigan Health System
Ann Arbor, Michigan

Amir A. Ghaferi
Class of 2005
Johns Hopkins School of Medicine
Baltimore, Maryland

Karen Goldstein, MD
Class of 2004
Duke University School of Medicine
Durham, North Carolina

Carla Keirns, MD, PhD
Resident, Internal Medicine
Hospital of the University of Pennsylvania
Philadelphia, Pennsylvania

Helen J. Kim, MD
Intern
Medical College of Virginia
Richmond, Virginia

Larissa Lee
Class of 2005
Harvard Medical School
Boston, Massachusetts

Anil Nair, MD
Class of 2004
University of Missouri-Kansas City School of Medicine
Kansas City, Missouri

Sachin S. Parikh, MD
PGY-1, Department of Internal Medicine
University of Michigan Hospitals
Ann Arbor, Michigan

Victor Rodriguez, MD, MS
Resident in Internal Medicine
Yale University School of Medicine
Bridgeport Hospital
Bridgeport, Connecticut

David E. Ruchelsman, MD
Resident, Department of Orthopaedic Surgery
NYU-Hospital for Joint Diseases Orthopaedic Institute
New York, New York

Jennifer Shane
Second year student
Physician Assistant Program
University of Oklahoma Health Science Center
Oklahoma City, Oklahoma

Hogan Shy, MD
Intern, PGY-2
Internal Medicine
Oregon Health and Sciences University
Portland, Oregon

Arleigh Trainor, MD
Emergency Medicine Resident
Hennepin County Medical Center
Minneapolis, Minnesota

Derek Wayman, MD
PGY-2
Rapid City Regional Health Family Practice Residency Clinic
Rapid City, South Dakota

Vivian Yu, MD
Resident, Otolaryngology
University of Minnesota
Minneapolis, Minnesota

Preface

In 1997, the first five books in the **Blueprints** series were published as board review for medical students, interns, and residents who wanted high-yield, accurate clinical content for USMLE Steps 2 & 3. Nearly a decade later, the **Blueprints** brand has expanded into high-quality, trusted resources covering the broad range of clinical topics studied by medical students and residents during their primary, specialty, and subspecialty rotations.

The **Blueprints** were conceived as a study aid created by students, for students. In keeping with this concept, the editors of the current edition of the **Blueprints** books have recruited resident contributors to ensure that the series continues to offer the information and the approach that made the original **Blueprints** a success.

Now in their second edition, each of the five specialty **Blueprints**—**Blueprints** *Emergency Medicine*, **Blueprints** *Family Medicine*, **Blueprints** *Neurology*, **Blueprints** *Cardiology*, and **Blueprints** *Radiology*—have been completely revised and updated to bring you the most current treatment and management strategies. The feedback we have received from our readers has been tremendously helpful in guiding the editorial direction of the second edition. We are grateful to the hundreds of medical students and residents who have responded with in-depth comments and highly detailed observations.

Each book has been thoroughly reviewed and revised accordingly, with new features included across the series. An evidence-based resource section has been added to provide current and classic references for each chapter, and an increased number of current board-format questions with detailed explanations for correct and incorrect answer options are included in each book. All revisions to the **Blueprints** series have been made in order to offer you the most concise, comprehensive, and cost-effective information available.

Our readers report that **Blueprints** are useful for every step of their medical career—from their clerkship rotations and subinternships to a board review for USMLE Steps 2 & 3. Residents studying for USMLE Step 3 often use the books for reviewing areas that were not their specialty. Students from a wide variety of health care specialties, including those in physician assistant, nurse practitioner, and osteopathic programs, use **Blueprints** either as a course companion or to review for their licensure examinations.

However you use **Blueprints**, we hope that you find the books in the series informative and useful. Your feedback and suggestions are essential to our continued success. Please send any comments you may have about this or any book in the **Blueprints** series to medfeedback@bos.blackwellpublishing.com.

Thank you for your willingness to share your opinions, offer constructive feedback, and to support our products.

The Publisher
Blackwell Publishing, Inc.

Acknowledgments

We would like to acknowledge and thank the authors of the first edition of Blueprints in Cardiology: Arjun Gururaj, Melanie Maytin, Michael Tsang, and Benoy Zachariah. Their contributions were invaluable and provided the framework for the current edition.

C. J.
M. W
E. A.
J. L.

Abbreviations

2D	two-dimensional
3D	three-dimensional
5-HIAA	5-hydroxyindoleacetic acid
A_2	aortic component of the second heart sound
ABE	acute bacterial endocarditis
ABI	ankle-brachial index
ACE	angiotensin-converting enzyme
ACE-I	ACE inhibitor
ACS	acute coronary syndrome
ADLs	activities of daily living
ADP	adenosine 5'-diphosphate
AF	atrial fibrillation
AI	aortic insufficiency
AIVR	accelerated idioventricular rhythm
AMI	acute myocardial infarction
AP	action potential
apo C-II	apolipoprotein C-II
AR	aortic regurgitation
ARB	angiotensin receptor blocker
AS	aortic stenosis
ASD	atrial septal defect
ASH	asymmetric septal hypertrophy
ASO	antistreptolysin O
ATP III	Adult Treatment Panel III
AV	aortic valve, atrioventricular
AVNRT	atrioventricular nodal reentrant tachycardia
AVRT	atrioventricular reentrant tachycardia
BNP	B-type natriuretic peptide
BP	blood pressure
BPM	beats per minute
BPV	biological prosthetic valve
BSA	body surface area
BUN	blood urea nitrogen
CABG	coronary artery bypass graft
CAD	coronary artery disease
cAMP	cyclic adenosine monophosphate
CBC	complete blood count
CCB	calcium channel blocker
CCU	coronary care unit
CEA	carotid endarterectomy
cGMP	cyclic guanosine monophosphate
CHB	complete heart block
CHD	coronary heart disease, congenital heart disease
CHF	congestive heart failure
CI	cardiac index
CK	creatinine kinase
CK-MB	creatine kinase MB isoenzyme
CMP	cardiomyopathy
CNS	central nervous system
CO	cardiac output
COPD	chronic obstructive pulmonary disease
COX-2	cyclooxygenase-2
CPET	cardiopulmonary exercise testing
CPK	creatine phosphokinase
CPR	cardiopulmonary resuscitation
CRP	C-reactive protein
CSM	carotid sinus massage
CSS	carotid sinus sensitivity
CT	computed tomography
CTPA	computed tomography of the pulmonary arteries with IV contrast
CVA	cerebrovascular accident
CVD	cerebrovascular disease
CXR	chest x-ray
DBP	diastolic blood pressure
DC	direct current
DCM	dilated cardiomyopathy
DM	diabetes mellitus
DVT	deep venous thrombosis
EBCT	electron-beam computed tomography
EBV	Epstein-Barr virus
ECG	electrocardiogram
ED	emergency department
EEG	electroencephalogram
EF	ejection fraction
ELISA	enzyme-linked immunosorbent assay
EMS	emergency medical services
EPS	electrophysiologic study
ESR	erythrocyte sedimentation rate
ETT	exercise tolerance test

FBS	fasting blood sugar	LMCA	left main coronary artery
GERD	gastroesophageal reflux disease	LMWH	low-molecular-weight heparin
GI	gastrointestinal	Lp(a)	lipoprotein (a)
GP IIB/IIIA	platelet glycoprotein IIB-IIIA inhibitor	LPL	lipoprotein lipase
HACEK	*Haemophilus parainfluenzae, Haemophilus aphrophilus, Actinobacillus actinomycetemcomitans, Cardiobacterium hominis, Eikenella corrodens,* and *Kingella kingae*	LSB	left sternal border
		LV	left ventricle
		LVEDP	left ventricular end-diastolic pressure
		LVEF	left-ventricular ejection fraction
		LVH	left ventricular hypertrophy
		LVOT	left ventricular outflow tract
HA1c	hemoglobin A1c	MAO	monoamine oxidase
HB	heart block	MAP	mean arterial pressure
HCM	hypertrophic cardiomyopathy	MAT	multifocal atrial tachycardia
HCTZ	hydrochlorothiazide	METs	metabolic equivalents
HDL	high-density lipoprotein	MI	myocardial infarction
HDLc	high-density-lipoprotein cholesterol	MPV	mechanical prosthetic valve
HF	heart failure	MR	mitral regurgitation
HIDA	hydroxyiminodiacetic acid	MRA	magnetic resonance angiography
HIV	human immunodeficiency virus	MRI	magnetic resonance imaging
HJR	hepatojugular reflux	MS	mitral stenosis
HOCM	hypertrophic obstructive cardiomyopathy	MSC	midsystolic click
		MUGA	multiple gated acquisition
HR	heart rate	MV	mitral valve
HSM	holosystolic murmur	MVA	mitral valve area
HTN	hypertension	MVO_2	myocardial oxygen demand
I	iodine	MVP	mitral valve prolapse
IABP	intraaortic balloon pump	NCEP	National Cholesterol Education Program
ICD	implantable cardioverter-defibrillator		
ICP	intracranial pressure	NPV	negative predictive value
ICS	intercostal space	NSAID	nonsteroidal anti-inflammatory drug
ICU	intensive care unit	NSR	normal sinus rhythm
IDL	intermediate-density lipoprotein	NSTEMI	non-ST-elevation myocardial infarction
IE	infective endocarditis		
IHSS	idiopathic hypertrophic subaortic stenosis	NSVT	nonsustained ventricular tachycardia
		NVE	native valve endocarditis
IMI	inferior myocardial infarction	NYHA	New York Heart Association
INR	international normalized ratio	OS	opening snap
IV NTG	intravenous nitroglycerin	P_2	pulmonic component of the second heart sound
IVC	inferior vena cava		
IVUS	intravenous ultrasound	PA	pulmonary artery
JNC-7	Seventh Report of the Joint National Committee on Prevention, Detection, Evaluation, and Treatment of High Blood Pressure	PAC	premature atrial complex
		PAD	peripheral arterial disease
		PCI	percutaneous coronary intervention
		PCN	penicillin
JVP	jugular venous pressure	PCWP	pulmonary capillary wedge pressure
LA	left atrium	PDA	patent ductus arteriosus, posterior descending artery
LAD	left anterior descending (artery)		
LBBB	left bundle branch block	PE	pulmonary embolism
LCx	left circumflex (artery)	PFT	pulmonary function test
LDL	low-density lipoprotein	PLA	posterolateral artery
LDLc	low-density-lipoprotein cholesterol	PMI	point of maximal impulse
LHC	left heart catheterization	PND	paroxysmal nocturnal dyspnea

PPD	purified protein derivative (test for TB)	SEM	systolic ejection murmur
PPH	primary pulmonary hypertension	SIDS	sudden infant death syndrome
PPV	positive predictive value	SL NTG	sublingual nitroglycerin
PS	pulmonic stenosis	SLE	systemic lupus erythematosus
PTA	percutaneous transluminal angioplasty	SND	sinus node dysfunction
		SPH	secondary pulmonary hypertension
PTCA	percutaneous transluminal coronary angioplasty	SSS	sick sinus syndrome
		STE	ST elevation (MI)
PTT	partial thromboplastin time	STEMI	ST-elevation myocardial infarction
PV	pulmonic valve	SV	stroke volume
PVC	premature ventricular contractions	SVR	systemic vascular resistance
Qp	pulmonary blood flow	SVT	supraventricular tachycardia
Qs	systemic blood flow	TAO	thromboangiitis obliterans
PVE	prosthetic valve endocarditis	TB	tuberculosis
PVR	pulmonary vascular resistance	TEE	transesophageal echocardiography
RA	right atrium	TG	triglycerides
RBBB	right bundle branch block	TIA	transient ischemic attack
RCA	right coronary artery	TLC	therapeutic lifestyle changes
RCM	restrictive cardiomyopathy	TMR	transmyocardial laser revascularization
RF	radiofrequency, rheumatic fever		
RFA	radiofrequency ablation	TOF	tetralogy of Fallot
RHC	right heart catheterization	TPA	tissue plasminogen activator
RHD	rheumatic heart disease	TR	tricuspid regurgitation
RIND	reversible ischemic neurologic deficit	TSH	thyroid-stimulating hormone
RPE	right pleural effusion	TTE	transthoracic echocardiography
RV	right ventricle	TV	tricuspid valve
RVEF	right ventricular ejection fraction	UA	unstable angina
RVG	radionuclide ventriculography	V/Q	ventilation/perfusion
RVH	right ventricular hypertrophy	VA	ventriculoatrial
RVI	right ventricular infarction	VAD	ventricular assist device
S_1	first heart sound	VDRL	Venereal Disease Research Laboratory (test)
S_2	second heart sound		
S_3	third heart sound	VF	ventricular fibrillation
S_4	fourth heart sound	VLDL	very low density lipoprotein
SA	sinoatrial	VPC	ventricular premature complex
SB	sternal border	VSD	ventricular septal defect
SBE	subacute bacterial endocarditis	VT	ventricular tachycardia
SBP	systolic blood pressure	VTE	venous thromboembolism
SCD	sudden cardiac death	WPW	Wolff-Parkinson-White syndrome

Part One

History & Physical Examination

1

The History

Despite major innovations in diagnostic technology and advances in medical therapy, a well-performed history and physical examination remains the cornerstone of good patient care. A thorough evaluation yields important clues about a patient's illness, helps to direct further diagnostic testing and therapy, and gives the physician an opportunity to establish rapport with the patient; strong physician-patient relationships establish trust and help to ensure compliance with treatment regimens. This chapter and the next provide an overview of important features of the history and physical examination of patients with cardiac diseases. Subsequent chapters provide specific details of historic and physical findings in particular cardiac disorders.

The cardinal symptoms of heart disease include chest pain, dyspnea, and palpitations. A thorough history of each symptom includes information regarding symptom duration, frequency, quality, severity, aggravating or alleviating factors, and associated symptoms. With regard to chest pain, location and radiation are also important features.

CHEST PAIN

◼ CLINICAL MANIFESTATIONS

History

Angina, the cardinal symptom of coronary artery disease (CAD), results from inadequate oxygen delivery to the myocardium. It is usually an uncomfortable sensation rather than a pain and may be described as:

- An ache
- Indigestion
- Constriction
- Heartburn
- A choking sensation
- Pressure

The sensation is generally substernal in location but may radiate or localize to the precordium, neck, jaw, shoulders, arms, or epigastrium. Patients with angina often use a clenched fist to indicate the site of discomfort (Levine's sign). Anginal pain is generally triggered by exertion and relieved by rest; it resolves more rapidly (within 1 to 5 minutes) with sublingual nitroglycerin. Other precipitating factors include cold weather, walking on an incline, emotional upset, fright, and the postprandial state. Occasionally it may occur spontaneously in the early morning hours.

Anginal chest pain may occur in several patterns:

- **Stable angina** is angina that occurs in a well-defined, reproducible pattern, usually on exertion.
- **Unstable angina** is angina that is new, occurs at rest, or occurs more frequently than had been usual.
- The pain of a **myocardial infarction** (MI) is usually more intense and longer-lasting than that of angina; it radiates more widely and is often accompanied by dyspnea, diaphoresis, palpitations, nausea, and/or vomiting.

Importantly, many patients, especially diabetics, do not have typical anginal chest pain during an ischemic episode or MI. Rather, they may present with atypical chest pain, restlessness, dyspnea, nausea, or diaphoresis.

Physical Examination

Physical findings can be quite helpful in the evaluation of chest pain and may occasionally implicate specific etiologies. A pericardial friction rub is pathognomonic for pericarditis. A late-peaking systolic murmur at the upper sternal border indicates aortic stenosis. Unequal pulses or blood pressure in the arms and the presence of an aortic insufficiency murmur strongly suggest aortic dissection.

Angina may be associated with a normal physical examination; however, an S_3, S_4, or murmur of mitral regurgitation is often heard during the ischemic episode.

Differential Diagnosis

The key to differentiating innocuous causes of chest pain from those that are potentially life-threatening lies in the history (see Table 1-1). The chest pain of aortic stenosis (AS), hypertrophic cardiomyopathy, and pulmonary hypertension may be indistinguishable from that of angina. **Aortic dissection** classically presents with severe substernal chest pain that is tearing in quality, comes on abruptly, and radiates to the interscapular or lumbar region. The sudden onset of chest pain associated with dyspnea may herald a **pulmonary embolism (PE)**; this pain is usually worse on inspiration (pleuritic) and may be substernal or more lateral in location. A similar pain can occur with **pneumonia** or a **spontaneous pneumothorax**. **Pericarditis** causes chest pain that is substernal or precordial; radiates to the shoulder; is often pleuritic, sharp, and worse on swallowing or lying supine; and improves when the patient leans forward.

Several gastrointestinal (GI) disorders (e.g., peptic ulcer disease, gastroesophageal reflux disease, pancreatitis, gallbladder disease) can present with chest pain, but there is frequently an abdominal component to the discomfort; these conditions may also be temporally associated with eating and may be relieved by antacids. **Esophageal spasm** may mimic angina in its quality and may be relieved by nitroglycerin; however, it is not related to exertion and is frequently provoked by food. Pain resulting from diseases of the muscles, ligaments, or bones of the chest tends to be localized and is exacerbated by movement or certain postures. Sharp, stabbing chest pains localized to the precordium and lasting only a few seconds are rarely cardiac in etiology and are usually associated with anxiety.

Several other historic factors are important to note in evaluating a patient with chest pain. These include:

- Risk factors for CAD (see Chapter 9) (suggest angina)
- Cocaine use (suggests coronary spasm)
- Recent viral illness (suggests pericarditis or pneumonia)
- Recent prolonged immobility (suggests PE)
- History of bullous lung disease (suggests pneumothorax)
- Recent injury (suggests musculoskeletal pain)
- History of Marfan syndrome (suggests aortic dissection)

Diagnostic Evaluation

The initial tests for patients with chest pain should include an electrocardiogram (ECG) and a chest x-ray (CXR). The ECG may demonstrate regional ST-segment depression/elevation, indicating myocardial ischemia/infarction, or it may reveal the diffuse ST-segment elevation of pericarditis. A CXR may reveal rib fractures, focal infiltrates of pneumonia, wedge-shaped peripheral infiltrates of pulmonary emboli, or the radiolucency of a pneumothorax. It may also suggest aortic dissection (widened mediastinum) or hiatal hernia (stomach in the thoracic cavity).

If an acute coronary syndrome (ACS) is suspected, medical therapy (see Chapters 12 and 13) should be started immediately and serial ECGs and cardiac enzymes (creatine kinase and troponin) checked to confirm or exclude a MI. For patients in whom the diagnosis remains uncertain but CAD is suspected, a stress test can be performed for clarification. Chest pain associated with ST-segment depression during a stress test is diagnostic of angina. Cardiac catheterization remains the "gold standard" for the diagnosis of CAD and may be necessary to rule out significant CAD in a subset of patients for whom other tests are unable to confirm or exclude the diagnosis.

In patients with pulmonary emboli, arterial blood gases usually reveal hypoxia and/or a widened A-a gradient, and ventilation/perfusion (V/Q) scanning or spiral computed tomography (CT) scanning may confirm the diagnosis. Patients suspected of having an aortic dissection should undergo urgent transesophageal echocardiography, CT scanning with intravenous contrast, or magnetic resonance imaging (MRI). Patients suspected of having a gastroesophageal cause of their chest pain may need a barium swallow (esophageal reflux or rupture), endoscopy (esophagitis, gastritis, peptic ulcer disease), hepatobiliary hydroxyiminodiacetic acid (HIDA) scan, or abdominal ultrasound (gallbladder disease), esophageal manometry (eso-phageal spasm), or continuous esophageal pH measurement (reflux) to confirm the diagnosis.

KEY POINTS

1. The initial evaluation of the patient with chest pain should focus on possible life-threatening causes, including acute cardiac ischemia, aortic dissection, and PE.
2. Angina classically causes chest pain that is substernal, precipitated by exertion, and relieved with rest or after sublingual NTG.
3. A variety of pulmonary, musculoskeletal, and GI disorders can present with chest pain and may be difficult to distinguish from true angina.

■ TABLE 1-1

Differential Diagnosis of Chest Pain

Diagnosis	Characteristic Features	Physical Findings	Diagnostic Tests (Finding)
Angina	Substernal, exertional, relieved with rest or NTG; lasts 5–15 min	S_3, S_4, or MR murmur during pain; vascular bruits	ECG, exercise stress test (ST depression)
MI	Similar to angina, only more severe and prolonged	S_3, S_4, CHF, tachycardia	ECG (ST depression or elevation); increased cardiac enzymes
AS	Similar to angina	Murmur of AS	Echocardiogram (stenotic AV)
Aortic dissection	Sudden, severe, tearing pain, radiating to the back	Unequal arm pulses and BP; hypertension; AI murmur	TEE, MRI, or CT scan (dissection flap); CXR (wide mediastinum)
Pericarditis	Sharp, pleuritic pain that is worse with swallowing and when lying down; may radiate to shoulder	Pericardial friction rub	ECG (diffuse ST elevation)
Pulmonary HTN	Similar to angina	Loud P_2, signs of right heart failure	Echocardiogram, Swan-Ganz catheter (increased PA pressure)
PE	Sudden onset of pleuritic chest pain associated with shortness of breath	Tachypnea, hypoxia, tachycardia, signs of acute right HF	V/Q scan, spiral CT scan, PA angiogram (perfusion or filling defect)
Pneumonia	Sharp, pleuritic pain associated with cough; shortness of breath	Rhonchi over affected lung area	CXR (pulmonary infiltrate)
Spontaneous pneumothorax	Sudden, sharp chest pain, dyspnea	Decreased breath sounds and hyperresonance over affected lung	CXR (air in pleural space; lung collapse)
Esophageal rupture	Follows vomiting or esophageal instrumentation, constant	Mediastinal crunch	CXR (pneumothorax, left pleural effusion), barium swallow
Gastroesophageal reflux	Burning substernal pain aggravated by eating or lying down	None	Upper GI series, endoscopy (reflux of gastric contents)
Esophageal spasm	Sudden, severe pain that can mimic angina	None	Esophageal manometry (increased esophageal pressure)
Musculoskeletal pain	Sharp or achy pain, worse with movement, tender to touch	Tenderness over involved area	None
Herpes zoster	Sharp, burning pain in dermatomal distribution	Vesicular rash over affected area	Tzanck prep of vesicular fluid (giant cells)
Anxiety	Variable quality and location of pain; stressful situations	Chest wall tenderness	Diagnosis of exclusion

■ DYSPNEA

Dyspnea is an uncomfortable awareness of breathing. It is a common symptom of cardiac and pulmonary diseases and may also result from neurologic conditions, chest wall problems, and anxiety states.

Differential Diagnosis (See Table 1-2)

Cardiac causes of dyspnea predominantly relate to increased pressure in the left ventricle (LV) and/or atrium. This pressure is transmitted back to the lungs, where it results in transudation of fluid into the interstitial and alveolar spaces and interferes with alveolar gas exchange. This can occur as a result of:

- Valvular heart disease (mitral or aortic regurgitation or stenosis)
- LV systolic dysfunction (ischemic or nonischemic cardiomyopathies)
- LV diastolic dysfunction (e.g., LV hypertrophy, acute myocardial ischemia, infiltrative cardiomyopathy)

- Pericardial diseases (pericardial constriction or tamponade)

Pulmonary causes of dyspnea may result from abnormalities of the tracheobronchial tree, alveolae, pulmonary vasculature, or pleura. These include:

- Pneumonia
- Chronic obstructive pulmonary disease (COPD)
- Asthma
- PE
- Pneumothorax
- Pulmonary fibrosis
- Pulmonary hypertension
- Pleural effusion
- Airway obstruction
- Diaphragmatic paralysis

Dyspnea may also be a feature of anemia, hyperthyroidism, obesity, neurologic disorders that affect the respiratory muscles, physical deconditioning, and anxiety.

■ TABLE 1-2

Differential Diagnosis of Dyspnea

Categorical Cause of Dyspnea	Specific Cause of Dyspnea	Diagnostic Test(s) of Choice
Cardiac	CHF	CXR, echocardiogram, metabolic stress test; BNP
	Ischemia	ECG, exercise stress test
	Valvular disease (AS, AI, MS, MR)	Echocardiogram
	Pericardial (tamponade, constriction)	Echocardiogram
	Restrictive heart disease (infiltrative or hypertrophic heart diseases)	Echocardiogram
Pulmonary	COPD	CXR, PFTs
	Asthma	PFTs, methacholine challenge
	Pneumonia	CXR
	Pleural effusion	CXR
	PE	V/Q scan, spiral CT scan, PA angiogram
	Pneumothorax	CXR
	Pulmonary fibrosis	CXR, high-resolution CT scan
	Pulmonary hypertension	Echocardiogram, PA catheter
	Airway obstruction	CXR, PFTs, bronchoscopy
Other	Anemia	Hematocrit
	Hyperthyroidism	TSH
	Diaphragmatic paralysis	PFTs, CXR

Clinical Manifestations

History

Several historic features may help to differentiate between causes of dyspnea. The sudden onset of dyspnea may occur with angina, pulmonary edema, pneumothorax, or PE. Slowly progressive dyspnea may result from COPD, pleural effusions, anemia, or chronic congestive heart failure (CHF). Other historic features that suggest specific causes of dyspnea include:

- chest pain (angina, MI, pneumonia, PE, pneumothorax)
- cough (pneumonia, bronchitis, asthma)
- fever (pneumonia, bronchitis)
- hemoptysis (PE, bronchitis)
- history of smoking (COPD)
- cardiac risk factors (angina, MI)
- chest wall trauma (pneumothorax)

It is also important to note the pattern of dyspnea. Dyspnea is frequently precipitated by exertion irrespective of its cause. Dyspnea that occurs at rest usually indicates severe cardiac or pulmonary disease. Paroxysmal nocturnal dyspnea suggests left heart failure; this usually occurs 2 to 4 hours into sleep and requires that the patient sit up or get out of bed to obtain relief. Orthopnea is often a symptom of heart failure, but it can also occur as a result of pulmonary disorders.

Physical Examination

The physical examination of the person with dyspnea usually demonstrates tachypnea. Patients may also be cyanotic, reflecting poor oxygenation or low cardiac output (CO). In patients with cardiac diseases causing dyspnea, examination may reveal evidence of valvular heart disease (e.g., murmurs, opening snap (OS) of mitral stenosis (MS), widened pulse pressure of aortic regurgitation) or evidence of CHF [S_3, pulmonary rales, elevated jugular venous pressure (JVP)]. Patients with pneumonia may have fever and focal lung findings, whereas patients with COPD may have diffusely reduced air entry and wheezes. Decreased breath sounds may indicate pleural effusion or pneumothorax, whereas a pleural rub indicates pleuritis associated with PE or pneumonia. Wheezes may be heard with heart failure or bronchospasm, while stridor indicates upper airway obstruction.

Diagnostic Evaluation

The approach to patients with dyspnea depends in part on the acuity of the problem. Patients with acute dyspnea require a rapid evaluation to exclude life-threatening causes, whereas patients with chronic dyspnea require less urgent evaluation.

The initial test of choice for most patients with dyspnea is the CXR. This can be diagnostic in a variety of settings including:

- Pneumonia (focal infiltrate)
- CHF (Kerley B lines, vascular cephalization, cardiomegaly, pulmonary edema)
- Pleural effusion (blunted costophrenic angle)
- Pneumothorax (mediastinal shift, loss of lung markings)

The CXR may also suggest the diagnosis in the setting of:

- PE (peripheral infiltrate, loss of vascular markings)
- COPD (hyperinflation, bullous changes)
- cardiac tamponade (large, "water bottle"-shaped cardiac silhouette)

If dyspnea is associated with chest pain or the patient has known or suspected CAD, an ECG should be obtained to exclude acute ischemia as the cause. Suspected cardiac causes of dyspnea should be investigated with an echocardiogram to evaluate ventricular systolic and diastolic function and exclude valvular heart disease.

A complete blood count should be obtained to evaluate for anemia. Arterial blood gas analysis rarely clarifies the underlying diagnosis, but it can be helpful in assessing the physiologic significance and severity of the disease. The extent to which dyspnea is attributable to lung disease can be assessed with pulmonary function tests (PFTs). During PFTs, flow-volume loops, lung volumes, and diffusion capacity can be measured to assess for restrictive or obstructive lung diseases. CT scanning is appropriate to evaluate patients suspected of having interstitial lung disease or pulmonary emboli; the latter may also be diagnosed with a V/Q scan.

Often it is not clear whether a patient's dyspnea is the result of cardiac or pulmonary disease. Measurement of the serum brain natriuretic peptide (BNP) level may be helpful in this setting; an increased level suggests CHF as the cause of dyspnea. Occasionally, metabolic exercise testing (see Chapter 4) or invasive assessment of intracardiac and pulmonary vascular pressures with a pulmonary artery catheter (Swan-Ganz catheter) is necessary to distinguish between the two possibilities.

KEY POINTS

1. Dyspnea is the uncomfortable awareness of one's breathing.
2. Dyspnea most commonly results from cardiac or pulmonary disease.
3. Life-threatening causes of dyspnea include PE, pneumothorax, pneumonia, and myocardial ischemia/infarction.

PALPITATIONS

The individual with palpitations has a subjective awareness of his or her heartbeats, usually because of a change in heart rate, heart rhythm, or the force of cardiac contraction. A wide variety of disorders can produce palpitations (Table 1-3). The most common causes are arrhythmias, medications, and psychiatric disorders.

Clinical Manifestations

History

The patient may describe palpitations as a fluttering, skipping, or pounding sensation in the chest and may have associated light-headedness, dizziness, or dyspnea. Arrhythmias are the predominant cause; they include supraventricular (SVT) and ventricular (VT) tachycardias as well as premature atrial (PAC) and ventricular (PVC) contractions. The pattern of palpitations may suggest the underlying cause. Patients can often reproduce the rhythm by tapping their fingers on a table—a rapid, regular rhythm suggests sinus tachycardia, SVT, or VT, whereas a rapid, irregular rhythm suggests atrial fibrillation (AF) or frequent premature beats.

Abrupt onset and termination suggest SVT or VT. Associated syncope is more likely with VT than SVT. Single "missed beats" or "flip-flops" are usually due to atrial or ventricular premature contractions. Rapid regular palpitations associated with a pounding sensation in the neck suggest a specific type of SVT called atrioventricular (AV) nodal reentrant tachycardia (AVNRT) (see Chapter 21). A very slow rate suggests sinus bradycardia or heart block. Palpitations trig-

TABLE 1-3

Common Causes of Palpations

Cardiac	Tachyarrhythmias (see Chapter 21) Bradyarrhythmias (see Chapter 22) Valvular heart disease (e.g., MV prolapse) Implanted pacemaker Cardiomyopathy (dilated or hypertrophic)
Metabolic disorders	Thyrotoxicosis Hypoglycemia Pheochromocytoma Electrolyte abnormalities (hyper- or hypokalemia, hypomagnesemia)
Medications/ drugs	Sympathomimetic agents (e.g., theophylline, albuterol) Vasodilators Cocaine Amphetamines Caffeine Nicotine
Psychiatric	Panic attacks Anxiety disorder Depression Emotional stress
Other	Pregnancy Anemia Fever

gered by mild exertion suggest underlying heart failure, valvular disease, anemia, thyrotoxicosis, or poor physical fitness. Occasionally, VT that arises from the right ventricular (RV) outflow tract may present as exercise-induced palpitations. Although anxiety can cause palpitations (typically owing to sinus tachycardia), other more worrisome diagnoses should be excluded. Many young women with SVT are wrongly labeled with anxiety or panic disorder as the cause of their palpitations.

A history of excessive caffeine intake or of cocaine use suggests SVT or PACs as the cause. A thorough review of the patient's medications should be performed to exclude proarrhythmic medications (e.g., antiarrhythmic agents, antipsychotic agents) or stimulants (e.g., beta agonists, theophylline).

Physical Examination

The examination of the person with palpitations is frequently unrevealing; however, clues to the underlying disease may be found and include:

• Murmurs (valvular heart disease)

- Elevated jugular venous pressure (JVP), rales (heart failure)
- Enlarged thyroid gland (thyrotoxicosis)

Diagnostic Evaluation (See Figure 1-1)

The most helpful diagnostic study in the evaluation of palpitations is a 12-lead ECG performed during the patient's symptoms. Unfortunately, a routine ECG performed in the absence of symptoms is rarely diagnostic. The routine ECG may, however, provide clues to the presence of cardiac conditions such as preexcitation syndrome (short PR, delta wave), cardiomyopathy (Q waves, ventricular hypertrophy), or valvular heart disease (ventricular hypertrophy, atrial enlargement).

Prolonged monitoring with a 24-hour ambulatory ECG, ambulatory event monitor, or an implantable loop recorder is usually necessary to determine the cause of infrequent palpitations. An echocardiogram should be performed if underlying heart disease is suspected. A serum level of thyroid-stimulating hormone (TSH) should be routinely obtained to exclude hyperthyroidism as a cause of PACs or SVT. A very aggressive diagnostic strategy should be pursued in those patients with a high likelihood of VT; this includes those with significant valvular disease, myocardial disease, or prior MI, and those with a family history of syncope or sudden death. Rarely, electrophysiologic studies may be necessary to determine the cause of palpitations.

> **KEY POINTS**
>
> 1. Although they are often the result of benign conditions, palpitations may indicate the presence of life-threatening disorders; the history is crucial to identifying possible etiologies.
> 2. An ECG (12-lead or rhythm strip) during an episode of palpitations is essential to confirm the diagnosis.
> 3. Prolonged ECG monitoring may be required before the diagnosis of palpitations is established.

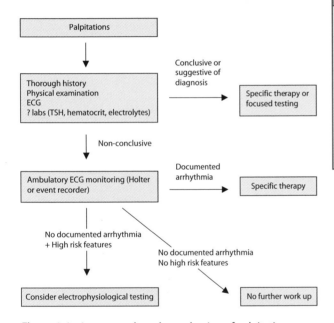

Figure 1-1 • An approach to the evaluation of palpitations.

Physical Examination of the Cardiovascular System

A thorough physical examination can provide clues to the presence and severity of cardiovascular disease as well as alert one to the presence of life-threatening conditions even before the results of any diagnostic workup are available.

GENERAL APPEARANCE

Dyspnea, tachypnea, use of accessory respiratory muscles, discomfort from pain, diaphoresis, and cyanosis may all indicate underlying cardiac disease.

PULSE

The pulse should be examined for rate, regularity, volume, and character. Some abnormalities in the character of the pulse may be diagnostic for certain cardiovascular conditions:

- **Irregularly irregular**: Atrial fibrillation, multifocal atrial tachycardia.
- **Water-hammer** (abrupt upstroke followed by rapid collapse): Aortic insufficiency
- **Bisferiens** (double impulse): Combined aortic stenosis (AS) and insufficiency
- **Pulsus parvus** (weak) **et tardus** (delayed): Severe aortic stenosis
- **Pulsus alternans** (alternating strong and weak pulse): Severe LV dysfunction
- **Pulsus paradoxus** (marked inspiratory decrease in strength of pulse): Cardiac tamponade, pericardial constriction, severe obstructive airway disease.

JUGULAR VENOUS PRESSURE

The jugular venous pulsation is best visualized with the patient lying with the head tilted up 30 to 45 degrees. As illustrated in Figure 2-1, the JVP is composed of characteristic waves. The "a wave" is the result of atrial contraction and occurs during late ventricular diastole. The "x descent" results from atrial relaxation during early ventricular systole and is interrupted by the "c wave," which reflects closure of the tricuspid valve. The "v wave" is the result of venous return to the atrium during late ventricular systole. The "y descent" occurs during early ventricular diastole and results from the opening of the tricuspid valve with subsequent passive emptying of the atrium into the ventricle. The central venous pressure can be estimated by adding 5 cm [the vertical distance between the center of the right atrium (RA) and the sternal angle] to the maximum vertical height of the pulsations above the sternal angle. The JVP is elevated in heart failure and not identifiable in volume depletion. When heart failure is present, firm pressure over the abdominal right upper quadrant will cause persistent elevation of the JVP (hepatojugular or abdominojugular reflux). Characteristic abnormalities of the jugular venous waveforms occur in a variety of cardiac disorders.

INSPECTION AND PALPATION OF THE CHEST

The point of maximal impulse (PMI) of the LV apex should be located and palpated. It is usually in the fifth intercostal space at the midclavicular line; it is displaced laterally with RV dilation and inferolaterally with LV dilation. It is diffuse with dilated cardiomyopathy or LV aneurysm and may demonstrate a double impulse with hypertrophic cardiomyopathy, AS, or hypertension (HTN). A left parasternal heave may be evident with RV hypertrophy.

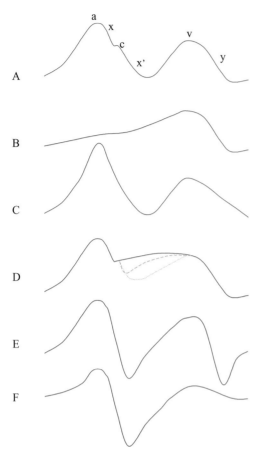

Figure 2-1 • Jugular venous waveforms. (a) Normal. (b) Absent a wave in atrial fibrillation. (c) Prominent a wave and shallow y descent in tricuspid stenosis. (d) CV wave in varying degrees of tricuspid regurgitation. (e) Rapid x and y descents in constrictive pericarditis. (f) Rapid x descent and absent y descent in pericardial tamponade.

TABLE 2-1

Abnormal Heart Sounds and Their Significance

Heart Sound	Associated Disease State
Loud S_1	MS
Variable-intensity S_1	AF, AV dissociation
Loud A_2	Hypertension
Soft A_2	AS
Loud P_2	Pulmonary hypertension
Fixed split S_2	ASD
Paradoxically split S_2	LBBB, severe AS, PDA
Widely split S_2 with normal variation	RBBB
S_3	Ventricular dysfunction, volume overload, high cardiac output (fever, anemia)
S_4	Hypertension, AS, HCM
Early systolic ejection click	Bicuspid aortic valve, pulmonary stenosis, pulmonary hypertension
Midsystolic click	MVP
Opening snap	MS
Pericardial knock	Constrictive pericarditis

Electrocardiogram

Timing of Heart Sounds

AUSCULTATION OF THE CHEST

Heart Sounds

The entire precordium should be systematically examined for normal heart sounds (S_1 and S_2), gallops (S_3 or S_4), and other additional sounds (e.g., clicks, snaps). These auscultatory findings are strongly correlated with specific cardiac disorders (see Table 2-1). Higher-pitched sounds (e.g., S_1, S_2, pericardial rubs, most murmurs) are best heard with the diaphragm of the stethoscope, whereas lower pitched sounds (e.g., S_3, S_4, diastolic rumbles) are best heard with the bell of the stethoscope.

The first heart sound reflects closure of the mitral and tricuspid valves (TVs), although TV events are frequently silent. S_1 is loud with mitral stenosis, soft or absent with mitral regurgitation, and variable with atrial fibrillation and complete heart block.

The second heart sound comprises the aortic valve (A_2) and pulmonic valve (P_2) closure sounds and is abnormal in a variety of disease states. Normally, P_2 follows A_2, and the split widens with inspiration secondary to a delay in P_2 as a result of an inspiratory increase in capacitance of the pulmonary vascular bed. A widely split S_2 that still varies normally with respiration may result from right bundle branch block (RBBB), severe RV failure, or severe pulmonary hypertension owing to the delayed emptying of the RV in these settings. Wide splitting that does not vary with respiration (**fixed splitting**) is characteristic of an atrial septal defect (ASD). Paradoxical splitting (splitting that narrows with inspiration) is a feature of left bundle branch block (LBBB), patent ductus arteriosus

■ TABLE 2-2

Classification of Murmurs

Category	Graphic Representation	Examples
Early-peaking systolic ejection murmur	S1 S2	Benign flow murmur, aortic sclerosis
Late-peaking systolic ejection murmur		AS, PS, HCM
Holosystolic murmur		MR, tricuspid regurgitation, VSD
Midsystolic murmur	MSC	MVP with MR
Decrescendo diastolic murmur	S1 S2	AI, pulmonic insufficiency
Diastolic rumble (with presystolic accentuation)	S1 S2 S1 OS	MS
Continuous murmur ("machinery" murmur)		PDA, AV fistulas
Pericardial friction rub		Pericarditis

(PDA), and severe AS and reflects either a delay in LV emptying (LBBB, severe AS) or premature pulmonary valve (PV) closure (PDA).

An S_3 gallop signifies rapid diastolic ventricular filling. This low-frequency heart sound is best heard over the apex (LV S_3) or the left sternal border (RV S_3) using the bell of the stethoscope. It may be heard normally in children and adolescents but is considered abnormal in people over 40 years of age, in whom it is associated with volume overload, ventricular dysfunction, or high-output states such as fever or anemia.

An S_4 gallop represents atrial contraction in late diastole. Like an S_3, this is a low-frequency sound heard best over the apex (LV S_4) or the left sternal border (RV S_4) with the bell of the stethoscope. An S_4 is never heard normally. It is associated with conditions in which the ventricles lose their compliance (e.g., LV hypertrophy, MI).

Murmurs

Murmurs usually arise from blood flow across an abnormal valve, but they can also be the result of increased blood flow across a normal valve. The origin of a murmur can often be inferred from its auditory character, its timing within the cardiac cycle (see Table 2-2), and its area of maximal intensity (see Figure 2-2). Various maneuvers may be performed at

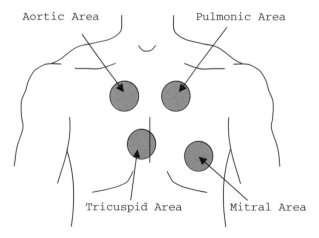

Figure 2-2 • Locations of maximal intensity of murmurs depending on the valve of origin.

■ TABLE 2-3

Differential Diagnosis of Systolic Murmurs

	Location	Character	Radiation	Accentuating Maneuvers	Attenuating Maneuvers	Other Findings
AS	Right upper SB	Ejection systolic	Neck, carotids	Leg raising, post-Valsalva, post-PVC	Handgrip	Paradoxically split S_2; soft A_2; S_4
HOCM	3rd–4th left ICS	Ejection systolic	Upper left SB	Sudden standing, Valsalva	Squatting, post-Valsalva	MR
MR	Apex	Holosystolic	Axilla	Handgrip	Inspiration, Valsalva	S_3
MVP with MR	Apex	Late systolic	Varies	Sudden standing, Valsalva	Supine posture, post-Valsalva	Midsystolic click
VSD	3rd–4th left ICS	Holosystolic	None	Handgrip	Valsalva	S_3
PS	Left upper SB	Ejection systolic	None	Inspiration, passive leg raising	Expiration, sudden standing	Ejection click
TR	Left lower SB	Holosystolic	None	Inspiration, passive leg raising	Expiration	Pulsatile liver

the bedside to clarify the nature of a particular murmur (see Table 2-3).

Murmur intensity can be graded on a scale of 1 to 6. A grade 1 murmur is barely audible, a grade 2 murmur is easily audible, and a grade 3 murmur is loud. Grade 4 to grade 6 murmurs are all loud murmurs that are associated with palpable precordial thrills. Grade 4 murmurs can be heard only with the stethoscope firmly on the chest, grade 5 murmurs can be heard with just the edge of the stethoscope on the chest, and grade 6 murmurs can be heard without the stethoscope.

Several general principles worth remembering during cardiac auscultation are:

- Aortic events are best heard with the patient leaning forward and at end-expiration.
- Mitral events are best heard in the left lateral position during expiration.
- With the exception of the pulmonary ejection click, all right-sided events are louder with inspiration.
- Left-sided events are usually louder with expiration.

Pericardial friction rubs may be mistaken for systolic and diastolic murmurs. They tend to have a scratchy quality and vary significantly with respiration. Classically there are three components of a pericardial rub:

- An atrial systolic component
- A ventricular systolic component
- A ventricular diastolic component

Frequently, however, only one or two components are heard.

■ THE LUNGS

It is essential to examine the lungs in every cardiac patient, paying special attention to the following features:

- Inspiratory crackles (rales): indicate left heart failure.
- Bronchospasm (wheezing): may indicate peribronchial edema ("cardiac asthma").
- Diminished breath sounds and dullness to percussion at the lung bases: may represent pleural effusions.

Several other physical findings are worth noting:

- Hepatomegaly, ascites, and peripheral edema may reflect RV failure.
- A pulsatile liver is seen with tricuspid regurgitation.
- Central cyanosis is commonly associated with congenital heart disease, whereas peripheral cyanosis is associated with diminished cardiac output.
- Digital clubbing may be seen with congenital cyanotic heart disease and endocarditis.

KEY POINTS

1. The jugular venous pressure should be estimated with the patient lying at a 30- to 45-degree angle.
2. The point of maximal impulse of the LV should be located in the fifth intercostal space at the mid-clavicular line.
3. Murmurs should be described by their location, character, intensity, and area of radiation.
4. High-pitched sounds (e.g., S_1, S_2, systolic murmurs) are best heard with the diaphragm of the stethoscope, whereas low-pitched sounds (e.g., S_3, diastolic rumble) are best heard with the bell of the stethoscope.

Part Two

Diagnostic Modalities

3 The Electrocardiogram

The electrocardiogram (ECG) is a visual representation of the electrical impulses generated by the heart with each beat. Ever since Willem Einthoven developed the ECG in the early 1900s, it has become an invaluable tool in the diagnosis of a variety of cardiac conditions. This section presents the fundamental electrophysiology of the cardiac cycle and the components and appearance of the normal ECG; it also briefly outlines criteria for some abnormal findings.

■ BASIC CARDIAC ELECTROPHYSIOLOGY

The mechanical process of ventricular contraction begins with an electrical impulse generated in a region of the superior right atrium known as the sinoatrial (SA) node (Figure 3-1). The sinus impulse quickly spreads through the atria, resulting in atrial contraction,

and then continues through the atrioventricular (AV) node, the His bundle, and the right and left bundle branches, eventually reaching the ventricular myocardium, where it results in synchronized biventricular contraction. If ventricular contraction results from impulses that originate in the SA node, normal sinus rhythm is said to be present. Abnormalities of this process result in various arrhythmias.

■ THE LEAD SYSTEM

The electrical impulses in the heart can be recorded by means of electrodes strategically placed on the surface of the body. The standard ECG has 12 leads: 6 limb leads and 6 precordial or chest leads. The limb leads (I, II, III, aVR, aVL, aVF) record cardiac electrical impulses in a vertical or frontal plane (Figure 3-2). The precordial leads (V_1 to V_6) are placed over the left chest and record elctrical impulses in a horizontal plane. Figure 3-3 demonstrates proper lead placement for recording a surface ECG.

The ECG is generated by simultaneously recording the electrical activity of the heart at each electrode or pair of electrodes. Any net electrical impulse directed toward the positive aspect of a lead is represented by an upward deflection of the ECG tracing in that lead. The magnitude of the deflection reflects the strength of the electrical signal, which depends in part on the mass of myocardium that is being depolarized and in part on the electrical impedance of interposed tissue. Each small box on the ECG paper represents 0.1 mV in amplitude (vertical axis) and 200 milliseconds in time (horizontal axis). A stepwise approach to analyzing an ECG is important so that no abnormality is missed (see Box 3-1). Details of rhythm analysis are covered in later chapters (see Chapters 20, 21, and 22).

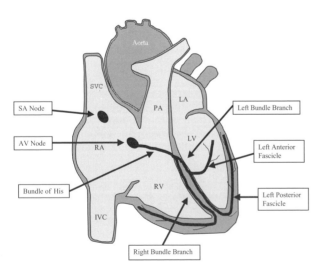

Figure 3-1 • The anatomy of the cardiac conduction system.

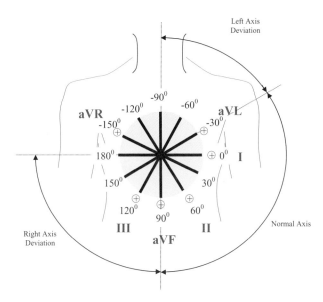

Figure 3-2 •Orientation of limb leads and axis. Positive pole of lead denoted by +.

CALCULATION OF HEART RATE (FIGURE 3-4) AND QRS AXIS (FIGURE 3-2)

Heart rate in beats per minute (bpm) can be determined from the 12-lead ECG. One approach is to count the total number of QRS complexes across the ECG and multiple by 6, since most standard ECGs reflect 10 seconds of time. Alternatively, if the rhythm is regular and the paper speed is standard (25 mm/sec), the heart rate can be calculated by dividing 300 (the number of large hatch marks per minute of ECG recording) by the number of large hatch marks between two QRS complexes. Thus, if a QRS complex occurs once every two hatch marks, the heart rate is 150 bpm, and so on (Figure 3-5).

The electrical axis is the overall direction of the electrical depolarization of the heart. If this direction is horizontal and to the right, the axis is assigned a value of zero. Axes directed more clockwise are assigned positive values, whereas axes directed more counterclockwise are assigned negative values. The axis can be estimated by identifying the limb lead in which the QRS is isoelectric (in which positive and negative deflections are of equal size); the axis is perpendicular to this lead. Because the ventricles depolarize predominantly from superior to inferior and from right to left, the QRS axis normally falls between −30 and +90 degrees.

THE NORMAL ECG (SEE FIGURE 3-4)

Every cardiac cycle's electrical impulse is inscribed on the ECG as a waveform with the following components: P wave, QRS complex, and T wave (Figure 3-5).

The P Wave

The onset of the P wave heralds the onset of atrial depolarization. The normal electrical impulse travels

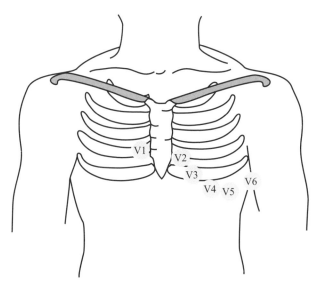

Figure 3-3 •Proper placement of precordial leads for recording a 12-lead ECG. Leads V_1 and V_2 are placed in the right and left fourth intercostal spaces (ICS), respectively. V_3 is placed between V_2 and V_4. V_4 is placed in the fifth ICS in the midclavicular line. V_5 is placed in the anterior axillary line and V_6 in the midaxillary line, both in the same horizontal plane as V_4.

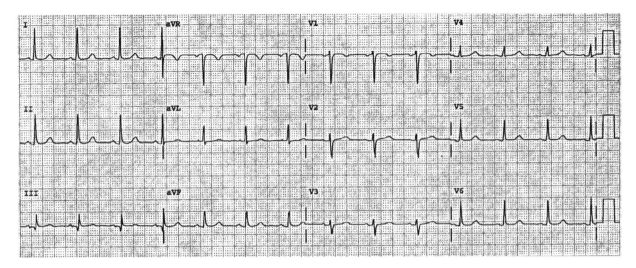

Figure 3-4 • Normal 12-lead ECG (see text for details).

from the SA node and depolarizes the atria in a superior-to-inferior direction, resulting in a P wave on the ECG that is upright (positive) in lead II and downward (negative) in lead aVR. An impulse arising from a site other than the SA node will depolarize the atria in a different direction and results in a different P-wave morphology. The normal P wave is ≤0.1 mV in

amplitude in lead V_1, ≤0.25 mV in amplitude in lead II, and ≤0.12 seconds in duration in lead II. Increases in these parameters occur with atrial enlargement.

The PR Interval

The PR interval is measured from the onset of the P wave to the onset of the QRS complex and is a measure of the time it takes for the sinus impulse to traverse the atria, AV node, and His-Purkinje system before depolarizing the ventricles. The normal PR interval can vary between 0.12 to 0.20 seconds; this variability is mainly the result of autonomic tone. A prolonged PR segment reflects slowing of the impulse through the conduction system. An abnormally short PR segment may represent accelerated conduction through the AV node or a "short circuit" between the atria and the ventricles (a **bypass tract**).

The QRS Complex

The QRS complex is measured from the onset of the Q or R wave to the end of the S wave. The initial 0.04 seconds of this complex represents depolarization of the septum, which occurs from left to right. This results in a small initial negative deflection ("septal q wave") in leads I and V_6 because the impulse is directed away from the positive poles of these leads. The remainder of the QRS complex reflects depolarization of the right and left ventricles. Because of its greater mass, the electrical forces from the left ventricle predominate, resulting in a QRS complex that is mainly positive in leads I and V_6 and negative in

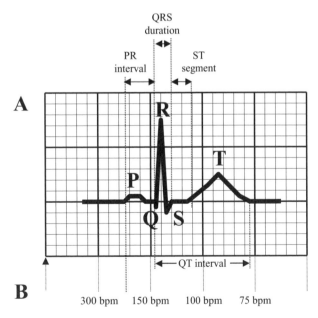

Figure 3-5 • (a) Normal ECG waveforms and intervals. (b) Calculation of heart rate based on paper speed of 25 mm/sec: if an initial QRS complex occurs at the dotted arrow, a subsequent QRS complex 0.2 seconds later (or at the next dark hatch mark) reflects a heart rate of 300 bpm. Longer intervals between QRS complexes reflect heart rates as noted.

aVR and V_1. Thus, the appearance of the QRS complex in normal sinus rhythm is characterized by:

- Initial "septal Q waves" in leads I and V_6
- Predominantly positive QRS complex in leads I and V_6
- Predominantly negative QRS complex in leads aVR and V_1
- Incremental increase in the amplitude of R waves from V_2 to V_5

The QRS duration is the total time required for ventricular depolarization; this is normally less than 100 milliseconds. A longer QRS duration suggests conduction block or delay.

The ST Segment

The ST segment corresponds to the time during which the ventricles have completely depolarized but have not yet begun to repolarize. During this time there is no net electrical activity in the heart and the ECG records a flat segment at the electrical baseline. This segment becomes abnormal during myocardial ischemia (ST-segment depression) and infarction (ST-segment elevation).

The T Wave

The onset of the T wave denotes the onset of ventricular repolarization. The T wave in most circumstances

▪ TABLE 3-1

Diagnostic Criteria for Common ECG Abnormalities

Abnormality	Diagnostic Criteria
LA enlargement	P-wave duration in lead II ≥ 0.12 seconds **OR** P wave in V_1 ≥ 0.1 mV deep and ≥ 0.04 seconds long
RA enlargement	P wave in V_1 > 0.15 mV in amplitude **OR** P wave in II > 0.25 mV in amplitude
LVH	S wave in V_1 + the R wave in V_5 or V_6 > 3.5 mV **OR** S wave in V_2 + the R wave in V_5 or V_6 > 4.5 mV **OR** R wave in V_5 > 2.6 mV **OR** R wave in lead aVL > 1.1 mV **OR** R wave in lead I > 1.4 mV
RVH	R/S ratio in V_1 >1 **OR** R wave in V_1 + the S wave in V_5 or V_6 ≥ 1.1 mV **OR** R wave in V_1 >0.7 mV **OR** R/S ratio in V_5 or V_6 ≤ 1
Left-axis deviation	Axis −30 to −105 degrees
Right-axis deviation	Axis > +100
Pathologic Q wave	Duration ≥ 0.04 seconds **AND** amplitude >1/3 the height of the R wave
Peaked T wave	T-wave amplitude >0.6 mV in limb leads **OR** T-wave amplitude > 1.0 mV in precordial leads
LBBB	QRS duration ≥ 0.12 seconds **AND** Broad monophasic R wave in leads I, V_5, and V_6
RBBB	QRS duration ≥ 0.12 seconds **AND** rsR pattern in V_1 **AND** wide S wave in V_5, V_6, and lead I
Left anterior fascicular block	QRS axis −45 to −90 degrees **AND** qR complex in leads I and aVL **AND** rS complex in leads III and aVF **AND** QRS duration ≤ 0.10 seconds
Left posterior fascicular block	QRS axis +100° to +180° **AND** deep S wave in lead 1, Q wave in lead III, **AND** QRS duration ≤ 0.10 seconds

follows the same direction (polarity) as the predominant portion of the QRS complex: normally upright in leads I and V_6 and inverted in lead aVR. However, the normal T wave can be either upright or inverted in leads V_1, aVL, and III. Changes in T-wave morphology may reflect myocardial ischemia or infarction and can also occur as a result of metabolic abnormalities.

QT Interval

The QT interval is measured from the onset of the QRS complex to the end of the T wave. The normal duration of the QT interval depends on many factors, including a person's age, gender, and heart rate. Nonetheless, a QT interval greater than 0.46 seconds or greater than 50% of the associated interval from R wave to R wave is abnormally long. A prolonged QT interval may reflect a primary congenital abnormality of myocardial repolarization or be secondary to medications or metabolic abnormalities and predisposes to malignant ventricular arrhythmias.

■ ABNORMAL ECG PATTERNS

A variety of cardiac disorders are associated with specific patterns on the ECG. Although it is beyond the scope of this text to provide a comprehensive discussion of this topic, the reader should be familiar with the ECG patterns associated with some common abnormalities, as outlined in Table 3-1.

4 Stress Testing

Stress testing is one of the most widely used tools in cardiology. It provides diagnostic and prognostic information in patients with suspected or known CHD and is a useful tool for assessing the adequacy of therapy. Stress testing can also objectively assess the exercise capacity of a patient and help determine the nature of his or her functional limitations.

INDICATIONS

The most common indication for stress testing is to determine whether a patient's symptoms relate to underlying CAD. For patients in whom the diagnosis of CAD is already certain, stress testing may be useful to:

- Assess risk of a cardiovascular event
- Determine long-term prognosis
- Assess exercise capacity
- Evaluate the efficacy of therapy
- Assist in therapeutic decision making (i.e., determine who may benefit from cardiac catheterization and revascularization)
- Localize a region of ischemia in order to target percutaneous revascularization
- Detect exercise-related arrhythmias

CONTRAINDICATIONS

Major complications associated with stress testing are rare, occurring in approximately 9 of every 10,000 tests performed. These complications include MI, serious arrhythmias, and death. Most of these complications occur in patients with certain high-risk features; therefore patients should be carefully screened for contraindicatons before undergoing exercise testing (see Table 4-1).

TESTING MODALITIES

Stress testing can be performed in several ways. The stress can be induced by exercise (either walking on a treadmill or riding a bicycle) or by pharmacologic means with dobutamine or coronary vasodilators. Treadmill exercise is the best-standardized modality and allows for more flexible protocols, as speed and incline can be varied independently. The Bruce protocol is the most commonly used and consists of incremental increases in the speed and slope of the treadmill every 3 minutes. Bicycle testing may be better tolerated by patients who have orthopedic or balance problems. The

TABLE 4-1

Absolute and Relative Contraindications to Exercise Stress Testing

Absolute	Acute MI (within 2 days)
	UA (until medically stabilized)
	Acute myocarditis, pericarditis, or endocarditis
	Uncontrolled HTN (resting SBP > 200 mm Hg or DBP > 120 mm Hg)
	Uncontrolled tachy- or bradyarrhythmias
	Decompensated symptomatic CHF
	Severe or symptomatic AS
	Acute/recent DVT or PE
	Acute aortic dissection
	Recent CVA
Relative	Moderate, asymptomatic valvular stenosis
	Hypertrophic obstructive CMP
	Suspected left main CAD
	High-grade AV block
	Acute illness, such as active infection, thyrotoxicosis, severe anemia
	Inability to exercise adequately

aim of the exercise is to increase myocardial oxygen demand (MVO_2). In patients with CAD, the increased MVO_2 may exceed the ability of the coronary arteries to supply oxygenated blood, resulting in ischemia.

Dobutamine produces an increase in heart rate, contractility, and blood pressure, thereby mimicking exercise and increasing MVO_2. Dipyridamole and adenosine cause coronary vasodilation preferentially in normal coronary arteries. This results in a flow mismatch: blood flow in normal coronary arteries increases relative to flow in diseased coronary arteries. Pharmacologic stress testing with these agents yields sensitivities and specificities comparable to those of exercise stress testing. As with exercise stress testing, pharmacologic stress is not without risk. Dobutamine can induce ventricular arrhythmias and precipitate myocardial ischemia, while dipyridamole and adenosine can cause bronchospasm. The coronary vasodilators are therefore contraindicated in patients with asthma or emphysema associated with a bronchospastic component. Of note, caffeine and adenosine compete for receptors; all caffeine products should therefore be avoided for 12 hours prior to an adenosine or dipyridamole stress test.

■ MONITORING MODALITIES

All patients who undergo stress testing are assessed for symptoms and have continuous ECG monitoring to evaluate for ischemic changes (ST-segment depression or elevation) or arrhythmias. The sensitivity and specificity of stress testing can be improved with the use of echocardiographic or nuclear imaging to further identify regional areas of myocardial ischemia.

During a stress test with echocardiographic imaging, LV function is assessed at both rest and peak stress. The finding of stress-induced deterioration of regional LV wall motion is consistent with inducible ischemia. If the entire ventricle becomes dysfunctional or dilates with stress (reflecting widespread ischemia), multivessel CAD is likely to be present.

The isotopes used in myocardial perfusion imaging are thallium-201 (^{201}Tl) and technetium-99m (^{99m}Tc) sestamibi. The imaging quality of sestamibi is superior to that of thallium; both allow for the assessment of LV function as well as ischemia. After intravenous injection, these isotopes are taken up by viable myocardial cells in quantities proportional to their regional blood flow. Regions of the myocardium that are well perfused appear brighter on nuclear imaging than regions that are poorly perfused because of CAD (Figure 4-1). As with echocardiographic imaging, nuclear imaging is performed both at rest and peak exercise and the results are compared.

■ CHOICE OF TESTING MODALITIES (PHYSIOLOGIC VS. PHARMACOLOGIC)

In general, if a patient can exercise, an exercise test is preferred over a pharmacologic stress test (see Figure 4-2) because it is a more physiologic study. Pharmacologic stress testing is employed when the patient is unable to exercise adequately. With exercise or dobutamine stress testing, the patient must

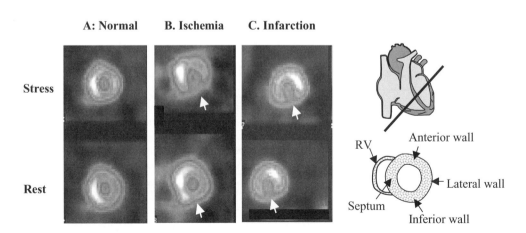

Figure 4-1 • Nuclear imaging during stress testing. (a) Normal scan. Both rest and stress images demonstrate homogeneous perfusion of the myocardium. (b) Ischemia. The stress image demonstrates a large inferior wall perfusion defect that "fills in" in the rest images. (c) Infarction. Both rest and stress images demonstrate a large inferior wall perfusion defect.

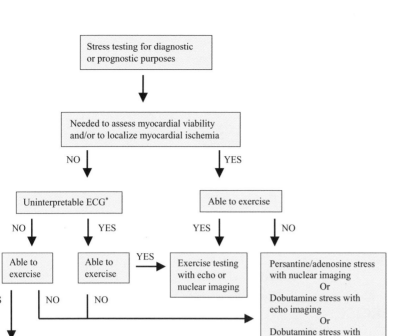

Figure 4-2 • Selection of stress test modality. *Uninterpretable ECG includes LVH, LBBB, intraventricular conduction delays, paced ventricular rhythms, digitalis effect, and resting ST-T-wave abnormalities.

attain at least 85% of his or her maximum predicted heart rate in order to achieve a sufficient level of myocardial stress to precipitate ischemia. The maximum predicted heart rate is calculated by subtracting the patient's age from 220. When dipyridamole or adenosine is used as the stress modality, it is presumed that maximum coronary vasodilation occurs with the standard dose, and a heart rate response is not required.

The level of physiologic stress achieved can be compared among different exercise protocols and related to routine daily activities by calculating the metabolic equivalents (METs) attained by the patient during the stress test (see Table 4-2). One MET equals the body's oxygen requirement at rest ($\sim$3.5 mL O_2/min/kg body weight).

■ CHOICE OF MONITORING MODALITIES (ECG ALONE VS. IMAGING)

If a patient can exercise and has no significant ST-segment abnormalities on his or her resting ECG, ECG monitoring alone is usually adequate. In patients with abnormal resting ECGs (LBBB, LVH, digoxin effect, paced rhythms, persistent ST-segment depression), the ECG is not adequate to identify ischemia and an additional imaging modality is necessary. When pharmacologic stress testing is used, an imaging modality is always necessary because of the low sensitivity of drug-induced ST-segment changes. The use of echocardiographic or nuclear imaging improves the sensitivity and specificity of the test in these settings. The decision

■ TABLE 4-2

Activities of Daily Living and Their Corresponding Metabolic Equivalent Level

METs*	Equivalent Workload
1	Eat, dress, use the toilet
3–4	Walk at 2.5-mph pace, bowl, do light housework
4–5	Push power lawn mower, play golf (walk, carry clubs), do moderate housework, walk downstairs
5–6	Carry anything up a flight of stairs without stopping, have sexual intercourse, garden, rake, weed, walk at 4-mph pace on level ground
7–10	Carry at least 24 lb up a flight of stairs, shovel snow, carry objects that weigh at least 80 lb, jog/walk at a 5-mph pace
>10	Strenuous sports, e.g., swimming, basketball, tennis
18	Elite endurance athlete
20	World-class athlete

*One MET = 3.5 mL O_2/kg.

TABLE 4-3

Comparison of the Diagnostic Value of Various Types of Stress Tests

Type of Stress Test	Sensitivity	Specificity	PPV	NPV
Exercise ECG	65–70%	80–84%	91%	41%
Dobutamine echocardiography	78–85%	70–88%	92%	69%
Nuclear imaging	80–90%	70–80%	85%	72%

*The reported values for exercise nuclear imaging include the average of both sestamibi and thallium studies.

as to which imaging modality should be employed depends on the expertise of the institution. The reported sensitivities among the various modalities are similar (see Table 4-3).

INTERPRETATION OF EXERCISE ECG TESTING

ST-segment depression is the most common ECG manifestation of ischemia. Other stress-induced ECG findings suggestive of ischemia include ST-segment elevation, ventricular ectopy or arrhythmias, QRS widening, and increased R-wave amplitude. Several different types of ST-segment changes may be seen, although horizontal or down-sloping ST-segment depressions are the most specific (see Figure 4-3). Although chest pain occurs in only about one-third of stress tests, its presence increases the likelihood of underlying CHD.

When echocardiographic testing or nuclear imaging is performed, ischemia is defined as a region of myocardium that appears normal at rest but abnormal with exercise. Infarction is a region that appears abnormal at both rest and exercise. Either of these findings is strong evidence of CAD.

Certain findings during stress testing are markers for adverse prognosis. These include:

- ST-segment depression of ≥2 mm or in ≥5 leads
- ST-segment elevation
- Angina pectoris
- Ventricular tachycardia
- Exercise-induced hypotension (>20-mm Hg drop in systolic BP)
- Low exercise capacity (≤5 MET level)

The theory of conditional probability, or Bayes theorem, is an integral component of the interpretation of stress testing when it is used for diagnosing ischemic heart disease. This theorem states that the posttest probability of a particular disease depends on the incidence of the disease in the population being

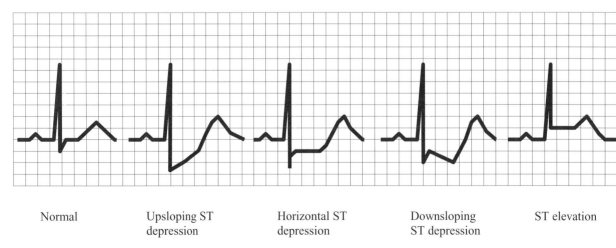

| Normal | Upsloping ST depression | Horizontal ST depression | Downsloping ST depression | ST elevation |

Figure 4-3 • Patterns of ST-segment changes during stress testing. Most physicians use the criteria of 1 mm ST-segment depression if the pattern is horizontal or downsloping, and 1.5 mm if upsloping. ST-segment elevation greater than 1 mm is a significant finding.

studied. That is, an abnormal stress test in a person with a very low likelihood of having CAD is probably a false-positive test, and a negative test in a person with a very high probability of having CAD is likely a false-negative test. Therefore stress testing for the diagnosis of CAD is most helpful in patients who have an intermediate probability of CAD.

■ STRESS TESTING IN WOMEN

Women under the age of 55 to 60 years often have "false-positive ST depression"—i.e., ST-segment depression in relation to exertion that is not due to epicardial CAD. Consequently other exercise variables, such as exercise time and hypotension, must be considered in diagnosing CHD in women. Given the lower prevalence of ischemic heart disease in women as compared with men, all modalities of stress testing are less accurate in this population.

■ CARDIOPULMONARY STRESS TESTING

Cardiopulmonary exercise testing (CPET) measures respiratory gas exchange during treadmill or bicycle exercise protocols. It uses these data to provide information regarding peak oxygen uptake, anaerobic threshold, and minute ventilation. Indications for CPET include:

- Objective assessment of functional capacity
- Determination of the appropriateness and timing of cardiac transplantation
- Determination of whether a patient's dyspnea or low exercise capacity is the result of cardiac disease, pulmonary disease, deconditioning, or poor motivation

KEY POINTS

1. Stress testing is a useful test for diagnosing CAD and determining cardiovascular prognosis.
2. Stress testing can be accomplished with exercise protocols or pharmacologic agents. If a patient can exercise, an exercise protocol is preferred.
3. During stress testing, ischemia can be identified by monitoring the patient's symptoms and ECG, with or without echocardiographic or nuclear imaging.
4. If a patient's ECG is abnormal at rest, an imaging modality is necessary to identify ischemia during stress.
5. The posttest probability of CAD depends in part on the pretest probability of CAD in the population being studied.

Chapter 5

Echocardiography

Echocardiography comprises a group of tests that utilize reflected ultrasonic waves (echoes) to generate images of the heart and related structures. Since its discovery and application to medicine over 30 years ago, it has become widely used and is an indispensable tool for the assessment of cardiac structure and function.

▓ PRINCIPLES AND TECHNIQUES

Two-dimensional (2D) echocardiography is the most common technique used clinically and produces 2D images of the heart in multiple planes (see Figure 5-1). The images can be obtained by either transthoracic or transesophageal techniques. In transthoracic echocardiography (TTE), the ultrasonic **transducer** is placed at various locations on the surface of the chest to obtain different views or planes of the heart. The probe emits an ultrasound beam that moves across a sector, so that a pie-shaped slice of the heart is interrogated and images are obtained. This technique allows the visualization of cardiac structures and measurement of wall thickness and chamber size.

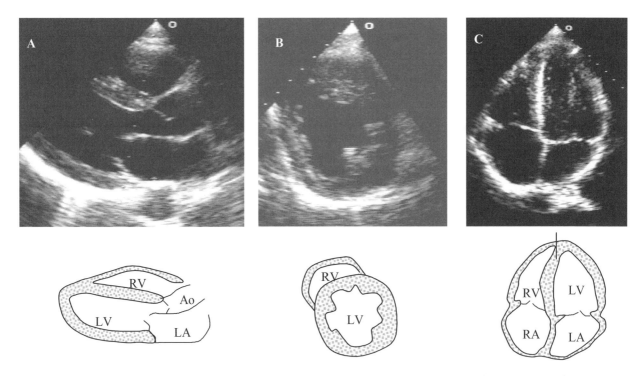

Figure 5-1 • Two-dimensional images of the heart from various transducer positions. (a) Parasternal long-axis view. (b) Parasternal short-axis view. (c) Apical four-chamber view.

During the study, the heart is imaged continuously throughout the cardiac cycle. By comparing images in systole and diastole, the motion of various regions of the heart can be assessed and overall systolic function (ejection fraction) estimated. Regions of the LV that do not contract well during systole provide evidence of prior MI or nonischemic injury. TTE is also an effective method with which to visualize the pericardium and identify and assess the significance of pericardial effusions.

Doppler echocardiography is often used in addition to 2D echocardiography to record blood flow within the cardiovascular system. It utilizes the principle of the Doppler effect to determine the direction and velocity of blood flow relative to the transducer. This information can also be recorded in a spatially correct format superimposed on a 2D echocardiogram. **Color Doppler echocardiography** takes such information and uses various shades of red to depict blood moving toward the transducer and various shades of blue for blood moving away from the transducer. Doppler techniques are used to assess the presence and severity of valvular stenosis or regurgitation and to identify intracardiac shunts. A summary of the uses and limitations of TTE is given in Box 5-1.

Transesophageal echocardiography (TEE) utilizes standard echocardiography principles; however, the transducer is placed at the end of a probe and inserted into the patient's esophagus. The distance from the transducer to the heart is thereby minimized, allowing for improved image resolution compared to TTE (see Figures 29-1 and 44-1). TEE is especially well suited for assessing valvular anatomy and function, identifying valvular vegetations in patients with endocarditis, visualizing aortic atherosclerosis and aortic dissections, and identifying potential cardiac sources of emboli in patients with embolic neurologic events. The advantages and disadvantages of TEE are listed in Box 5-2.

Other techniques and applications of echocardiography include:

- **Intravascular ultrasound** (IVUS): A miniaturized ultrasound transducer is placed on the tip of a vascular catheter, allowing for imaging of atherosclerotic plaques from within an artery.
- **Contrast echocardiography**: Agitated saline or microbubbles are injected intravenously. The bubbles are highly refractory under ultrasound and opacify the cardiac chambers, allowing better definition of LV and RV wall motion, identification of intracardiac shunts, and assessment of myocardial perfusion.
- **Three-dimensional (3D) echocardiography**: Allows visualization of cardiac structures in a 3D format. Currently its utility is limited to congenital heart disease (CHD), valvular abnormalities, and research protocols.

BOX 5-1 USES AND LIMITATIONS OF ECHOCARDIOGRAPHY

Used for the assessment of
LV systolic and diastolic function
LV segmental wall motion (e.g., post-MI)
RV systolic function
Wall thickness (e.g., LV hypertrophy)
Valvular disease (acquired or congenital)
Infective endocarditis
CHD
Cardiac shunts (ASD, VSD, PDA)
Cardiomyopathies (hypertrophic, dilated, or infiltrative)
Pericardial disease (effusion, tamponade)
Cardiac tumors and thrombi
Aortic aneurysm
Aortic dissection

Limitations
Poor transmission of ultrasound waves through bone or air (lung).
Images from obese patients or those with COPD may be of limited value.
Study quality is operator-dependent.

BOX 5-2 ADVANTAGES AND DISADVANTAGES OF TRANSESOPHAGEAL ECHOCARDIOGRAPHY

Advantages
Image quality superior vs. transthoracic echo
Better visualization of valves and atria
Particularly useful in assessing prosthetic valves, vegetations, aortic disease, and intracardiac masses
Can be used during cardiac surgery

Disadvantages
Invasive
Requires conscious sedation
Risk of aspiration
Risk of trauma to teeth, pharynx, and esophagus

KEY POINTS

1. Echocardiography utilizes ultrasonic waves and their reflected signals to generate images of the heart.
2. Echocardiography permits the assessment of cardiac structure, valvular function, ventricular systolic and diastolic function, and estimation of LV ejection fraction. Serial images can be obtained over time, allowing for the assessment of disease progression.
3. TEE provides higher image resolution than TTE. TEE is well suited for imaging valvular structures and thoracic aortic pathology and for the identification of potential intracardiac sources of emboli.

6 Cardiac Catheterization

Cardiac catheterization involves the percutaneous placement of catheters into the vasculature and cardiac chambers. This allows for the measurement of intracardiac pressures, assessment of ventricular function, and visualization of the coronary anatomy. This information is an essential part of the assessment of a variety of cardiac disorders.

full diagnostic cardiac catheterization encompasses several techniques, including right heart catheterization (RHC), left heart catheterization (LHC), assessment of oxygen saturation, measurement of cardiac output, coronary angiography, and contrast ventriculography. The specific techniques performed during a particular procedure depend on the information required.

TECHNIQUES

Access to the vasculature is most often obtained via the femoral artery and vein, although the brachial or radial arteries and the subclavian or internal jugular veins may also be used. A sheath with a one-way valve is placed in the vessel; through it, various catheters may be advanced and positioned into the desired cardiac chamber or vessel (see Figure 6-1). A

■ RIGHT HEART CATHETERIZATION

Hemodynamics

During RHC, a balloon-tipped catheter is advanced through the right-sided cardiac structures, allowing for the direct measurement of pressure in the RA, RV, and pulmonary artery (PA) (see Figures 6-1b and 6-2). The catheter can then be advanced as far as possible

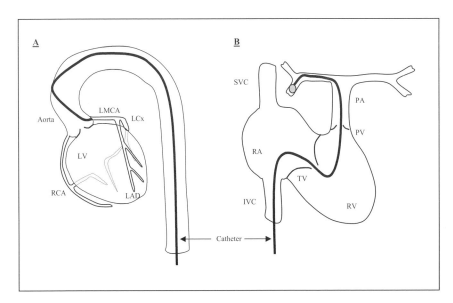

Figure 6-1 • (a) Left heart catheterization and coronary angiography. An intravascular catheter is advanced from the femoral artery through the aorta and placed into the ostium of the left main coronary artery. Catheters can also be placed into the ostium of the right coronary artery and across the aortic valve into the LV chamber. (b) Right heart catheterization. A balloon-tipped catheter is advanced through the IVC, into the RA, across the TV, into the RV, and across the PV; it is then "wedged" into a branch of the PA.

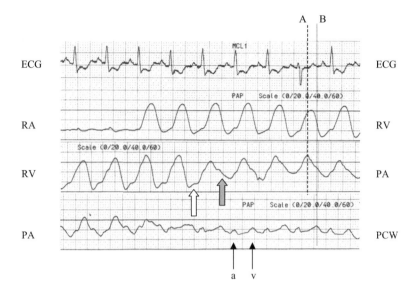

Figure 6-2 • Continuous pressure recording during right-heart catheterization.

Line 1: An ECG rhythm strip (similar to lead V_1).

Line 2: Demonstrates the rise in pressure from the RA to the RV.

Line 3: Demonstrates the change in pressure as the catheter is advanced from the RV to the PA. Note the similar systolic pressure and the rise in diastolic pressure. Also note that the pressure rises during diastole in the RV (white arrow) but falls during diastole in the PA (gray arrow).

Line 4: As the catheter is advanced from the PA to the PCW position, the systolic pressure falls and distinct a and v waves are seen. Note that the peak of the PA waveform occurs during the ST segment on the ECG (line A); whereas the peak of the v wave in the PCW tracing occurs after the peak of the T wave on the ECG (line B). This feature may help to distinguish the two pressure waveforms in patients with large V waves on the PCW pressure tracing.

in the PA (the PCW position); pressure measured in this position is an indirect measurement of the left atrial (LA) pressure.

Oximetry

Blood samples can be drawn sequentially from the various right-sided cardiac chambers and vessels (vena cavae to PA). If a sudden increase in saturation is noted, it identifies the location where oxygenated blood from the left side of the heart is entering the right heart circulation (i.e., intracardiac shunting through an ASD, VSD, or PDA). The magnitude of the oxygen "stepup" can be used to quantify the size of the shunt.

Cardiac Output

CO can be measured by two methods. The thermodilution technique consists of injecting a known volume of saline at a known temperature into the RA and monitoring the temperature changes distally in the PA. The Fick method calculates CO using the patient's oxygen consumption as measured with a

metabolic rate meter or as assumed based on the patient's body surface area (O_2 consumption = 125 mL/min × BSA). Using these techniques, the following formula applies:

$$\text{Cardiac output} = O_2 \text{ consumption} \div AV\ O_2 \text{ difference}$$

The AV O_2 difference is the difference in the oxygen content between arterial and venous blood and is derived using the following equation:

$$AV\ O_2 \text{ difference} = (13.6\ \text{mL}\ O_2/\text{g Hgb/liter of blood}) \times (\text{serum Hgb}) \times (\%\ \text{arterial}\ O_2\ \text{saturation} - \%\ \text{venous}\ O_2\ \text{saturation})$$

For example, if a patient's measured Fick O_2 consumption is 300 mL/min, his serum hemoglobin is 15 g/dL blood, and arterial and venous O_2 saturations are 0.99 and 0.75 respectively, then:

$$300 \div [13.6 \times 15 \times (0.99 - 0.75)] = 6.1\ \text{L/minute}$$

SVR can be calculated from the CO and arterial blood pressure (BP) using the following formula:

$$SVR = [(\text{mean arterial BP} - \text{RA pressure}) \div \text{CO}] \times 80$$

SVR is expressed in units of dynes-sec-cm^{-5}. Measurement of the CO, SVR, and chamber pressures can be very useful in delineating the cause of a patient's hemodynamic abnormalities and determining the appropriate treatment (see Table 6-1).

Indications for Right Heart Catheterization

Right heart catheterization may be performed alone or as part of a complete diagnostic cardiac catheterization. The major indications for right heart catheterization include:

- Assessment of filling pressures and cardiac output in patients with HF, especially when complicated by hypotension or renal failure
- Assessment of volume status and vascular resistance in patients with sepsis
- Evaluation of intracardiac shunts
- Evaluation of pericardial disease (e.g., tamponade, constrictive physiology)
- Perioperative monitoring of patients with a high risk of periprocedural HF

■ LEFT HEART CATHETERIZATION

Hemodynamics

During LHC, a catheter is passed through the femoral artery and advanced retrograde through the aorta, across the aortic valve, and into the LV. LV pressure can then be measured, as can the pressure gradient across the AV, thereby allowing for the assessment of AS (see Figure 27-1). Simultaneous right and left heart catheterization permits measurement of the gradient across the mitral valve (MV), allowing for the assessment of MS (see Figure 28-1).

Coronary Angiography

Catheters can be placed directly into the coronary ostia (Figure 6-1a) and radiopaque contrast material injected. The contrast fills the lumina of the coronary arteries and their branches and allows for the fluoroscopic visualization of the coronary anatomy and identification of stenoses or occlusions (Figures 6-3 and 13-3).

Ventriculography and Aortography

The LV can be visualized by injecting contrast directly into the LV cavity. Contractility and wall motion of the ventricle can be assessed and MR quantified. Injection into the ascending aorta may help to

■ TABLE 6-1

Characteristic Hemodynamic Profiles

Diagnosis	Systemic BP	RA Pressure	PA Pressure	PCW	CO	SVR	Treatment
Normal	120/80 mm Hg	0–5 mm Hg	12–30/5–15 mm Hg	8–12 mm Hg	5 L/min	800–1200 dynes-sec-cm^{-5}	
Cardiogenic shock	↓	↑	↑	↑	↓	↑↑	Vasopressors, inotropes
Septic shock	↓	↓	Normal or ↓	↓	↑	↓↓	Vasopressors, IV fluids, antibiotics
Hypovolemia	↓	↓	↓	↓	↓	↑	Volume resuscitation
Pulmonary HTN/cor pulmonale	Normal	↑	↑↑↑	Normal	Normal	Normal	Pulmonary vasodilators, diuretics
Pericardial tamponade*	↓	↑	↑	↑	↓	↑	Pericardiocentesis

*In pericardial tamponade, the RA, PA diastolic, and PCW pressures are not only elevated but also equal.

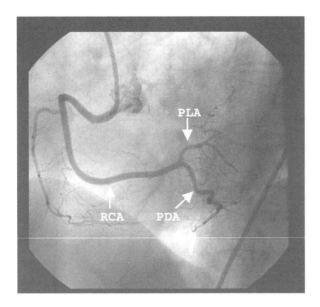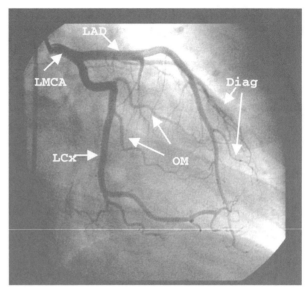

Figure 6-3 • Normal coronary angiogram. (a) Normal RCA showing bifurcation into the PDA and the PLA. (b) Normal LMCA and its bifurcation into the LAD and LCx arteries. The diagonal branches (Diag) arise from the LAD and the obtuse marginal (OM) branches arise from the LCx.

assess the severity of aortic regurgitation (AR) and identify an aortic aneurysm or dissection.

Indications for LHC

LHC may be performed for diagnostic or therapeutic purposes. Indications for **diagnostic** LHC include the following:

- To define the coronary anatomy in patients with:
  - Acute ST-elevation MI (with a view to immediate angioplasty)
  - Unstable angina or non–ST elevation MI with high-risk markers (especially if there is elevated troponin or concomitant heart failure)
  - Postinfarction angina
  - Stable angina refractory to medical therapy or with a high-risk stress test result
  - Previous cardiac arrest
  - Recurrent chest pain for which noninvasive testing is equivocal or nondiagnostic
- To measure hemodynamics and quantify valvular abnormalities in patients with aortic or mitral valve disease
- To assess LV systolic function
- To evaluate proximal aortic disease (i.e., dissection or aneurysm)
- To assess hemodynamics in patients with suspected pericardial constriction or restriction

Therapeutic applications of cardiac catheterization include:

- Balloon angioplasty and stent placement for the treatment of CAD
- Intraaortic balloon pump (IABP) placement for cardiogenic shock and as a bridge to surgery in patients with refractory ischemia or mechanical complications of MI
- Balloon valvuloplasty for valvular stenosis
- Percutaneous closure of intracardiac shunts

▆ PERCUTANEOUS CORONARY INTERVENTION (PCI)

Patients with coronary or thrombosis often atheroslerosis require revascularization of the narrowed coronary artery. This can be performed via catheter-based systems whereby equipment can be delivered through the catheters and directly to the site of coronary stenosis or occlusion. The stenosis can then be dilated with a balloon (angioplasty) to restore normal blood flow. Arteries treated in this fashion are prone to renarrowing (restenosis). Placement of an intracoronary stent—a hollow tube made of stainless steel scaffolding—significantly reduces the risk of restenosis. A variety of stents are currently available, some of which are impregnated with medications such as sirolimus or paclitaxel, which reduce the rate of vessel restenosis by decreasing the proliferation of smooth muscle cells. The choice of stent size and type depends on the anatomy of the specific coronary lesion being treated. For patients who do develop restenosis, repeat angioplasty or stenting and the application of intracoronary radiation (brachytherapy) may be used to prevent recurrence.

COMPLICATIONS OF CARDIAC CATHETERIZATION

The most frequent complication of cardiac catheterization is bleeding; this requires transfusion in ~1% of patients. Major complications such as death, MI, stroke, ventricular fibrillation (VF), anaphylactic reactions to contrast, and emergent need for coronary artery bypass grafting (CABG) are rare (<1% incidence). Contrast nephropathy occurs in as many as 15% of patients and is much more common in diabetics and patients with preexisting renal insufficiency. Vascular injury at the access site (arterial laceration, thrombosis, distal embolization, pseudoaneurysm, AV fistula, hematoma, retroperitoneal hemorrhage), cholesterol embolization, non–life threatening allergic reactions, infection at the access site, atrial arrhythmias, and HB are also well-recognized complications.

CONTRAINDICATIONS TO CARDIAC CATHETERIZATION

Relative contraindications to catheterization include:

- Active infectious processes
- Ongoing major bleeding
- Recent (<1 month) stroke
- Worsening renal impairment
- Severe anemia
- Severe electrolyte and/or acid–base disturbances
- Severe active noncardiac systemic illness
- Severe uncontrolled psychiatric illness
- Digitalis toxicity
- Severe systemic hypertension

KEY POINTS

1. Cardiac catheterization is a safe and effective tool for the diagnosis of cardiovascular diseases.
2. Important information provided by cardiac catheterization includes right and left heart pressures, oxygen saturations, CO, LV function, and coronary artery anatomy.
3. Cardiac catheterization is the "gold standard" for assessing the severity of valvular heart disease, especially valvular stenosis.
4. Treatment of coronary lesions can be accomplished with balloon angioplasty and/or stents.

Diagnostic Modalities for Arrhythmias

Several diagnostic modalities are available for use in patients with known or suspected arrhythmic disorders. These include ambulatory ECG monitoring, tilt-table testing, and electrophysiologic study (EPS).

■ AMBULATORY ECG MONITORING

An ambulatory ECG monitor is a portable telemetric device that allows ECG recording in the outpatient setting. A Holter monitor is a specific device that records for 24 to 48 hours continuously. Patients perform their usual activities while wearing the device and record any symptoms they experience. The device is interrogated for the presence of arrhythmias, which can then be correlated with the patient's symptoms. Holter monitors are useful to:

- Evaluate for an arrhythmic cause of unexplained syncope, near syncope, or dizziness
- Evaluate for an arrhythmic cause of palpitations
- Assess a patient's response to antiarrhythmic therapy

Twenty-four-hour monitoring may be helpful for patients who have frequent symptoms; however, infrequent symptoms are unlikely to occur during the short duration of recording. Loop monitors (or event monitors) are similar to the 24-hour monitors but can be worn for weeks or months at a time and record a person's ECG when the device is activated. This device may be useful for the evaluation of infrequent symptoms. Devices are now available that are implanted under the skin of the chest wall and can remain in place for many months. These may be useful to evaluate very infrequent symptoms.

■ TILT-TABLE TESTING

During this test, a patient is strapped onto a level table and then tilted to an upright position (usually 60 degrees from supine) for 15 to 30 minutes. The patient's blood pressure and heart rate (HR) are monitored and the patient is assessed for symptoms of presyncope or syncope.

Indications

The main indication for tilt-table testing is to evaluate patients with suspected neurocardiogenic (vasovagal) syncope. It may also be useful in patients with recurrent syncope of unclear cause.

Pathophysiology of the Response

Theoretically, rapid assumption of the upright position results in a sudden decrease in venous return to the right heart. This evokes a sudden increase in ventricular contractility and stimulates ventricular mechanofibers (C fibers). In patients with neurocardiogenic syncope, a parasympathetically mediated, paradoxical reflex ensues (the Bezold-Jarisch reflex), in which systemic vascular resistance and HR both drop precipitously, resulting in cerebral hypoperfusion and syncope.

Interpretation of the Test

Three abnormal responses may be seen:

- Cardioinhibitory response: sudden HB and/or drop in HR without significant change in BP
- Vasodepressor response: a dramatic reduction in BP with little change in the HR (less common)

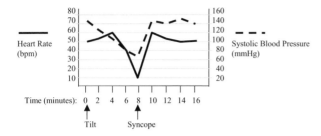

Figure 7-1 · Abnormal response to tilt-table testing. Following initial tilt to 60 degrees, the patient rapidly developed hypotension and bradycardia (mixed vasodepressor and cardioinhibitory response) and subsequently lost consciousness. This resolved after placing the patient supine.

- Mixed response: a combination of the cardioinhibitory and vasodepressor responses (most common abnormal response)

The test is considered positive if it precipitates a syncopal episode or elicits presyncopal symptoms in the face of a significant reduction in HR and/or BP (Figure 7-1). The sensitivity of this test for the detection of vasovagal syncope is approximately 70%. Unfortunately, serial testing of an individual patient may not elicit the same response, and 20 to 25% of patients without a history of syncope will have an abnormal test.

ELECTROPHYSIOLOGIC STUDY

EPS involves the introduction of multiple catheter-based electrodes through the femoral veins and into the RA and ventricle. These electrodes are then strategically positioned in the heart and used to measure endocardial electrical activity (Figure 7-2). Each segment of the cardiac conduction system (from the sinoatrial node to the His-Purkinje fibers) can be systematically studied to assess its ability to conduct electrical impulses normally. Additionally, the atrial and ventricular myocardium and the conduction system can be evaluated to determine their ability to generate and maintain tachyarrhythmias.

Indications

EPS is primarily indicated in the evaluation of certain tachyarrhythmias. It may also occasionally be useful in assessing certain bradyarrhythmias. Specific indications include the evaluation of:

- Nonsustained VT in patients with prior MI and LV ejection fraction (LVEF) <35%

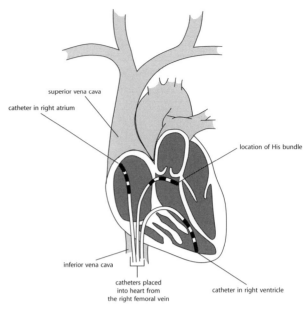

Figure 7-2 · Intracardiac position of catheters for EPS. The catheters are positioned to allow measurement of electrical activity in the RA, RV, and the bundle of His.

- Sustained VT or cardiac arrest in the absence of a precipitating cause (e.g., ischemia, hypokalemia)
- SVT of uncertain mechanism
- Wide-complex tachycardia of uncertain origin
- HB of unclear etiology (especially second-degree HB type 2)
- Unexplained syncope in patients with decreased LVEF
- Possibly to risk stratify patients with symptomatic hypertrophic cardiomyopathy

Once the EP catheters are in place, attempts are made to induce the tachyarrhythmia by electrically stimulating certain areas of the heart (programmed electrical stimulation). Once the arrhythmia is induced, its conduction sequence can be mapped. In certain arrhythmias, the electrical circuit by which the arrhythmia is perpetuated can be interrupted with the use of radiofrequency (RF) energy. This energy is used to make a focal burn in the endocardium overlying a part of the abnormal circuit. This **ablates** the conductive tissue where the energy was applied, thereby destroying the circuit and preventing recurrences of the arrhythmia (**RF ablation**). Examples of arrhythmias that are frequently amenable to RF ablation include:

- Atrioventricular reentrant tachycardia [e.g., Wolff-Parkinson-White (WPW)]
- AV-nodal reentrant tachycardia

- Atrial flutter (occasionally AF may be amenable)
- Certain forms of VT

Patients who have inducible ventricular tachyarrhythmias during an EP study may be candidates for implantation of a cardioverter-defibrillator (see Chapter 25).

KEY POINTS

1. Twenty-four-hour ambulatory ECG monitoring may be helpful in identifying arrhythmias that occur on a relatively frequent basis. Event monitors are useful in evaluating less frequent arrhythmias.
2. Tilt-table testing is indicated for the evaluation of suspected neurocardiogenic syncope.
3. EPS may be used to determine the mechanism of both tachy- and bradyarrhythmias and to localize the source or pathway of a tachyarrhythmia so that RF ablation can be performed.

8 Other Imaging Modalities

Although the vast majority of cardiac imaging is performed with echocardiography, nuclear perfusion imaging, or coronary angiography, several other imaging modalities are currently in clinical use or may be so in the future.

▨ CHEST RADIOGRAPHY (SEE FIGURE 8-1)

Chest radiography provides an image of various cardiac and vascular structures and remains an important tool in the initial evaluation of patients with suspected heart disease. In reviewing a CXR for evidence of cardiovascular disease, attention should focus on the following:

- Cardiac size (normally less than half the thoracic diameter)
- Evidence of individual chamber enlargement (see Table 8-1)
- The pulmonary vasculature (see Table 8-2)
- Aortic and mediastinal size
- Evidence of prior cardiothoracic surgery (sternotomy wires, surgical clips, prosthetic rings and/or valves, pacemaker, implantable defibrillator)
- Calcification of the vasculature, valves, or pericardium

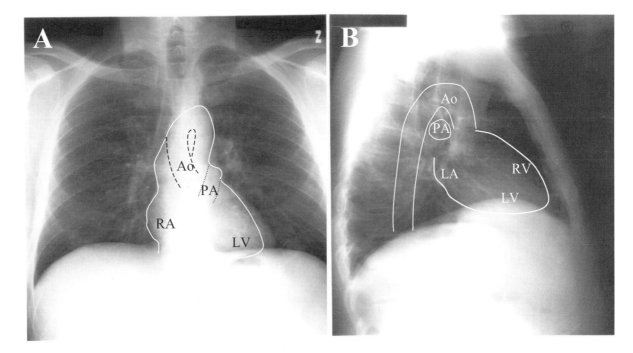

Figure 8-1 • Normal CXR and location of cardiac structures. (a) Posteroanterior view. (b) Lateral view.

■ TABLE 8-1

Characteristic Radiographic Findings of Specific Cardiac Abnormalities

Cardiac Abnormality	Associated Radiographic Finding
LA enlargement	Straightening or lateral bulging of left heart border, widening of the carinal angle to >75 degrees
RA enlargement	Bulging of right heart border
LV hypertrophy	Rounding of LV apex
LV enlargement	Downward and lateral displacement of LV apex, globular appearance, loss of retrocardiac air space (on lateral view)
RV enlargement	Loss of retrosternal airspace (on lateral view)

■ MULTIPLE GATED ACQUISITION (MUGA)

MUGA, or multiple gated blood-pool imaging, is a form of radionuclide ventriculography (RVG); it is among the most reliable methods of quantifying ventricular systolic function. In performing MUGA, the patient's blood is labeled with a radioactive tracer and the radioactivity subsequently emitted from the heart is measured with a gamma camera. The quantity of radiation emitted at any instant reflects the amount of blood in the heart at that point in time. By "gating" the measurement of radioactivity to the person's ECG, systolic and diastolic radiation emission can be measured separately and compared; the difference reflects the amount of blood ejected from the heart with each contraction [the **ejection fraction** (EF)]. Both RVEF and LVEF can be accurately measured.

Advantages

- High degree of accuracy
- Reproducible
- Provides information about both RV and LV function
- Assessment of function not limited by body habitus
- Easy to perform and requires less than 30 minutes

Disadvantages

- Exposes the patient to radiation.
- Provides essentially no information about valvular structure and function.
- Is less accurate in patients with arrhythmias.

■ TABLE 8-2

Abnormal Radiographic Findings in Selected Cardiovascular Disorders

Cardiovascular Disorder	Abnormal CXR Finding	Radiographic Appearance
CHF	Vascular cephalization	Prominent vessels in upper lung fields
	Kerley B lines	Horizontal, linear densities in the lateral lung fields reflecting engorged lymphatic vessels
	Blunting of the costophrenic angle (i.e., pleural effusion)	Concave upward radiopacity of the costophrenic angle
Pulmonary hypertension	Pruning of the pulmonary vasculature	Prominent central pulmonary arteries with loss of peripheral pulmonary vasculature
Pericardial effusion with or without tamponade	"Water bottle" heart	Enlarged cardiac silhouette with broad inferior diameter
Constrictive pericarditis	Pericardial calcification	Thin, radiopaque outline of the cardiac silhouette
Aortic aneurysm/dissection	Widened mediastinum	Wide mediastinal shadow
Congenital cardiac shunts (ASD, VSD)	Shunt vascularity	Increased pulmonary vascular markings; atrial enlargement

Clinical Utility

MUGA/RVG is frequently used when accurate, serial measurements of ventricular function are needed and slight changes in EF are clinically significant. Such situations include monitoring for cardiotoxicity in patients receiving chemotherapy and evaluation before and after cardiac transplantation to monitor for acute allograft rejection. MUGA is also useful to determine LV and RV systolic function when technical limitations (e.g., extreme obesity, severe COPD) impair the quality of the images obtained by other modalities, such as echocardiography.

▇ ELECTRON-BEAM COMPUTED TOMOGRAPHY (EBCT)

EBCT, formerly known as **ultrafast** or **cine** CT, provides high-resolution imaging of the heart that is gated to the cardiac cycle. It differs from standard CT in that the imaging source does not have to be rotated around the patient, thus allowing for faster image acquisition. EBCT can provide both anatomic and functional data, including the assessment of ventricular volumes, myocardial mass, EF, regional cardiac function, contractility, infarct size, valvular function, and pericardial disease. In addition, it can detect and quantify coronary artery calcification, a surrogate marker of coronary atherosclerosis (see Figure 8-2).

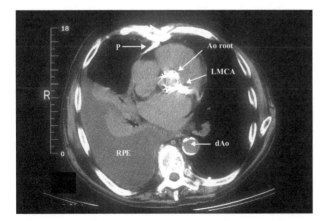

Figure 8-2 • EB CT in a patient with severe CAD and constrictive pericarditis. There is dense calcification of the aortic root (AO root), left main coronary artery (LMCA), descending thoracic aorta (dAo), and the pericardium (P). A large right pleural effusion (RPE) is also noted.

Advantages

- Superb image resolution
- Not limited by patient's body habitus
- Rapid acquisition time
- Relatively inexpensive (about $475)

Disadvantages

- Provides anatomic but not physiologic information.
- Movement during image acquisition can lead to artifact.
- Patient must hold his or her breath for 20 to 50 seconds so as to reduce motion artifact.
- Radiation exposure.
- Intravenous contrast (typically required for image acquisition) may be nephrotoxic.
- 25% of coronary segments cannot be imaged owing to respiratory motion artifact, excessive calcification, or small vessel caliber.

Clinical Utility

Currently, the main utility of cardiac EBCT is in the evaluation of pericardial diseases and cardiac tumors. It is the test of choice for the visualization of the pericardium in suspected constrictive pericarditis and for anatomic delineation of invasive cardiac tumors. EBCT may also play a role in the noninvasive assessment of CAD. Coronary arterial calcification is an early component of atherosclerotic plaque formation and its measurement may reflect total atherosclerotic burden. EBCT can accurately detect and quantify coronary calcium; it can therefore be used as a screening test to identify CAD in asymptomatic patients. A calcium score can be derived (range from 0 to >400); high scores (>400) have a strong correlation with the presence of obstructive CAD (sensitivity: 80 to 100%) but low specificity (40 to 60%). Nonetheless, the finding of coronary calcification in an asymptomatic patient does not warrant any specific therapy aside from risk-factor modification, and controversy exists regarding the appropriate use of this modality in predicting clinical outcome or guiding preventive therapy.

▇ CARDIAC MRI

Cardiac MRI offers great potential as a new modality for noninvasive cardiac imaging (Figure 8-3); however, its application in clinical medicine has been limited by

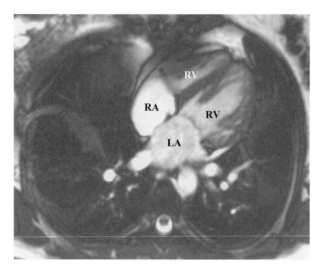

Figure 8-3 • Cardiac MRI.
(Image courtesy of Frederick Ruberg, MD, Division of Cardiology, Boston Medical Center, Boston, Massachusetts.)

the complex nature of the technology and its high cost. Images are obtained in the same way as with routine MRI, and image acquisition is gated to the person's ECG, so that systole and diastole can be distinguished. Patients must be able to hold their breaths for 20 to 50 seconds to eliminate respiratory motion during image acquisition. Cardiac MRI provides a variety of anatomic and functional information including LVEF and RVEF, myocardial mass, intracardiac volumes, regional wall motion analysis, myocardial ischemia, myocardial viability, coronary anatomy, valvular structure and function, anatomic abnormalities, pericardial diseases, infiltrative disorders of the myocardium, and myocardial wall thickness.

Advantages

- Superb image resolution without interference from lung, bone, or fat.
- Absence of radiation exposure.
- Images can be obtained in any orientation or geometric plane.
- Provides for assessment of almost every aspect of cardiac anatomy and performance.

Disadvantages

- Not available at all facilities.
- Costly.
- Involves sophisticated technology that requires additional extensive training.

- Requires gating of images to the ECG (may be difficult in patients with AF).
- Cannot be used in patients with pacemakers, defibrillators, or other metallic foreign bodies.
- Patients with claustrophobia may not be able to tolerate the study.
- Motion during image acquisition can result in artifacts.
- Patients must be able to hold their breath for 20 to 50 seconds.

Clinical Utility

Currently, cardiac MRI is used predominantly for research purposes. However, over the past few years, it has become more clinically useful for the assessment of myocardial and valvular function, delineation of coronary anatomy, detection of myocardial ischemia, detection of postinfarction complications (e.g., VSD, LV aneurysms), assessment of myocardial viability, and diagnosis of myocardial and pericardial diseases.

KEY POINTS

1. Chest radiography remains a valuable tool in the assessment of a variety of cardiac disorders. It should be evaluated with regard to size and morphology of the cardiac silhouette, mediastinal size, presence of vascular calcification, and evidence of pulmonary vascular congestion.
2. MUGA scanning provides an accurate and highly reproducible assessment of LV and RV function.
3. Electron-beam CT is the test of choice for visualizing pericardial thickening and invasive cardiac tumors. It may also play a role as a screening test for CAD.
4. Currently, cardiac MRI is mainly investigational; however, it may soon play a role in the diagnostic evaluation of a variety of cardiac disorders.

Part Three

Coronary Artery Disease

Coronary Artery Disease— Pathophysiology

CAD is the leading cause of death in the United States, accounting for half of the nearly one million deaths resulting from cardiovascular disease each year. The term *atherosclerosis* is derived from the Greek "athero" (gruel) and "sclerosis" (hardening). Atherosclerosis of the coronary arteries is the major cause of CAD; intracoronary thrombosis (atherothrombosis) also plays an important role. CAD is a progressive degenerative process that begins in childhood and manifests itself in middle to late adulthood as an acute coronary syndrome, or ACS [i.e., unstable angina and acute myocardial infarction (AMI)] or chronic ischemic heart disease (e.g., chronic stable angina, ischemic cardiomyopathy). Epidemiologic studies have identified multiple risk factors for atherosclerosis and CAD; the modification of these risk factors holds promise for the prevention and treatment of this disease.

■ NORMAL CORONARY ARTERIES

Anatomy

The heart receives blood through the left and right coronary arteries, which are the first branches of the aorta (Figure 9-1). The right coronary artery (RCA) gives off acute marginal branches to the RV and, in 85% of people, it also gives off branches to the inferior aspect [posterior descending artery (PDA)] and posterior aspect (posterolateral branches) of the LV. This is referred to as **right-dominant circulation**.

The left main coronary artery is quite short and bifurcates into the left anterior descending (LAD) and the left circumflex (LCx) arteries. The LAD gives off diagonal branches that supply blood to the anterior aspect of the left ventricle, and the LCx artery gives off obtuse marginal branches that supply blood to the lateral aspect of the left ventricle. In 10% of people,

the LCx gives rise to both the posterior descending and posterolateral arteries (**left-dominant circulation**). In 5% of people, the RCA gives rise to the posterior descending artery and the LCx gives rise to the posterolateral arteries (**codominant circulation**).

Small collateral vessels interconnect the coronary arteries. These collaterals are nonfunctional in the normal setting but provide an alternate route for blood flow if the coronary artery becomes stenosed.

Physiology

The coronary arteries are conductance vessels and offer very little resistance to coronary blood flow in their normal state. They can, however, constrict or dilate in response to vasoactive substances, thereby allowing the heart to maintain a fairly constant level of coronary blood flow despite changes in perfusion pressure. This phenomenon is referred to as **autoregulation** and allows coronary blood flow to increase in the face of increased myocardial oxygen demand (e.g., exercise). The difference between the resting coronary blood flow and the maximal coronary blood flow is referred to as the **coronary flow reserve** (Figure 9-2).

The normal arterial wall consists of the endothelium, intima, media, and adventitia. The endothelium plays an important role in autoregulation. It synthesizes and releases powerful vasodilators such as endothelium-derived relaxing factor (nitric oxide) and prostacyclin in response to various stimuli, including platelet-derived factors [acetylcholine, serotonin, and adenosine 5'-diphosphate (ADP)], thrombin, and increased shear stress (**flow-mediated vasodilation**). The endothelium is also intimately involved in the prevention of intravascular thrombosis via its production of antiplatelet (heparan, prostacyclin) and

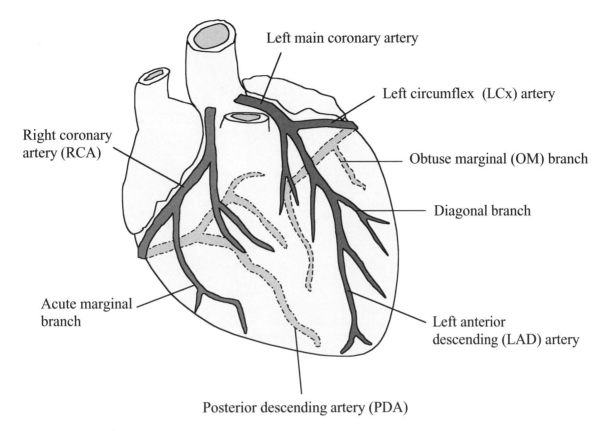

Figure 9-1 • Anatomy of the coronary arteries.

thrombolytic [tissue plasminogen activator (TPA)] factors. Thus, a normal, intact endothelium is crucial in regulating coronary vascular tone and maintaining adequate coronary blood flow.

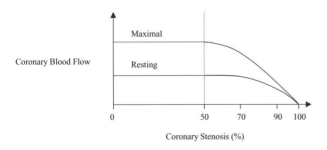

Figure 9-2 • Coronary flow reserve and alterations in coronary blood flow in relation to the degree of coronary artery stenosis present. *Maximal* refers to the maximal coronary blood flow possible in response to increased myocardial oxygen demand. The difference between the maximal and resting flows is the coronary flow reserve. Maximal coronary blood flow is significantly reduced in the face of a stenosis of > 70%. Resting coronary blood flow is not significantly affected until the stenosis is > 90%.

ATHEROSCLEROSIS

Pathogenesis

The initiating event of atherosclerosis is an injury to the vascular endothelium; the response to this injury leads to the development of atherosclerotic lesions. The initial injury can be mechanical (shear stress), biochemical (e.g., lipoproteins, tobacco), and possibly infectious (e.g., viruses, *Chlamydia*). This injury results in alterations in endothelial permeability, increased adhesiveness of leukocytes to the endothelium, and altered release of vasoactive and hemostatic substances from endothelial cells. These changes, collectively referred to as **endothelial dysfunction**, are the earliest measurable changes of atherosclerosis and result in a local prothrombotic state and impaired ability of the endothelium to modify vascular tone.

Following the initial injury, circulating monocytes adhere to the endothelial surface and migrate into the vascular intima, where they become macrophages. Low-density lipoprotein (LDL) is transported through the endothelial cells and ingested by the macrophages,

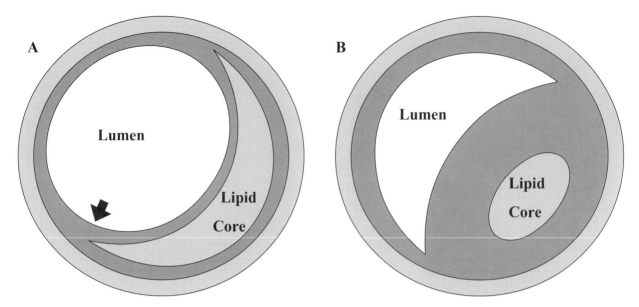

Figure 9-3 • Morphology of atherosclerotic plaques. (a) Lipid-rich plaque. This type of plaque is prone to rupture at the shoulder region (arrow), resulting in coronary thrombosis and acute coronary syndromes. (b) Predominantly fibrous plaque. This type of plaque is relatively stable but tends to progressively narrow the arterial lumen, thereby limiting blood flow and causing exertional angina (see text for details).

thus producing "foam cells." Collections of these foam cells produce the earliest visible lesion of atherosclerosis, a yellowish deposit in the vascular wall known as a "fatty streak."

The activated macrophages produce and release toxic substances (e.g., superoxide anion, oxidized LDL) that result in endothelial denudation and subsequent platelet adhesion to the site of injury. Platelets and activated macrophages also release various cytokines and growth factors, resulting in the migration and proliferation of T cells, smooth muscle cells, and fibroblasts. This process eventually creates a neointima with a fibrous cap overlying the lipid core.

The Atherosclerotic Plaque

Atherosclerotic plaques may be predominantly fibrotic or consist of a large lipid core with a thin fibrous cap (Figure 9-3). Fibrotic plaques generally appear during early adulthood, are white in appearance, and may progressively protrude into the lumen of the artery, thus narrowing it and resulting in decreased coronary blood flow. In response, the vessel distal to the stenosis dilates in the resting state to allow for normalization of resting blood flow. This, however, decreases the vessel's ability to augment flow in response to increased metabolic demand

(decreased coronary flow reserve). Once the metabolic demand exceeds maximal coronary blood flow, ischemia and angina develop. In general, a 70% decrease in the diameter of the artery is enough to

BOX 9-1 RISK FACTORS FOR ATHEROSCLEROSIS

Positive risk factors
Major
  HTN
  Hyperlipidemia
  Smoking
  DM
  Male gender
  Advanced age
  Family history of premature atherosclerosis
Minor
  Obesity
  Physical inactivity
  Hyperhomocysteinemia
  Elevated Lp(a)
  Elevated fibrinogen levels
  Elevated plasminogen activator inhibitor
Negative risk factors
Elevated HDL

limit blood flow in the face of increased demand (e.g., exercise) and produce exertional angina. A 90% decrease in the arterial diameter may limit blood flow and result in angina even in the resting state (see Figure 9-2).

In largely lipid-laden plaques, the accumulating lipid causes necrosis of the macrophages, resulting in the release of digestive enzymes such as collagenase and gelatinase (matrix metalloproteinases). These enzymes weaken the fibrous cap and a "vulnerable plaque" is formed. This type of plaque is prone to fissure or rupture, especially at the edge (or "shoulder") of the lesion (Figure 9-3b). Such plaque rupture exposes the lipid core and vascular collagen to the circulating blood, leading to platelet activation and aggregation. A thrombus is then formed at the site of plaque rupture, causing partial or complete occlusion of the coronary artery and resulting in the clinical syndromes of unstable angina and AMI (refer to Chapters 12 and 13).

RISK FACTORS

Many epidemiologic studies have demonstrated an association between CAD and certain risk factors, some of which clearly play a causal role (e.g., hypertension, hyperlipidemia, diabetes, smoking) (see Box 9-1). High-density lipoprotein (HDL) is a negative risk factor; higher levels of HDL cholesterol (>60 mg/dL) are associated with a decreased risk of CAD. Some risk factors (e.g., diabetes, hypercholesterolemia, smoking, etc.) can be modified, whereas others (age, gender, and family history) cannot. Modification of risk factors decreases the future risk of CAD, stabilizes existing CAD, and potentially stimulates regression of atherosclerotic plaques in patients with established disease.

KEY POINTS

1. CAD is the leading cause of death in the United States.
2. CAD is caused by atherosclerosis of the coronary arteries and has both acute and chronic manifestations (refer to Chapters 11, 12, and 13).
3. Atherosclerosis is characterized by endothelial injury, inflammation, lipid deposition, plaque formation, and thrombosis.
4. A 70% stenosis of a coronary artery will limit blood flow in the face of increased demand (e.g., exercise), while a 90% stenosis is sufficient to limit blood flow at rest.
5. Risk factors for CAD can be identified and modified to reduce the risk of this disease.

10 Dyslipidemia

Dyslipidemia comprises a group of disorders characterized by abnormal circulating levels of lipid or lipoprotein fractions. They are caused by genetic and/or environmental conditions that alter the metabolism of these lipoproteins.

■ NORMAL LIPID AND LIPOPROTEIN METABOLISM (SEE FIGURE 10-1)

The major plasma lipoproteins are distinguished by their lipid content and density and their constituent proteins (Table 10-1). **Chylomicrons** (formed within the intestine from dietary fat) and **very low density lipoproteins** (VLDL) (produced in the liver) are both rich in **triglycerides** (TG). They are metabolized to **chylomicron remnants** and **intermediate-density lipoproteins** (IDL), respectively, after acquiring apolipoprotein C-II (apo C-II) from **high-density lipoproteins** (HDL) and then undergoing hydrolysis by lipoprotein lipase (LPL) in muscle and adipose tissue. The liver clears chylomicron remnants, and IDL undergoes further conversion to **low-density lipoproteins** (LDL), which can circulate for 3 to 5 days. LDL accounts for approximately 70% of the total plasma cholesterol and is cleared mainly by the liver.

Lipoprotein (a) [Lp(a)] is secreted by the liver and makes up less than 10% of the total plasma lipoprotein mass. LDL, together with Lp(a), has been shown to be atherogenic, and elevated levels are associated with increased risk of cardiovascular disease. HDL is secreted by both the liver and intestine; it readily accepts cholesterol from cells and other lipoproteins and is believed to be cardioprotective.

■ DYSLIPIDEMIA

Epidemiology

Approximately 32% of American men and 27% of American women have hypercholesterolemia requiring treatment. More than half of the CHD in the United States is attributable to lipid abnormalities, predominantly elevated LDL cholesterol. An individual's cholesterol or LDL is, on average, intermediate between that of his or her parents, reflecting genetic influences.

Etiology

In the majority of people, elevated lipid levels result from a combination of factors that include obesity, inactivity, a diet high in fats and cholesterol, and genetic predisposition. A minority of patients have dyslipidemia resulting purely from genetic mutations in the genes involved in lipid metabolism (primary dyslipidemias). The underlying metabolic defects and associated lipid profiles of these primary dyslipidemias are outlined in Table 10-2. Of these primary dyslipidemias, **polygenic hypercholesterolemia** is the most common.

A variety of conditions can produce elevated lipoprotein levels in the absence of an underlying genetic defect (**secondary hyperlipidemia**). These conditions are outlined in Box 10-1.

Diagnostic Evaluation

Every adult over the age of 20 years should have a complete fasting lipid profile [total serum cholesterol, HDL cholesterol (HDLc), and TGs] measured

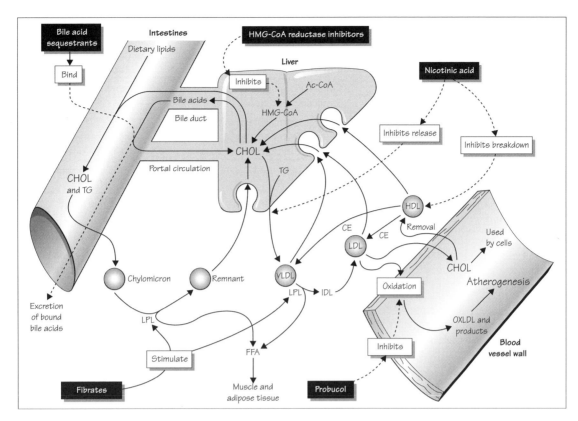

Figure 10-1 • Normal metabolism of lipoproteins and sites of action of lipid-lowering agents.
(Reproduced by permission from Aaronson PI, Ward J, Wiener CM. The Cardiovascular System at a Glance. Oxford, UK: Blackwell Publishing, 2003.)

every 5 years. If TG levels are <400 mg/dL, LDL-cholesterol (LDLc) can be calculated as follows:

$$LDLc = total\ cholesterol - (HDLc + TG/5)$$

Clinical Manifestations

History

Most patients with hyperlipidemia are asymptomatic, although patients with severe hypertriglyceridemia

(TG > 1,000 mg/dL) may present with acute pancreatitis. Patients should be thoroughly questioned regarding symptoms of cardiovascular disease [angina, claudication, transient ischemic attack (TIA), cerebrovascular accident (CVA)]. Measurement of lipid levels should be performed in concert with a search for other major risk factors for CAD, including:

• Current cigarette smoking.
• Hypertension (BP > 140/90 mm Hg, or on antihypertensive medications).

■ TABLE 10-1

Properties of Lipoproteins

Lipoprotein Class	Origin	Major Surface Apoproteins	Major Core Lipid
Chylomicrons	Intestine	B-48, C, E	Dietary TG, cholesterol esters
VLDL	Liver	B-100, C, E	Hepatic TG
LDL	VLDL catabolism	B-100	Cholesterol esters
Lp(a)	Liver	B-100, (a)	Cholesterol esters
HDL	Liver, intestine	A, C	Cholesterol esters

TABLE 10-2

Classification of Primary Dyslipidemias

Class	Lipid Profile	Phenotypes	Metabolic Defect(s)
I, V	↑ Chylomicrons (class I) ↑ VLDL (class V)	Familial LPL deficiency Familial apo CII deficiency	Impairment/absence of LPL Functional deficiency of LPL
IIa	↑ LDL	Familial hypercholesterolemia; Familial defective apo B100; Polygenic hypercholesterolemia	LDL receptor defects (↓ receptor number or ↓ affinity for LDL)
IIb	↑ VLDL, ↑ LDL	Familial combined hyperlipidemia	↑ VLDL secretion +/− LPL defect
III	↑ VLDL, ↑ IDL	Dysbetalipoproteinemia	Defective apo E
IV	↑ VLDL	Familial hypertriglyceridemia	↑ VLDL production or ↓TG metabolism

- Diabetes.
- Age (men ≥45 years, women ≥55 years).
- Family history of premature CAD (in males <55 years or females <65 years). A strong family history of dyslipidemia or cardiovascular disease suggests a primary lipid disorder.
- HDL: low HDL (<40 mg/dL) is a risk factor for CAD, whereas high HDL (>60 mg/dL) is considered protective and negates the effect of one other risk factor.

Physical Examination

Corneal arcus (a gray ring around the cornea), xanthelasmas (yellowish periorbital plaques), xanthomas (subcutaneous nodules on extensor tendons), and hepatosplenomegaly are sometimes present in patients with dyslipidemias. Manifestations of atherosclerosis, including diminished peripheral pulses and arterial

bruits, should be looked for in patients with a dyslipidemia or suspected of having one.

Treatment

Goals (See Table 10-3)

For the vast majority of hyperlipidemic patients, the goal of therapy is reducing CAD risk by lowering LDLc. The National Cholesterol Education Program (NCEP) has developed guidelines (Adult Treatment Panel III, or ATP III) for treating hyperlipidemia based on a person's absolute lipid levels, the presence of CAD or CAD equivalents (other atherosclerotic disease, including symptomatic carotid artery disease, peripheral arterial disease, and abdominal aortic aneurysm; and diabetes mellitus), and the presence of other coexisting cardiac risk factors (refer to "History," above). In patients without CAD and with fewer

TABLE 10-3

LDL Treatment Recommendations

Risk Profile	LDL Level at Which to Initiate Drug Therapy	Goal LDL
Without CAD, fewer than two other risk factors	≥190	<160
Without CAD, two or more risk factors	≥160	<130
With CAD or CAD equivalent*	≥130[‡]	<100
Patients at very high risk[†]	≥100	<70

*CAD *equivalent* refers to other atherosclerotic disease or diabetes mellitus.
[†]Patients at very high risk are those who have had a recent heart attack, or have CAD combined with either diabetes or severe/poorly controlled risk factors or with metabolic syndrome.
[‡]Physician should exercise clinical judgment in patients with LDLs of 101 to 129 mg/dL to determine whether drug therapy should be initiated.

BOX 10-1	SECONDARY CAUSES OF HYPERLIPIDEMIA

Secondary causes of hypercholesterolemia
High-fat diet
Obstructive liver disease
Nephrotic syndrome
Hypothyroidism
Medications (corticosteroids, anabolic steroids, progestins)

Secondary causes of hypertriglyceridemia
Type II diabetes mellitus
Obesity
Hypothyroidism
Alcohol use
Medications (beta blockers, diuretics, estrogen)

than two other cardiac risk factors, the goal of treatment is an LDLc < 160 mg/dL; in patients with two or more risk factors, the goal LDLc is < 130 mg/dL. Patients with known CAD or CAD equivalents should have an LDLc of < 100 mg/dL. In patients at very high risk, including those who have had a recent heart attack, or have CAD combined with either diabetes or poorly controlled risk factors, a goal of attaining a lower LDL should be considered (< 70 mg/dL).

Hypertriglyceridemia (TG ≥ 150 mg/dL) is usually associated with elevated LDLc, and this responds to treatment. For persistently elevated TGs, therapy should be instituted to lower the non-HDL cholesterol (total cholesterol – HDLc) to no greater than 30 mg/dL above the respective LDLc goal.

Nonpharmacologic Therapy

Primary treatment for hypercholesterolemia and hypertriglyceridemia involves dietary therapy in concert with

TABLE 10-4

Lipid-Lowering Agents

Drug Class	Mechanism of Action	Lipid Effects	Side Effects
Bile-acid sequestrants	↑ Fecal bile acid excretion ↑ LDL-receptor activity	↓↓ LDL ↑ HDL ?↑ TG	Constipation Abdominal bloating ↓ Absorption of other drugs
Nicotinic acid (niacin)	↓ Plasma free fatty acids ↓ Hepatic VLDL synthesis	↓ LDL ↑ HDL ↓↓ TG	Elevated LFTs Increased uric acid GI upset, flushing, and pruritus
HMG-CoA reductase inhibitors (statins)	↓ Cholesterol biosynthesis ↑ LDL-receptor activity	↓↓ LDL ↑ HDL ↓ TG	Elevated LFTs Myositis (↑ CK; rare) Mild GI symptoms
Fibric-acid derivatives (fibrates)	↓ Hepatic VLDL synthesis ↑ LPL activity	+/−LDL ↑ HDL ↓↓ TG	Elevated LFTs Cholelithiasis Myositis (rare) Diarrhea, nausea
Probucol	Enhances scavenger pathway removal of LDL	↓ LDL ↓↓ HDL −TG	Prolonged QT Ventricular arrhythmias (rare) Nausea, diarrhea Flatulence
Ezetimibe	Inhibits intestinal absorption of cholesterol	↓ LDL-C ↓TG ↑HDL	Headaches Nausea Fever Myalgias
Fenofibrate	Activates LPL and decreases production of apo C-III, resulting in increased lipolysis	↓ LDL-C ↓TG ↑HDL	GI symptoms, myalgias, fevers

weight loss and regular exercise. These measures are collectively referred to as therapeutic lifestyle changes (TLC) under ATP III. The TLC diet derives less than 7% of total calories from saturated fat and contains < 200 mg/day of cholesterol. Intake of soluble fiber (10 to 25 g/day) and plant stanols/sterols (2 g/day) should also be considered as therapeutic options to enhance LDL lowering. On average, dietary therapy lowers lipid levels by about 10 to 20%. Secondary causes of dyslipidemia should also be corrected or treated.

Pharmacologic Therapy (See Table 10-4)

Drug therapy for hypercholesterolemia should be considered when the LDLc level remains above the initiation level for drug therapy despite 3 to 6 months of maximal dietary therapy. Pharmacologic treatment may also be considered as initial therapy in addition to diet in patients with elevated lipid levels and known CAD, atherosclerotic vascular disease, or diabetes. The preferred first-line agent for hypercholesterolemia is an HMG-CoA reductase inhibitor, or "statin," because of its efficacy in reducing both LDL and cardiovascular events (MI or death). With use of escalating doses, statins can reduce LDLc by 10 to 50%. Ezetimibe is a useful alternative in patients who are intolerant of statins. This drug lowers LDLc by as much as 40% by decreasing the absorption of cholesterol in the intestines. Other useful agents include niacin and bile acid sequestrants (e.g., cholestyramine). These agents may also be added to a statin for refractory patients, in which case close monitoring for liver toxicity is required.

Drug therapy for hypertriglyceridemia is recommended if TG levels remain high (≥200 mg/dL) for any patient or borderline high (150 to 199 mg/dL) for patients with CAD risk factors despite an adequate trial of lifestyle modification. A statin is usually sufficient therapy in patients with borderline elevations of TG; niacin or a fibric-acid derivative (fibrate) may be necessary for patients with higher TG levels. Patients should be monitored closely when statins and fibrates are used in combination, as this regimen is associated with a higher risk of myositis and rhabdomyolysis.

A fasting lipid profile should be obtained 1 to 3 months after starting or changing lipid therapy. If goal lipid levels are not achieved, more aggressive lifestyle modifications or pharmacologic therapy should be employed. LFTs and the serum creatine kinase (CK) level should also be checked several months after initiation of pharmacologic therapy to assess for occult toxicity.

KEY POINTS

1. The major serum lipids are LDL, HDL, and TGs.
2. Dyslipidemias usually result from the combined effects of diet, inactivity, obesity, and genetic factors.
3. Elevated LDL cholesterol and, to a lesser extent, elevated TGs are associated with increased risk of CAD and cardiovascular events.
4. Low HDL (<40 mg/dL) is a risk factor for CAD, whereas increased HDL (>60 mg/dL) is protective.
5. The treatment of dyslipidemias is based on the absolute level of lipids, the presence of other CAD risk factors, and the presence of established cardiovascular disease or diabetes mellitus.

Chronic Stable Angina

Angina is the clinical manifestation of myocardial ischemia (MI). It is overwhelmingly the result of a limitation in coronary blood flow induced by atherosclerotic narrowing of the coronary arteries. Angina that is long standing and reproduced by a predictable amount of exertion is referred to as chronic stable angina.

Pathophysiology

Normal coronary arteries mediate changes in coronary blood flow in response to changes in MVO_2. When the demands of the heart increase (as during exercise), the coronary arteries dilate to allow increased blood flow to meet these demands (see Figure 9-2). This system of autoregulation occurs at the level of the arterioles, requires an intact vascular endothelium, and is mediated by by-products of metabolism including adenosine, acidosis, low oxygen tension, and high levels of carbon dioxide. When a coronary artery becomes narrowed by greater than 70%, its blood flow is decreased by approximately 90%. In this setting, maximal coronary vasodilation occurs, allowing for enough blood flow to meet the metabolic demands of the resting heart. However, during periods of increased myocardial demand (e.g., exercise), the artery is unable to dilate further, resulting in inadequate coronary blood flow and ischemia. Higher-grade stenoses (>90% reduction in diameter) may cause ischemia in the resting state. The narrowing of coronary arteries is overwhelmingly the result of atherosclerosis, the pathogenesis of which is described in Chapter 9.

Clinical Manifestations

History

The term *angina pectoris* (see also Chapter 1) is used to describe a discomfort in the chest or adjacent areas caused by myocardial ischemia without myocardial necrosis. In chronic stable angina, the discomfort is usually precipitated by physical or emotional stress. It is frequently not described as painful but rather as "pressure-like" or "squeezing." It is usually retrosternal in location but can radiate to the neck and the arms, and it can be associated with dyspnea, diaphoresis, nausea, or vomiting.

Typical angina begins gradually and reaches maximal intensity over a few minutes; then it gradually subsides with rest or after the administration of nitroglycerin. The resolution of the discomfort with nitroglycerin can be a helpful diagnostic feature of angina; however, it is a relatively nonspecific response—esophageal pain and other syndromes may also be alleviated by nitroglycerin. Characteristics that are not suggestive of angina include fleeting chest pain, chest pain that is localized to a discrete point, discomfort that is brought on or worsened by breathing or arm movement, or discomfort that is reproducible by palpation on examination. Identification of risk factors for atherosclerosis is crucial in the assessment and treatment of patients with chronic stable angina (see Box 9-1).

PHYSICAL EXAMINATION

The physical examination of patients with CAD and chronic stable angina is often entirely normal. However, evidence of hypertension (HTN—elevated blood pressure, retinal changes), hyperlipidemia (xanthomas, xanthalasma), and vascular disease (diminished pulses, vascular bruits) should raise the suspicion of underlying CAD. Examination of the heart is often normal, but in patients with prior MI, signs of LV dysfunction (dyskinetic apical impulse, third heart sound, elevated jugular venous pressure, or pulmonary edema) may be present. A transient murmur of mitral regurgitation may be heard during an episode of angina and results from ischemic papillary muscle dysfunction.

Differential Diagnosis

A wide variety of disorders can mimic anginal chest pain; they are outlined in Chapter 1.

Diagnostic Evaluation

The diagnosis of angina (and thus of CAD) can often be made by history alone. Further objective testing may be confirmatory or may be necessary to clarify the diagnosis when the cause of the patient's symptoms is not clear. In approximately 50% of patients with chronic stable angina, the resting ECG is normal or demonstrates nonspecific ST-T changes. Q waves, conduction abnormalities, or premature ventricular complexes may be present in patients with a prior MI.

Stress testing is frequently used to establish the diagnosis and estimate prognosis of patients with chronic stable angina (see Chapter 4). Exercise-induced ST-segment depression is the hallmark of exertional ischemia. Features on stress testing that reflect a poorer prognosis in patients with chronic stable angina include:

- A greater magnitude of ST depression (>2 mm)
- Ischemic changes occurring in multiple (>5) ECG leads
- Ischemia occurring at a low level of stress
- Exercise-induced hypotension
- Multiple areas of ischemia on nuclear or echocardiographic imaging

Echocardiography (see Chapter 5) can also be used to identify evidence of a prior MI and assess LV function in these patients. A definitive diagnosis of CAD can be made by performing coronary angiography. This procedure allows precise determination of the number and severity of coronary stenoses, which can be used to estimate prognosis and to guide therapy.

Treatment

General Approach

There are several key aspects of the management of chronic stable angina, which are often considered and applied simultaneously.

TABLE 11-1	
Modifiable Risk Factors for Coronary Artery Disease and the Goals of Modification	
Risk Factor	**Goal of Modification**
HTN	SBP < 130, DBP < 80
DM	FBS < 120, HA1c < 8
High LDLc	LDL < 160 if there are no other risk factors
LDL < 130 if there are one or two risk factors
LDL < 100 if known CAD or DM
LDL < 70 in patients at very high risk (see Chap. 10)
Low HDLc	HDL > 35
Cigarette smoking	Total cessation
Physical inactivity	30 min of exercise ≥ 3 times per week
Obesity	<120% ideal body weight
Hyperhomocysteinemia	Normalize homocysteine level

1. Symptomatic relief of angina can be achieved by either decreasing MVO_2 (with medications) or increasing myocardial oxygen supply/coronary blood flow (with medications or with percutaneous or surgical revascularization).
2. Any concomitant disorders such as anemia, fever, tachycardia, thyrotoxicosis, CHF, and infections increase the metabolic demands on the heart and should be identified and treated.
3. Aggressive risk-factor modification (including cholesterol lowering, control of HTN, treatment of diabetes mellitus, smoking cessation, weight loss, dietary changes, and regular exercise) should be undertaken to lower the subsequent risk of future adverse cardiac events (Table 11-1).

Pharmacologic Therapy (Table 11-2)

Several different classes of medications are useful as antianginal therapy, including nitrates, beta blockers, calcium channel blockers, and antiplatelet therapy. Nitrates are potent vasodilators that reduce both preload and afterload, thus reducing MVO_2. They also dilate the coronary vasculature to some extent, thereby improving supply. Nitrates can be used either to treat symptoms or as chronic prophylactic therapy; however, it is important to have a nitrate-free period when long-acting nitrates are being used so as to prevent the development of tolerance.

■ TABLE 11-2

Effect of Antianginal Agents on Determinants of Myocardial Oxygen Supply and Demand

	Preload	Afterload	HR	Contractility	MVO_2	Supply
Nitrates	↓↓	↓	—	—	↓	↑
Beta blockers	—	↓	↓↓	↓↓	↓↓↓	—
Calcium channel blockers	—	↓↓	↓	↓	↓↓	↑

Beta blockers and calcium channel blockers both reduce MVO_2 by decreasing heart rate, BP, and contractility; they are effective in relieving symptoms of angina and improving exercise tolerance. Beta blockers are the agents of choice for the treatment of patients who have had a prior MI or have known LV dysfunction (refer to Chapters 12, 13, and 17) and produce a significant mortality benefit in these settings. Aspirin inhibits platelet aggregation and prevents thrombosis at the site of a coronary stenosis, an effect that is essential in the treatment of all forms of CAD. All patients with symptoms of CAD should therefore be placed on daily aspirin therapy. Patients who are intolerant of aspirin may be treated with other antiplatelet agents, such as clopidogrel. Combined antiplatelet therapy with aspirin and clopidogrel may be beneficial in patients with persistent symptoms despite pharmacologic therapy who are not felt to be candidates for revascularization.

Revascularization Therapies

When angina persists despite optimal medical management or when patients with "high-risk" stress tests are identified, cardiac catheterization should be recommended in order to define the coronary anatomy and determine the feasibility of coronary revascular-ization. Revascularization may be performed by either percutaneous transluminal coronary angioplasty (PTCA), with or without coronary stenting, or CABG (see Table 11-3).

Percutaneous revascularization has been shown to be more effective than medical therapy in relieving symptoms of angina, but without a clear mortality benefit. CABG can provide complete revascularization, is effective for the control of angina, and has been shown to be superior to both medical therapy and percutaneous approaches in terms of reducing mortality in a subset of high-risk patients. Patients in whom bypass surgery is of particular benefit include those with left main CAD and those who have LV dysfunction and either three-vessel CAD or two-vessel CAD with involvement of the proximal LAD. This is especially true for diabetic patients.

PRINZMETAL VARIANT ANGINA

In 1959, Prinzmetal described a syndrome of anginal chest pain that occurs almost always at rest and is associated with ST-segment elevation on the ECG. It may be associated with acute MI, ventricular arrhythmias, or sudden death.

■ TABLE 11-3

Percutaneous vs. Surgical Coronary Revascularization

	PTCA	CABG
Advantages	Less invasive; shorter hospital stay; lower initial cost; easily repeated	May improve long-term survival; more complete revascularization; improved outcome in diabetic patients; may reduce the need for medications
Disadvantages	Less complete revascularization; no clear mortality benefit; need for repeat procedures	Higher initial morbidity and mortality; higher initial cost

Etiology

Variant angina is caused by coronary artery spasm leading to complete occlusion of the vessel. This tends to occur in areas adjacent to atheromatous plaques, but it can also occur in normal arterial segments (pure coronary vasospasm). Cigarette smoking is an important risk factor for variant angina. Cocaine use can precipitate coronary vasospasm even in individuals without a prior history of this syndrome.

Clinical Manifestations

Patients with variant angina tend to be younger than those with chronic stable angina, and the chest pain with which they present tends to occur at rest rather than with exertion. In contrast to the ST-segment depression associated with classic angina, the ECG during episodes of variant angina demonstrates ST-segment elevation. The diagnostic hallmark of variant angina is the finding of spasm of a proximal coronary artery with resultant ischemia during coronary arteriography. Intracoronary infusion of ergonovine or acetylcholine can be used to induce coronary vasospasm in patients with suspected variant angina.

Treatment

Coronary vasospasm responds very promptly and completely to nitrates. Short-acting nitrates are useful in abolishing acute attacks, while long-acting nitrates can prevent recurrent episodes. Calcium channel blockers, especially nifedipine, are also very effective. Beta blockers have a variable effect and may be detrimental—selective inhibition of the beta-adrenergic receptors leaves alpha-adrenergic receptors unopposed, thereby predisposing to alpha-adrenergic–mediated vasoconstriction and aggravating coronary spasm. The overall long-term prognosis is good unless there is coexisting CAD, MI, or significant arrhythmias.

KEY POINTS

1. Chronic stable angina is caused by obstructive, flow-limiting atherosclerotic stenoses within the epicardial coronary arteries.
2. Chronic stable angina is characterized by exertional chest pain that is relieved with rest or after the administration of nitroglycerin.
3. Exercise stress testing is helpful in clarifying the diagnosis and prognosis of patients with suspected angina; cardiac catheterization remains the "gold standard" for diagnosing CAD.
4. Aspirin, risk-factor reduction, and antianginal medications are the mainstays of medical therapy; percutaneous or surgical revascularization is indicated for patients with refractory angina or high-risk results of noninvasive tests.
5. Prinzmetal's angina is the result of coronary artery spasm, usually at the site of an atherosclerotic plaque. It is associated with ST-segment elevation on ECG and responds to nitrates or calcium channel blockers.
6. Beta blockers are relatively contraindicated in the treatment of vasospastic angina owing to their potential to induce unopposed alpha-adrenergic vasoconstriction.

Unstable Angina and Non-ST-Elevation Myocardial Infarction

The term *acute coronary syndrome* (ACS) refers to unstable angina (UA), non-ST-elevation myocardial infarction (NSTEMI; previously referred to as non-Q-wave MI), and ST-elevation MI (STEMI; previously referred to as Q-wave MI). The first two of these syndromes (UA and NSTEMI) are discussed in this chapter and STEMI is discussed in Chapter 13.

Epidemiology

In the United States alone, there are nearly 1.5 million hospital admissions for UA and NSTEMI each year. Additionally, NSTEMI accounts for 30 to 40% of all MIs.

Etiology (See Also Chapter 9)

Slowly progressive, high-grade coronary stenoses can cause angina and may progress to complete occlusion; however, they rarely precipitate ACS because of the development of collateral circulation. Rather, most ACS result from rupture of nonocclusive lipid-laden atherosclerotic plaque with subsequent intravascular thrombosis (see Figure 9-3). If the thrombus is flow-limiting but not occlusive or is only transiently occlusive, UA or NSTEMI results. In addition to atherosclerosis, several other disorders may result in myocardial ischemia and infarction. These include:

- Coronary vasospasm (of normal coronary arteries or at the site of an atherosclerotic plaque)
- Severe hypertension
- Disorders that increase MVO_2 (e.g., hyperthyroidism, pheochromocytoma, sepsis) or decrease oxygen delivery (anemia)

Clinical Manifestations

History

Unstable angina encompasses a broad range of anginal presentations, including:

- Crescendo angina superimposed on chronic stable angina
- New-onset angina (within 2 months) brought on by minimal exertion
- Rest angina of >20 minutes in duration
- Post-MI angina (occurring >24 hours after MI)

An NSTEMI presents with features similar to those of UA except that the anginal symptoms tend to be more severe and prolonged. CHF may accompany UA or NSTEMI if severe ischemia or underlying LV dysfunction is present. Ischemia-induced arrhythmias [sinus tachycardia, premature ventricular complexes (PVCs), nonsustained ventricular tachycardia (VT)] may also occur (see Chapter 14).

Physical Examination

Physical examination during an ACS may demonstrate:

- Tachycardia
- Hypertension or hypotension (secondary to cardiogenic shock)
- Transient S_3 or S_4
- Transient or increased murmur of MR (resulting from papillary muscle ischemia)

Diagnostic Evaluation

The diagnosis of UA is primarily based on clinical symptoms and confirmed by ancillary tests. The ECG obtained during chest pain typically demonstrates ST

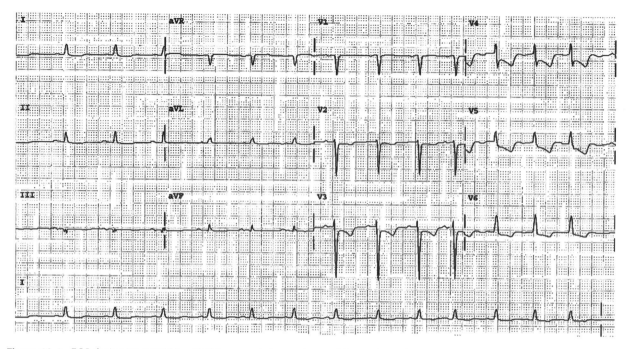

Figure 12-1 • ECG during UA/NSTEMI, with ST-segment depression and T-wave inversions seen in leads V_2 to V_6.

segment depression or symmetric T-wave inversions (Figure 12-1); however, it may be normal in approximately 5% of patients. These ECG changes are often labile during UA (present during angina but normalized after resolution of angina), whereas they persist or evolve following an NSTEMI.

Cardiac enzymes [creatine kinase-MB isoenzyme (CK-MB) and troponins] are highly sensitive and specific markers of myocardial necrosis and distinguish NSTEMI (elevated enzyme levels) from UA (normal enzyme levels). Serial measurements (on admission and every 8 hours for 24 hours) of CK-MB and troponin are usually performed to differentiate between UA and NSTEMI and to estimate infarct size. Serum CK levels begin to normalize after 24 to 48 hours, whereas troponin levels remain elevated for 7 to 10 days; the latter provides a useful test for diagnosing MI several days after the event (see Figure 12-2).

Differential Diagnosis

The complete differential diagnosis of chest pain is reviewed in Chapter 1. The most important diagnoses to consider include:

• Pulmonary embolism
• Aortic dissection
• Pneumothorax
• Pneumonia
• Pericarditis
• Gastrointestinal disorders (gastroesophageal reflux disease, cholelithiasis, pancreatitis)

Prognosis

UA progresses to MI in about 10% of cases and to death in about 5%. The presenting symptoms, ECG findings, and serum markers of myocardial necrosis all affect the risk of MI or death in patients with UA and NSTEMI. Elevated troponins are independently

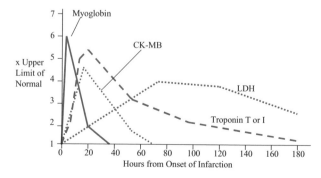

Figure 12-1 • Time course of appearance of serum markers of myocardial injury.

BOX 12-1	RISK* CATEGORIES OF PATIENTS WITH UNSTABLE ANGINA

High risk
At least one of the following features must be present:
   Prolonged (> 20 min), ongoing rest pain
   Pulmonary edema
   Rest angina with dynamic ST changes (>1 mm)
   Angina with new MR murmur
   Angina with S_3 or rales
   Angina with hypotension
   Positive cardiac troponin[†]

Intermediate risk
No high-risk feature but must have any of the following:
   Resolved prolonged rest pain
   Rest angina (> 20 min) relieved with SL NTG
   Angina with dynamic T-wave changes
   New-onset class III to IV angina within past 2 weeks
   Nocturnal angina
   Q waves or resting ST depression < 1 mm in multiple
      leads
   Age >65 years

Low risk
No high- or intermediate-risk features but any of the following:
   Increased anginal frequency, severity, or duration
   Angina provoked at lower than usual threshold
   Normal or unchanged ECG
   New-onset angina within past 2 months

*Risk refers to the risk of progression to MI or death.
[†]May be classified as NSTEMI.

predictive of MI and death; hence, elevation of this marker is considered a high-risk feature in patients with UA or NSTEMI. Factors that identify a patient as being at high risk are summarized in Box 12-1. The presence of one or more of these factors suggests the need for more aggressive therapy.

Treatment

The primary goals of treatment are to control symptoms and preserve myocardial function. These goals are accomplished by:

- Administration of analgesia
- Reduction of MVO_2
- Improvement in coronary blood flow
- Prevention of intracoronary thrombosis

Additionally, long-term prevention of recurrent ischemic events through risk-factor modification is essential.

Liberal use of anxiolytics (benzodiazepines) and analgesia (morphine) helps to relieve pain and anxiety, thus decreasing heart rate, BP, and MVO_2.

Antiplatelet therapy should be initiated as soon as the diagnosis of UA or NSTEMI is suspected. At least 160 mg of aspirin should be given acutely, followed by 81 to 325 mg daily. The first dose should be chewed to ensure rapid absorption. Clopidogrel (300 mg initial dose followed by 75 mg daily) appears to decrease morbidity when added to aspirin and is an alternative antiplatelet agent for patients with an aspirin allergy.

Antithrombotic therapy with either unfractionated heparin or low-molecular-weight heparin (LMWH) (enoxaparin or dalteparin) should be administered for 48 to 72 hours to patients with intermediate- or high-risk features. LMWHs are more effective than unfractionated heparin but are contraindicated in the setting of renal insufficiency or marked obesity. Direct antithrombin agents such as hirudin and hirulog may be considered as alternatives for those in whom heparin cannot be used. These agents are more potent inhibitors of clot-bound thrombin than heparin and have been shown to be equivalent to heparin in preventing adverse ischemic events. Glycoprotein (GP) IIb-IIIa inhibitors, which block platelet activation and aggregation, have been shown to be of benefit in the treatment of UA and NSTEMI. GP IIb-IIIa inhibitors should be used in patients with high-risk clinical features and in those for whom cardiac catheterization and percutaneous intervention are planned.

Beta blockers decrease MVO_2 and are therefore effective in controlling ischemia. They should be used in all patients with UA/NSTEMI unless contraindicated. Nondihydropyridine calcium channel antagonists may be used in patients without heart failure and with preserved LV systolic function; they may prevent recurrent infarction in this setting. Nitrates, in oral, transdermal, or intravenous forms are effective in relieving anginal symptoms and for prophylaxis against further ischemic episodes, but they do not affect mortality. Angiotensin-converting enzyme (ACE) inhibitors appear to decrease morbidity and mortality in some patients with UA/NSTEMI and should be added if hemodynamically tolerated.

Thrombolytic therapy has no role in the treatment of UA and NSTEMI, as it is associated with higher mortality due to intracranial hemorrhage in these patients.

After the patient with UA or NSTEMI has been stabilized, cardiac catheterization and coronary revascularization should be considered. Clopidogrel should be started immediately in patients who undergo PCI and should be continued for at least 1 month following balloon angioplasty or placement of an uncoated stent, 3 to 6 months following placement of a drug-eluting stent, and up to 9 months in patients without a high risk of bleeding. Initial studies comparing **conservative therapy** [medications, risk stratification with exercise tolerance testing (ETT)] to an **early invasive strategy** (cardiac catheterization and revascularization) found a higher morbidity in the invasive group. More recent studies using intracoronary stenting have favored the early invasive strategy. Thus, the decision to proceed to cardiac catheterization is made case by case, based on an individual patient's risk profile, comorbidities, and patient/physician preference. A generally accepted approach follows:

- Low-risk patients: noninvasive stress testing for further risk stratification (may be done off medications if diagnosis is uncertain)
- Intermediate-risk patients: noninvasive stress testing after stabilization with medications
- High-risk patients: cardiac catheterization and revascularization if anatomically indicated

Patients who undergo noninvasive testing and have moderate to severe ischemia should undergo cardiac catheterization and revascularization, either percutaneously (PTCA with or without stent implantation) or surgically (CABG), depending on their anatomy.

Risk-Factor Modification

Risk factor modification is a key component of long-term therapy. Goals of risk factor modification are outlined in Box 11-1.

KEY POINTS

1. ACS comprises UA, NSTEMI, and STEMI.
2. An ACS results from atherosclerotic plaque rupture and intracoronary thrombosis.
3. Initial treatment of UA/NSTEMI includes analgesia, antiplatelet agents, heparin, beta blockers, and nitrates.
4. Low- and intermediate-risk patients should undergo risk stratification with stress testing and, if the test is very abnormal, cardiac catheterization. High-risk patients should undergo cardiac catheterization and revascularization.
5. All patients with ACS should undergo aggressive risk-factor modification.

ST-Elevation Myocardial Infarction

STEMI, previously referred to as **Q-wave** or **transmural** MI, is an ACS in which there is persistent, complete occlusion of the involved coronary artery.

Pathogenesis (See Also Chapter 9)

STEMI is most often the result of atherosclerotic plaque rupture with subsequent coronary thrombosis. Rarely, STEMI may be the result of another disorder including:

- Coronary emboli (from intracardiac thrombi or valvular vegetation)
- In situ thrombosis (due to a hypercoagulable state)
- Vasculitis (e.g., Kawasaki disease)
- Coronary artery dissection (either primary or as a result of aortic dissection)

Clinical Manifestations (See Also Chapter 1)

The majority of patients with STEMI report severe, persistent substernal chest pain that is commonly associated with nausea, vomiting, diaphoresis, dyspnea, and apprehension. Approximately 25% of patients are asymptomatic or have atypical symptoms. Large infarctions may present with CHF or cardiogenic shock. Patients with an inferior MI may present with hypotension if the infarct involves the right ventricle. Ventricular tachyarrhythmias are common and account for most of the deaths during the first hours following a STEMI (see Chapter 14).

Diagnostic Evaluation

The hallmark of STEMI is STE on the ECG (Figure 13-1). Serial 12-lead ECGs should be performed to confirm the diagnosis and localize the area of infarction. A characteristic evolution of ECG changes occurs (Figure 13-2): STE is present initially, followed sequentially by loss of R-wave height, development of Q waves, T-wave inversion, and finally return of the ST segments to baseline. Patients with extensive anterior wall MI may present with a new LBBB, which limits the interpretation of ST-segment deviation.

Cardiac enzymes have a similar pattern of elevation in STEMI as they do during non-STE MI (see Figure 13-2); however, the absolute increase tends to be greater. Echocardiography during a STEMI demonstrates focal hypokinesis or akinesis of the LV in the distribution of the occluded vessel. This finding can be helpful in the assessment of patients with suspected AMI but with a nondiagnostic or borderline abnormal ECG.

Treatment

Acute Therapy

Time is a key factor during a STEMI, because therapies are more beneficial when administered early. Therefore rapid assessment and treatment should be the goal. Initial management should include:

1. A brief targeted history.
2. Directed physical examination to identify complications and comorbid conditions (e.g., neurologic findings that might preclude thrombolytic therapy or signs suggestive of aortic dissection).
3. 12-lead ECG to confirm the diagnosis (within 10 minutes of presentation) and an ECG using right-sided leads in patients with an inferior STEMI.
4. Institution of analgesia, oxygen, antiplatelet agents, antithrombotic agents, and beta blockers.
5. Determination of the need for reperfusion therapy.

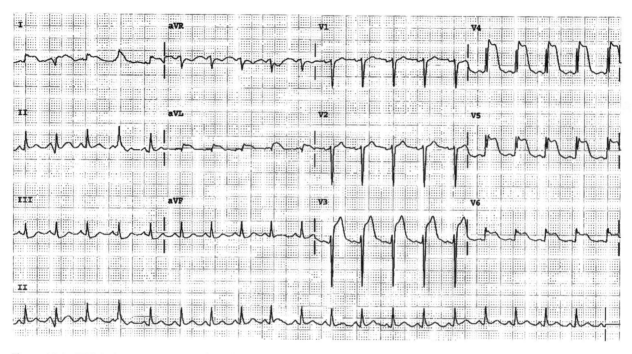

Figure 13-1 • ECG during an acute anterolateral STEMI. Note the marked STE in leads V_3 to V_6, I, and aVL.

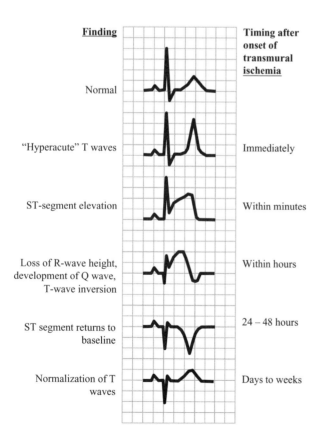

Figure 13-2 • Evolution of ECG changes during and after a STEMI.

The initial management of STEMI is similar to that of UA/NSTEMI. Antiplatelet therapy with aspirin and antithrombotic therapy with unfractionated heparin should be started as soon as STEMI is diagnosed. The first dose of aspirin should be chewed to ensure rapid absorption. Oxygen should be administered by nasal cannula or face mask. Analgesia, generally with morphine sulfate, and anxiolytics should be given as needed to provide comfort. SL NTG should be administered and IV NTG started if ischemic chest pain persists. Beta blockers decrease mortality, reinfarction, and ventricular arrhythmias after a STEMI and should be administered intravenously or orally to all patients unless contraindications exist (e.g., hypotension, bradycardia, bronchospasm). Calcium channel blockers are generally not indicated in this setting.

If the patient has evidence of persistent ischemia (continued angina, persistent STE) after initial medical treatment, reperfusion therapy with thrombolysis or primary angioplasty should be considered. Eligibility and exclusion criteria for thrombolytic therapy are outlined in Box 13-1. Time is a key issue, because thrombolysis is of minimal benefit beyond 6 hours after onset of symptoms.

Thrombolytic therapy with TPA (alteplase) establishes patency of the infarct-related artery in 75 to 80% of cases and has been proven to decrease mortality,

BOX 13-1 CRITERIA FOR THROMBOLYSIS IN AMI

Indications

1. Chest pain consistent with AMI, and
2. ST-elevation >0.1 mV in >2 contiguous leads or new LBBB, and
3. <6 hours from onset of symptoms (consider if within 6–12 hours), and
4. If primary PCI is not available

Absolute contraindications

1. Active internal bleeding (excluding menses)
2. Suspected aortic dissection
3. Prior hemorrhagic stroke at any time; other stroke within 3 months
4. Known intracranial neoplasm or vascular lesion
5. Significant head trauma within 3 months

Relative contraindications

1. Uncontrolled HTN on presentation (BP > 180/110 mm Hg)
2. History of ischemic stroke > 3 months prior
3. INR >2–3; known bleeding diathesis
4. Recent trauma, surgery, or CPR (within 3 weeks)
5. Noncompressible vascular punctures
6. Recent (within 2–4 weeks) internal bleeding
7. Pregnancy
8. Active peptic ulcer
9. History of chronic severe hypertension
10. For streptokinase: prior exposure (within 5 days to 2 years) or prior allergic reaction

decrease infarct size, improve LV function, and reduce HF in patients suffering a STEMI. Other thrombolytic agents (rPA/reteplase and TNK-tPA/tenecteplase) yield similar results and are easier to administer. Streptokinase is somewhat less effective but is associated with a lower rate of intracranial hemorrhage. Since streptokinase is isolated from *Streptococcus*, it elicits an antigenic response and should not be administered to patients who have previously received it.

Primary percutaneous coronary intervention (PCI) offers an alternative reperfusion technique by directly opening the infarct-related artery with catheter-directed balloons (angioplasty) and/or coronary stents (Figure 13-3; see Chapter 6). It is more effective at restoring flow in the affected coronary artery (>95% success rate) than is thrombolytic therapy,

and it poses a lower risk of intracranial hemorrhage. Comparative trials have demonstrated the superiority of primary angioplasty with regard to mortality, reinfarction, recurrent ischemia, and stroke. If angioplasty is planned, adjunctive use of a GP IIb-IIIa inhibitor should be considered and clopidogrel administered.

The main limitation to primary PCI is its lack of widespread availability. At institutions where it is available, it is the preferred strategy. If primary PCI is not available, the patient should be immediately transferred to an angioplasty-capable hospital or be given thrombolytic therapy. Patients with contraindications to thrombolytic therapy and those failing to reperfuse after attempted thrombolysis should be transferred to a nearby hospital with angioplasty facilities for either primary or rescue PCI (see Figure 13-4).

Post-MI Management

All patients should be continued on aspirin indefinitely after a STEMI. Low-dose aspirin (81 mg) is adequate and effective therapy after successful thrombolysis; however, full-dose aspirin (325 mg) should be used for the first month following PCI. Clopidogrel (75 mg daily) should be continued for 1 month following balloon angioplasty and for at least 3 months following placement of an intracoronary stent. Heparin should be continued for 24 to 48 hours after administration of thrombolytics but is not routinely warranted after PCI. Patients with anterior MIs should remain on anticoagulation (with warfarin) for 3 to 6 months to prevent the development of mural thrombi within the LV and the associated thromboembolic complication

Beta blockers should be continued and increased to the highest dose tolerated. ACE inhibitors should be initiated, especially if significant LV systolic dysfunction is present. An aldosterone antagonist (e.g., eplerenone) should be considered in patients with an LV ejection fraction (LVEF) less than 40% who have symptoms of heart failure (HF) or are diabetic. These agents should be used only if significant renal dysfunction is not present, serum potassium is normal, and the patient is tolerating therapeutic doses of an ACE inhibitor. Lipid levels should be checked within 24 hours of admission and appropriate lipid-lowering therapy with a statin started, with a target LDL of <70 mg/dL. As with NSTEMI, aggressive risk-factor modification should be undertaken.

Echocardiography is generally performed several days after AMI to assess LV function. It can also identify LV mural thrombi, valvular disease such as mitral regurgitation, ventricular septal defects, and ventricular aneurysms.

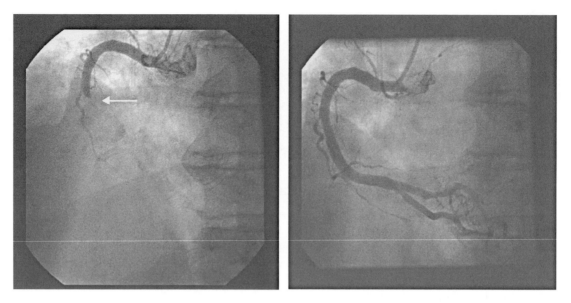

Figure 13-3 • Coronary angiogram during an acute inferior MI. (a) Initial angiogram reveals an occluded right coronary artery (arrow). (b) Same artery after angioplasty and placement of an intracoronary stent at the site of occlusion.

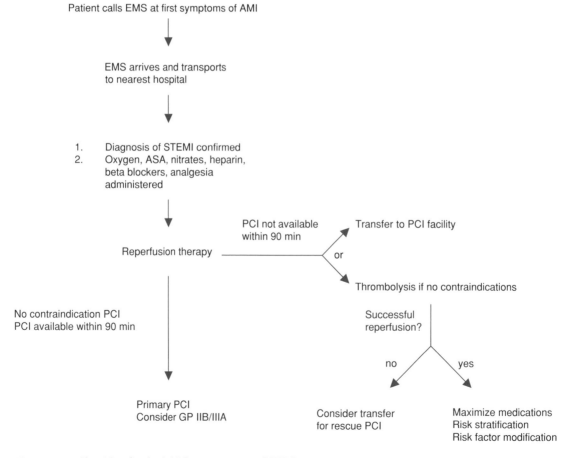

Figure 13-4 • Algorithm for the initial management of STEMI.

Patients who have undergone primary PCI with successful reperfusion, have no residual high-grade stenoses, and have had an uncomplicated course are usually discharged home 3 to 4 days after admission without further testing. Patients who are managed conservatively, including those who received thrombolytic therapy, should undergo low-level exercise tolerance testing (ETT) 3 to 5 days after infarction to assess for ischemia and for risk stratification. A symptom-limited ETT is recommended 3 to 6 weeks after discharge. If a patient is unable to exercise, a pharmacologic stress test such as dobutamine echo or adenosine nuclear perfusion scanning can be performed (see Chapter 4). If these tests reveal significant inducible ischemia or the patient develops recurrent angina, cardiac catheterization and revascularization should be performed. Treatment for complications of MI is described in Chapter 14.

KEY POINTS

1. STEMI usually results from atherosclerotic plaque rupture and subsequent coronary thrombosis.
2. Initial therapy for STEMI includes analgesia, oxygen, aspirin, heparin, nitrates, and beta blockers.
3. Patients with persistent angina and STE should undergo cardiac catheterization and PCI if available. If PCI is not available, thrombolytic therapy should be administered.
4. Following a STEMI, all patients should receive long-term therapy with aspirin, beta blockers, ACE inhibitors, and statins.
5. Aggressive risk-factor modification is essential following an MI.

Complications of Myocardial Infarction

Despite recent major advances in its treatment, AMI is still associated with significant morbidity and mortality. This is in large part a result of infarct-related complications, including:

- HF (both left and right ventricular dysfunction)
- Cardiogenic shock
- Arrhythmias
- Mechanical complications [ventricular free wall rupture, ventricular septal defect (VSD), papillary muscle rupture]

HEART FAILURE

Pathogenesis

Ischemic heart disease can result in heart failure through a variety of mechanisms. Acute ischemia results in an immediate rise in LV diastolic pressure owing to the impairment of myocardial relaxation. Continued ischemia results in acute systolic dysfunction, thereby decreasing cardiac output and further elevating intracardiac pressure. Both the systolic and diastolic dysfunction may precipitate heart failure during an AMI.

MI results in myocardial necrosis with a resultant loss of LV systolic function. Following the acute phase of an MI, ventricular remodeling occurs and results in LV dilation. This altered ventricular morphology produces a further fall in LV systolic function. The development of CHF following an MI also relates to infarct size (the larger the infarction, the more severe the degree of LV dysfunction), and infarct location (an anterior wall MI results in more severe dysfunction than does an inferior or lateral wall MI).

Diagnostic Evaluation

Patients with significant LV dysfunction following an MI may have symptoms and signs of CHF, including dyspnea, orthopnea, tachypnea, tachycardia, pulmonary rales, and an S_3 or S_4 gallop. CXR frequently demonstrates pulmonary vascular congestion and cardiomegaly. An echocardiogram will demonstrate hypokinesis or akinesis of the affected areas of the LV and allow for estimation of the overall LVEF. Invasive assessment of intracardiac pressures with a pulmonary artery catheter can definitively establish the diagnosis of CHF; however, this is usually required only in patients with hemodynamic instability.

Treatment

The management of mild to moderate HF in the setting of AMI includes treatment of the underlying ischemia as well as preload reduction, afterload reduction, and avoidance of hypoxia. Preload reduction with diuretics (e.g., furosemide) and nitrates is effective in reducing symptoms of pulmonary congestion. Care must be taken to avoid overdiuresis, as most patients presenting with AMI and mild CHF are not volume-overloaded. Aggressive diuresis in this setting can result in intravascular volume depletion and precipitate hypotension. Afterload reduction with ACE inhibitors improves both symptoms and mortality. Beta blockers reduce long-term mortality in CHF and should be given to most post-MI patients irrespective of LV function; however, they must be used with caution in patients with decompensated HF.

CARDIOGENIC SHOCK

The most severe form of acute HF is referred to as **cardiogenic shock**. It affects approximately 7% of patients with AMI.

Definition

Cardiogenic shock is characterized by:

- Reduced cardiac output [cardiac index (CI) <2.2 L/kg/min]
- Hypotension (SBP <90 mm Hg)
- Elevated PCWP (>18 mm Hg)
- Organ hypoperfusion

Pathogenesis

Approximately 80% of MI patients with cardiogenic shock have an extensive infarction with severe LV dysfunction (~40% of the LV must be infarcted to result in cardiogenic shock); the remaining patients have mechanical complications (see below) or hypovolemia. Patients with advanced age, prior infarction, diabetes mellitus (DM), large infarction size, and known preexisting LV dysfunction are at increased risk of developing cardiogenic shock after an infarction.

Diagnostic Evaluation

Patients with cardiogenic shock are hypotensive, have signs of pulmonary edema, and have poor organ perfusion (e.g., mental status changes, decreased urine output, cold extremities). The ECG frequently demonstrates signs of acute (STE or ST-segment depression) or chronic (pathologic Q waves) ischemic heart disease. The hemodynamic abnormalities can be confirmed with invasive monitoring (pulmonary artery catheterization).

Treatment

Management of cardiogenic shock requires continuous hemodynamic monitoring as a guide to optimizing LV filling pressure and cardiac output (CO). Medical management includes the use of vasopressors (e.g., dopamine) to maintain adequate BP, inotropes (e.g., dobutamine) to augment CO, and diuretics to decrease pulmonary congestion. Patients who develop cardiogenic shock within 36 hours of presentation of an AMI have improved survival if they undergo revascularization by either PTCA or CABG and should be considered for emergent cardiac catheterization. Placement of an IABP is sometimes necessary to augment systemic BP, improve organ perfusion, augment diastolic coronary artery perfusion, and improve HF. Despite aggressive therapy, the mortality of cardiogenic shock resulting from an AMI approaches 60%.

RIGHT VENTRICULAR INFARCTION

Right ventricular infarction (RVI) usually occurs in association with an inferior LV infarction because both these territories are supplied by the RCA. Isolated RV infarction is rare.

Clinical Manifestations

Patients with significant RVI have signs of RV failure, namely elevated JVP, hepatic congestion, and hypotension. The Kussmaul sign (an inspiratory increase in JVP) may be present. Pulmonary congestion is usually absent unless there is concomitant LV dysfunction. Bradycardia (either sinus bradycardia or AV-nodal block) may be present, generally as a result of increased vagal tone.

Diagnostic Evaluation

Any patient with a suspected inferior MI (and therefore possible associated RVI) should have a right-sided ECG. This is a 12-lead ECG with precordial electrodes placed across the right side of the chest, in the corresponding anatomic position as with left-sided leads V_1 to V_6 (see Chapter 3). STE of >1 mm in any right precordial lead (especially V_4R) is suggestive of RVI. This finding may be transient and usually resolves within 12 to 24 hours after infarction; the absence of right-sided STE does not rule out RV infarct. An echocardiogram will demonstrate RV hypokinesis and usually reveals an associated inferior wall-motion abnormality of the LV. Right heart catheterization demonstrates a low cardiac output, low PCWP, and elevated right heart pressures. The differential diagnosis of RVI includes PE and cardiac tamponade.

Treatment

Acute treatment of an RVI includes reperfusion therapy (thrombolysis or angioplasty) for the associated inferior MI. Hypotensive patients require volume resuscitation (to maintain adequate RV preload) and inotropic support with dobutamine. Nitrates should be avoided.

MECHANICAL COMPLICATIONS OF AMI (FIGURE 14-1)

Following an AMI, disruption of necrotic myocardium may occur and result in rupture of the LV free wall, VSD, or rupture of a papillary muscle with resultant acute MR. These conditions are summarized in Table 14-1.

Clinical Manifestations

Mechanical complications usually occur 3 to 5 days after an AMI. Patients suffering from free-wall rupture may present with recurrent chest pain, pericardial tamponade, or sudden death. Patients with an acute VSD or papillary muscle rupture usually have a new, harsh holosystolic murmur associated with a precordial thrill and rapidly develop PE and hemodynamic collapse.

Diagnostic Evaluation

The diagnosis of a mechanical complication following an AMI can be confirmed by echocardiography and pulmonary arterial catheterization (see Table 14-1).

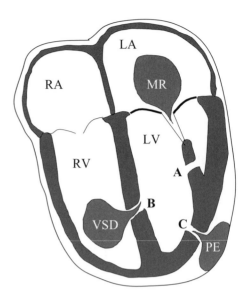

Figure 14-1 • Mechanical complications of AMI. (A) Papillary muscle rupture results in acute, severe MR. (B) Rupture of the interventricular septum produces an acute VSD, resulting in left-to-right shunt flow. (C) Ventricular free-wall rupture causes the rapid development of a pericardial effusion, resulting in pericardial tamponade.

Treatment

The treatment of LV free-wall rupture includes pericardiocentesis if the patient is in tamponade and emergent surgical LV repair. Treatment of an acute VSD or papillary muscle rupture includes inotropic

■ TABLE 14-1

Mechanical Complications of Myocardial Infarction			
Variable	Free-Wall Rupture	Ventricular Septal Defect	Papillary Muscle Rupture
Days post-MI	3–6	3–5	3–5
New murmur	25%	90%	50%
Palpable thrill	No	Yes	Rare
Previous MI	25%	25%	30%
Findings on echocardiography	Pericardial effusion	Shunt flow across septal defect	Flail or prolapsing mitral valve leaflet with severe regurgitation
PA catheterization	Equalization of diastolic pressures (tamponade)	Oxygen saturation stepup in RV-prominent V waves seen on PCW tracing	
Mortality			
Medical	90%	90%	90%
Surgical	Case reports	50%	40–90%

SOURCE: Modified from Braunwald E, Zipes DP, Libby P. Heart Disease: A Textbook of Cardiovascular Medicine, 6th ed. Philadelphia: Saunders, 2001:1183.

■ **TABLE 14-2**

Arrhythmias in Acute Myocardial Infarction

Arrhythmia	Mechanism	Goal of Treatment	Therapy
Ventricular premature beats	Electrical instability	Correct electrolyte abnormalities; reduce sympathetic tone.	Potassium, magnesium repletion; beta blockers.
VT	Electrical instability	Restore sinus rhythm; prophylaxis against VF.	Cardioversion/defibrillation acutely if sustained or hemodynamically unstable. Consider antiarrhythmic agents (amiodarone) if prolonged or recurrent. Anti-ischemic treatment with beta blockers, IABP, and revascularization.
VF	Electrical instability	Restore sinus rhythm.	Immediate defibrillation.
Accelerated idioventricular rhythm	Electrical instability	Restore sinus rhythm.	Observation unless hemodynamically unstable. Increase sinus rate (atropine or atrial pacing) if symptomatic. Avoid antiarrhythmic agents.
Sinus tachycardia	↑ Sympathetic tone	Correct underlying cause; control heart rate.	Antipyretics, analgesics, volume repletion, diuretics, or transfusion if needed. Beta blockers unless CHF present.
AF or atrial flutter	↑ Sympathetic tone, pericarditis	Control heart rate; restore sinus rhythm.	Beta blockers, nodally acting calcium channel blockers (diltiazem or verapamil), or digoxin for rate control. Consider cardioversion.
SVT	↑ Sympathetic tone	Control heart rate; restore sinus rhythm.	Vagal maneuvers, adenosine, beta blockers, or calcium channel blockers. Consider cardioversion.
Sinus bradycardia	↑ Vagal tone; SA nodal ischemia	↑ HR if hemodynamically unstable.	Observe if stable. Atropine or atrial pacing if hemodynamically unstable.
AV block	↑ Vagal tone; AV-node ischemia	Treatment dependent on severity of block and hemodynamic compromise.	1st degree block and Wenckebach: observe if stable. Higher degrees of block: atropine. Consider temporary pacemaker (especially if anterior MI with new BBB).
Intraventricular block (e.g., LBBB or RBBB)	Ischemia/infarction of conduction tissue	Observe.	Consider temporary pacemaker for new LBBB, especially if high-degree AV block also present.

agents, vasodilators, and placement of an IABP as a bridge to emergent surgery. Despite rapid surgical intervention, survival after LV free-wall rupture is rare. Survival after an acute VSD or papillary muscle rupture is generally <50%; rapid recognition and initiation of therapy are paramount.

ARRHYTHMIAS

A wide variety of arrhythmias may occur during an AMI. Some are relatively benign, but many are life-threatening and account for the majority of infarct-associated sudden cardiac deaths (SCDs). The advent of coronary care units and continuous telemetry monitoring has allowed for the early recognition and treatment of these arrhythmias and resulted in a significant reduction in mortality in the peri-infarct period. The genesis, diagnosis, and treatment of these arrhythmias are more fully discussed in Chapters 20 to 22. The specific etiology and treatment of various rhythm disturbances as related to the specific setting of AMI are listed in Table 14-2.

OTHER COMPLICATIONS OF ACUTE MI

Pericarditis (see Chapter 31) frequently occurs in the peri-infarct period as a result of pericardial inflammation adjacent to regions of myocardial necrosis. An autoimmune pleuropericarditis associated with fever and an elevated erythrocyte sedimentation rate (ESR) can also occur, usually weeks after the initial infarction (Dressler syndrome). Treatment is with aspirin or other nonsteroidal anti-inflammatory drugs (NSAIDs). Anticoagulants should be avoided owing to the associated increased risk of hemorrhagic pericarditis.

Ventricular aneurysms are areas of focal myocardial dilation that occur as a result of ventricular remodeling following an AMI. They are readily detected by echocardiography and may produce persistent STE on the surface ECG. True aneurysms are made up of scar tissue, rarely rupture, and require no specific therapy. False aneurysms, or pseudoaneurysms, represent ventricular wall rupture with containment by the pericardium and pose a high risk of spontaneous rupture. Surgical repair is the treatment of choice.

Both arterial and venous emboli may occur in patients with AMI. Venous emboli result from the hypercoagulable state as well as physical inactivity, manifest as deep venous thromboses or pulmonary emboli, and can be prevented by early ambulation or administration of prophylactic anticoagulants. Arterial emboli originate from left ventricular mural thrombi and can result in stroke, renal failure, mesenteric infarction, or limb ischemia. These occur more frequently following anterior-wall infarctions, especially with associated aneurysm formation. Mural thrombi may be identified by echocardiography and require systemic anticoagulation with warfarin for 3 to 6 months to lower the thromboembolic risk.

KEY POINTS

1. CHF in the setting of AMI or infarction results from both diastolic and systolic dysfunction. It is treated with afterload reduction (ACE inhibitors), preload reduction (nitrates), and diuresis.

2. Most patients with mild to moderate CHF complicating an AMI are not volume-overloaded. Overly aggressive diuresis in this setting may precipitate hypotension.

3. Cardiogenic shock is characterized by systemic hypotension (SBP <90 mm Hg), low cardiac output (CI <2.2 L/kg/min), elevated PCWP (>18 mm Hg), and evidence of organ hypoperfusion.

4. Treatment of cardiogenic shock includes pressors, inotropes, and diuretics. Patients with cardiogenic shock complicating an AMI should be considered for emergent cardiac catheterization and coronary reperfusion and may require hemodynamic support with an IABP.

5. Right ventricular infarction is characterized by hypotension, elevated neck veins, and lack of pulmonary congestion. It usually occurs in conjunction with an inferior LV infarction. Treatment consists of volume expansion, inotropic support, and reperfusion therapy for the associated inferior MI.

6. Mechanical complications following an AMI include ventricular free wall rupture, VSD, and papillary muscle rupture. These are all surgical emergencies and are associated with excessive mortality.

7. True aneurysms of the LV rarely rupture, whereas pseudoaneurysms are prone to rupture and require surgical resection.

Part Four

Heart Failure

15 Cardiovascular Hemodynamics

The four cardiac chambers comprise two separate pumps (the right and left sides of the heart) that function together in series. The efficiency of these pumps depends in part on their inherent contractile properties (contractility), as well as on the rate at which the pumps fill (preload) and the resistance against which they must pump (afterload). These and other hemodynamic variables are important measures of cardiac function and are altered in characteristic ways in the setting of HF. Assessment of the hemodynamic status of the failing heart allows for the recognition of specific disease states, quantification of disease severity, tailoring of specific therapy, and evaluation of the therapeutic response.

■ HEMODYNAMIC PARAMETERS

Intracardiac Pressures

The assessment of intracardiac pressure is discussed at length in Chapter 6 but is reviewed briefly here with regard to the assessment of HF. The normal pressure in each of the cardiac chambers is shown in Table 15-1. Changes in these pressures may reflect alterations in a person's volume status or the functional state of their heart. Most of these pressures can be directly measured by placing a catheter into the chamber of interest.

The pressure required to fill the LV (the **filling pressure**) is an important measure of ventricular function. It can be measured directly via placement of a catheter within the LV cavity (LVEDP), or it can be assessed indirectly by measuring the PCWP. In the absence of pulmonary vascular disease, the PCWP reflects LA pressure. Furthermore, in the absence of MS, the LA pressure reflects LVEDP. Thus, the PCWP can be used as an accurate surrogate for LVEDP.

■ TABLE 15-1

Summary of Normal Intracardiac Pressures and Hemodynamic Values

Hemodynamic Parameter	Range of Normal Values
HR	60–80 bpm (at rest)
CVP*	0–4 mm Hg
RV pressure	15–30/0–4 mm Hg
PA pressure	15–30/8–12 mm Hg
PCWP	8–12 mm Hg
LV pressure	120–140/8–12 mm Hg
CO	4–6 L/m
CI	2.5–4.0 L/min/m^2
SVR	800–1200 dynes-sec-cm^{-5}
EF	60%

* Note that central venous pressure and right atrial pressure are interchangeable.

Cardiac Output

The CO is the volume of blood pumped by the heart in 1 minute and is the product of the HR and the SV, or the amount of blood the heart pumps with each beat:

$$CO = HR \times SV \text{ (units: L/min)}$$

The CI is a method of normalizing the CO to body size and is obtained by dividing the CO by the body surface area [BSA, in meters squared (m^2)]:

$$CI = CO/BSA \text{ (units: L/min/m}^2)$$

The normal CO is approximately 4 to 6 L/min; however, this may increase greater than fivefold as a result of increases in HR and SV. The HR (also referred to as chronotropy) is largely controlled by the autonomic nervous system. The SV depends on three hemodynamic factors: preload, afterload, and contractility.

Preload

Preload refers to the volume of blood in the LV just prior to systole (**LV end-diastolic volume**). This volume, however, cannot easily be measured, and LV filling pressure (LVEDP, LA pressure, or mean PCWP) is therefore used as a surrogate.

Afterload

Afterload is the force against which the LV must pump. According to the law of LaPlace, afterload is directly proportional to blood pressure and LV diameter and inversely proportional to LV thickness. Clinically, however, SBP alone is often used as a measure of afterload. Afterload can also be quantified by assessment of the SVR, which can be calculated as:

$$SVR = [(MAP - CVP)/CO] \times 80 \text{ (units: dynes-sec-cm}^{-5})$$

Where MAP is the mean arterial pressure and CVP the central venous pressure. In general, as afterload increases, SV and cardiac output decrease.

Contractility

Contractility (also referred to as **inotropy**) is the inherent strength of ventricular contraction independent of preload and afterload. Contractility can be augmented by increased activity of the sympathetic nervous system and by sympathomimetic medications (e.g., dopamine or dobutamine). Contractility can be decreased by beta-blocking agents and calcium channel antagonists.

Pressure-Volume Relationships

The relationship between LV filling pressure and SV is described by the Frank-Starling curve (Figure 15-1). As can be seen, over a wide range of volumes, an increase in preload results in an increase in SV. At extremely high preload (not shown in figure), the relationship fails and SV falls (likely the result of overstretching of myocardial contractile elements).

As can be seen in Figure 15-1, HF is associated with decreased contractility, resulting in a lower SV for a given preload. In an attempt to augment SV, the

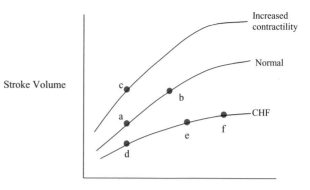

Figure 15-1 • Frank-Starling curve in various hemodynamic settings. In the normal setting, as filling pressure (preload) increases, stroke volume (SV) increases (point a → point b). Increased contractility (i.e., infusion of inotropic agents) is associated with an increased SV at any level of preload (point a → point c). In contrast, decreased contractility (i.e., heart failure) is associated with a decrease in SV at a given level of preload (point a → point d). In this setting, an increased preload is required to maintain the same SV (point a → point e). Additionally, further increases in preload (point e → point f) result in relatively minimal augmentation of SV at the expense of a marked elevation in filling pressure.

preload increases substantially. This increased pressure is transmitted to the pulmonary vasculature, resulting in pulmonary edema.

The relationship between LV pressure and volume can be represented graphically by a pressure-volume loop (Figure 15-2a). As can be seen, LVSV (i.e., LV performance) is affected by changes in preload, afterload, and contractility (Figure 15-2b). Abnormalities in any of these factors can result in impaired myocardial performance and alterations of normal cardiac filling pressures.

The end-diastolic pressure-volume curve defines the compliance, or distensibility, of the ventricle. A highly compliant ventricle is one that can accommodate a large volume of blood with only a small rise in pressure (as occurs with chronic aortic insufficiency). In contrast, a poorly compliant ventricle (as occurs with ventricular hypertrophy or acute ischemia) is one in which a small increase in volume results in a significant increase in pressure.

Ejection Fraction

The overall systolic function of the heart is reflected in the EF. This is the proportion of blood in the ventricle at the end of diastole that is subsequently

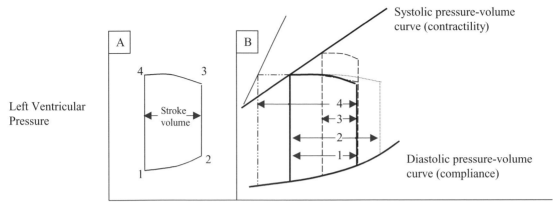

Figure 15-2 • LV pressure-volume loops. (a) Normal pressure-volume loop. The mitral valve opens at point 1 followed by LV filling. The LV reaches a maximum volume at point 2 (LV end-diastolic pressure/volume, or **preload**), followed by isovolumic contraction (line 2 to 3). The aortic valve opens at point 3, allowing for LV ejection (line 3 to 4). The volume of blood ejected represents the SV. Maximum pressure is generated at point 4 (LV end-systolic pressure, or **afterload**) and is followed by AV closure and isovolumic relaxation (line 4 to 1). (b) Effect of changing hemodynamic parameters on SV. (1) Normal SV. (2) Increasing preload results in increased SV. (3) Increasing afterload results in decreased SV. (4) Increasing contractility results in increased SV.

ejected during systole. The normal EF is approximately 60% and can be measured by echocardiography, nuclear scanning, contrast ventriculography, or MRI. Normal hemodynamic values are summarized in Table 15-1.

ALTERATIONS OF HEMODYNAMIC PARAMETERS IN HEART FAILURE

Most forms of HF are associated with a fall in cardiac output, frequently as a result of a decrease in contractility (systolic dysfunction). SBP may also fall, since BP is proportional to the product of the CO and SVR. Vasoconstriction occurs as a compensatory mechanism to maintain an adequate BP and accounts for the increase in SVR that is usually present in patients with HF (frequently >1,500 dynes-sec-cm^{-5}). However, this increase in afterload results in a further fall in SV (see Figure 15-2b).

HF is also associated with an increase in LV preload. The increased LVEDP is transmitted back to the pulmonary vasculature, resulting in a rise in the PCWP. A PCWP of >18 mm Hg may alter the local Starling forces such that fluid enters the extravascular space and pulmonary edema develops. Chronic elevation in the PCWP results in pulmonary vasoconstriction, thereby elevating the pulmonary vascular resistance and resulting in pulmonary HTN. This results in RV pressure overload and eventually RV failure, with elevation of RA pressure and CVP.

The therapy of heart failure is aimed at correcting these hemodynamic abnormalities—specifically decreasing afterload, decreasing preload, and increasing contractility.

KEY POINTS

1. The CO is the volume of blood that is pumped by the heart in 1 minute; it is the product of the HR and SV.
2. The PCWP is an indirect measure of LVEDP and thus of preload.
3. Afterload is proportional to BP and is estimated by the SVR.
4. Over a wide range of volumes, increases in preload result in increases in SV.
5. HF is associated with a fall in SV, frequently resulting from a decrease in contractility. A compensatory increase in preload and afterload helps to maintain SV and BP but results in pulmonary vascular congestion.

16 Mechanisms of Heart Failure

Clinically, HF can be defined as the inability of the heart to pump sufficient blood to meet the metabolic demands of the body. The term *cardiomyopathy* refers to a disorder of the myocardium that may or may not be associated with clinical HF.

■ CLASSIFICATIONS

HF may be classified as systolic or diastolic, right-sided or left-sided, high-output or low-output, and acute or chronic. These classifications reflect either the underlying pathophysiology of HF or the pattern of the patient's symptoms.

Systolic HF is characterized by impaired myocardial contractility. The heart becomes weakened and cannot pump blood effectively during systole. Consequently, blood backs up into the pulmonary system, resulting in pulmonary vascular congestion. This is the primary mechanism of HF in both ischemic and nonischemic dilated cardiomyopathies. The severity of LV systolic dysfunction can be assessed by echocardiography, contrast ventriculography, nuclear imaging, or MRI and can be quantified by calculation of the LVEF:

- Normal LVEF: ≥50%
- Mildly reduced LVEF: 40 to 50%
- Moderately reduced LVEF: 30 to 40%
- Severely reduced LVEF: <30%

Diastolic HF is characterized by impaired ventricular relaxation (i.e., decreased ventricular compliance). In this setting, any given volume of blood that enters the LV cavity will result in a higher-than-normal LV pressure. This leads to impairment of diastolic ventricular filling and an increase in LVEDP. The increased pressure is transmitted to the pulmonary system, resulting in pulmonary vascular congestion. This is the primary mechanism of CHF in hypertensive, hypertrophic, and infiltrative heart diseases.

Many HF patients, particularly those with advanced disease, have both systolic and diastolic HF. Advanced systolic dysfunction results in a rise in LVEDP, resulting in diastolic dysfunction. Many patients with diastolic dysfunction develop systolic dysfunction late in their disease (see Table 16-1).

Left-sided HF results from disorders that predominantly affect the LV (e.g., MI, HTN, valvular heart disease) or produce global myocardial dysfunction (i.e., nonischemic cardiomyopathy). Left-sided HF produces symptoms of pulmonary venous congestion (dyspnea, orthopnea, and paroxysmal nocturnal dyspnea).

Right-sided HF is most commonly the result of left-sided HF but can occur independently (e.g., right RV infarction, acute PE) and produces signs of systemic venous congestion (edema, ascites, congestive hepatomegaly, jugular venous distention). Right-sided HF resulting from primary lung disease (e.g., pulmonary HTN, COPD) is referred to as **cor pulmonale**. Both right- and left-sided HF frequently coexist (**biventricular HF**).

Low-output HF results when the heart is unable to pump enough blood to meet the body's normal metabolic demands; it can be seen with various forms of both systolic and diastolic failure. **High-output HF** results when a relatively normally functioning heart is unable to keep up with the body's abnormally increased metabolic demand, as may occur with thyrotoxicosis, anemia, and arteriovenous fistulas.

Acute HF refers to the sudden development of HF symptoms in a person who was either previously asymptomatic or whose HF was well controlled. It commonly occurs in the setting of:

- Myocardial ischemia or infarction
- Severe hypertension

TABLE 16-1

Common Causes of Heart Failure and Their Major Pathophysiologic Abnormalities

Cause of Heart Failure	Major Pathophysiologic Abnormality	
	Systolic Dysfunction	*Diastolic Dysfunction*
Acute ischemia	+	++
Ischemic cardiomyopathy	++	+
Nonischemic cardiomyopathy	++	+
AS	With advanced disease	++
MR	++	With advanced disease
HTN	With advanced disease	++
Infiltrative heart disease (i.e., amyloid, sarcoid)	+	++
HCM	With advanced disease	++

- Sudden valvular dysfunction (e.g., ischemic MR, ruptured mitral or aortic valve).

Chronic HF is that which has existed for a period of time. The patient may be chronically symptomatic or have well-controlled symptoms on medical therapy.

Frequently, several classifications can be used to describe HF in a single individual. For example, a person may have chronic left-sided systolic HF.

■ COMPENSATORY MECHANISMS

In response to the decreased CO that accompanies CHF, several adaptive processes occur that help to maintain adequate CO and tissue perfusion by augmenting stroke volume and HR. These include:

- Activation of the renin-angiotensin-aldosterone system, which results in improved BP and tissue perfusion through angiotensin-induced vasoconstriction and aldosterone-induced sodium and water retention.
- Increased activity of the sympathetic nervous system, which results in vasoconstriction, increased ventricular contractility, and increased HR.
- The release of vasopressin and natriuretic peptides, which results in fluid retention, increased preload, and thereby increased stroke volume.
- The release of endothelin, which produces further vasoconstriction.

Although these responses are initially adaptive, they eventually have deleterious effects (see Table 16-2). The increased afterload induced by angiotensin, norepinephrine, and endothelin may decrease stroke volume and result in a further decline in CO. The volume expansion results in fluid overload and elevated intracardiac pressure. If the LVEDP (and therefore the

TABLE 16-2

Compensatory Responses to Heart Failure

Compensatory Mechanism	Beneficial Effect	Detrimental Effect
Renin-angiotensin activation	↑ SVR to maintain BP and tissue perfusion	↑ SVR results in ↓ CO
↑ Aldosterone	Volume retention leads to ↑ preload, ↑ SV, and ↑ CO	Volume overload
↑ Sympathetic tone	↑ HR and contractility result in ↑ CO; ↑ SVR maintains BP	May induce ischemia; ↑ SVR results in ↓ CO
Natriuretic peptides	Volume retention leads to ↑ preload, ↑ SV, and ↑ CO	Volume overload
Endothelin	↑ SVR to maintain BP and tissue perfusion	↑ SVR results in ↓ CO

mean PCWP) acutely exceeds ~18 to 20 mm Hg, pulmonary edema develops. In patients with chronic HF, increased pulmonary lymphatic drainage partially compensates for the increased intrapulmonary pressure and may allow patients to remain relatively asymptomatic despite a PCWP of >25 mm Hg.

The failing heart also undergoes structural changes in response to myocyte loss (i.e., MI), increased afterload, or chronic volume overload. As a first response, the LV initially hypertrophies; this may be followed by LV dilation. These changes help to normalize the wall stress and lower the LVEDP. However, the progressive hypertrophy and dilation eventually alter the shape of the heart, producing a spherical LV cavity. This process is known as ventricular remodeling and eventually results in a further increase in wall stress and LVEDP as well as a decrease in LV systolic function.

KEY POINTS

1. HF may be classified as systolic or diastolic, left-sided or right-sided, low-output or high-output, and acute or chronic.
2. Systolic HF is characterized by impaired ventricular contraction, whereas diastolic HF is characterized by impaired ventricular relaxation.
3. Vasopressin, endothelin, aldosterone, natriuretic peptides, the renin-angiotensin system, and the sympathetic nervous system all contribute to the compensatory response to HF.
4. Although compensatory responses to HF are initially adaptive, they eventually have deleterious effects and may perpetuate or worsen HF.
5. The failing heart often undergoes a process of remodeling, whereby it assumes a spherical configuration. This change of shape results in mechanical inefficiency and worsening of LV systolic function.

Clinical Manifestations and Treatment of Heart Failure

Epidemiology

HF affects nearly 5 million Americans; it is the leading discharge diagnosis for persons over age 65 and accounts for almost $38.1 billion in health care costs annually. It is expected that these numbers will continue to rise as the population ages.

Etiologies

In the United States, the most common cause of systolic HF is ischemic heart disease. However, HF may also result from a variety of other primary cardiac disorders, including congenital or acquired valvular abnormalities, HTN, and infiltrative or inflammatory diseases of the myocardium (Table 17-1). A variety of metabolic abnormalities and several toxins may also result in HF. A thorough evaluation will usually implicate one of these disorders in the etiology of CHF; however, the exact cause cannot be determined in a significant number of cases. In such cases, the etiology is referred to as idiopathic. The major causes of diastolic HF include systemic HTN, acute ischemia, hypertrophic cardiomyopathy, and the restrictive cardiomyopathies.

Clinical Manifestations

History

HF may cause a variety of symptoms, most of which reflect either vascular congestion or poor cardiac output.
  Classic symptoms of **left HF** include:

- **Dyspnea**—the most common symptom of left-sided HF. May occur at rest or with exertion.
- **Orthopnea**—dyspnea that worsens immediately after lying down; it results from a sudden increase in venous return.

- **Paroxysmal nocturnal dyspnea**—dyspnea that occurs several hours after the patient lies down to sleep; it results from the central redistribution of extravascular fluid.
- **Wheezing and nocturnal cough**—these reflect pulmonary congestion.
- **Fatigue**, **lethargy**, and **poor exercise tolerance**— these reflect poor CO.

TABLE 17-1

Etiologies of Heart Failure

Etiologic Category	Examples
Ischemia	Acute ischemia Ischemic CMP
Valvular heart disease	Aortic stenosis or regurgitation Mitral stenosis or regurgitation
Hypertensive heart disease	Acute HTN Hypertensive CMP
Toxins	Alcohol, cocaine, doxorubicin
Metabolic abnormalities	Hyper- or hypothyroidism Thiamine deficiency (beri-beri) Selenium deficiency (Keshan disease)
Infiltrative diseases	Amyloidosis Hemochromatosis Sarcoidosis
Infectious diseases	Viral myocarditis
High-output failure	Arteriovenous shunts Paget disease Beri-beri Anemia
Idiopathic CMP	Cause unknown (presumed viral)
Hypertrophic CMP	Various genetic mutations

BOX 17-1	THE NEW YORK HEART ASSOCIATION CLASSIFICATION

Class 1: Symptoms only at levels of exertion that would limit normal individuals
Class 2: Symptoms with ordinary exertion
Class 3: Symptoms with less-than-ordinary exertion
Class 4: Symptoms with any activity or at rest

- **Chest discomfort**—may result from elevated intracardiac or intrapulmonary pressures or may reflect underlying CAD.

Classic symptoms of **right sided HF** include:

- **Lower extremity edema** that is exacerbated by prolonged standing and improved by elevation of the legs.
- **Abdominal discomfort** and **nausea**, resulting from intestinal edema and hepatic congestion.

The functional status of a patient with HF can be defined by the New York Heart Association (NYHA) classification (Box 17-1).

Physical Examination

Signs of HF are the same regardless of its cause. Signs of left-sided CHF include:

- Pulmonary rales (fine inspiratory crackles)
- Dullness at the lung bases (resulting from pleural effusions)
- Left-sided S_3 (systolic dysfunction)
- Left-sided S_4 (diastolic dysfunction)
- LV heave

Signs of right-sided CHF include:

- Elevated JVP
- Ascites
- Hepatomegaly
- Edema

Patients who have symptoms or signs of vascular congestion (e.g., pulmonary edema, lower extremity edema) or organ hypoperfusion (e.g., worsening renal function with decreased urine output, hypotension) are said to have decompensated HF, whereas patients without these features are said to be compensated.

Differential Diagnosis

The main differential diagnosis of left-sided HF includes pneumonia, PE, angina, and COPD. The differential diagnosis of right-sided HF includes cirrhosis, nephrotic syndrome, pericardial disease, venous stasis, and deep venous thrombosis (DVT).

Diagnostic Evaluation

The evaluation of the patient with CHF should include a search for the cause and an assessment of the severity of the HF. Routine laboratory examination should include a hematocrit and measures of thyroid, renal, and hepatic function. A CXR may reveal pulmonary vascular congestion (vascular redistribution, Kerley B lines, etc.), cardiomegaly, or pleural effusions. An ECG should be performed to evaluate for evidence of underlying CAD or LVH.

In urgent care settings where it is difficult to differentiate acute dyspnea due to CHF from pulmonary disease, a plasma B-type natriuretic peptide (BNP) level may be helpful. Plasma BNP appears to be the only natriuretic peptide that is specific to the cardiac ventricles and correlates in a positive way with PCWP, LVEDP, and the degree of LV systolic dysfunction. A low plasma BNP level (<100 pg/mL) can rapidly rule out decompensated CHF, whereas a high plasma BNP level (>400 pg/mL) supports a diagnosis of abnormal ventricular function or symptomatic CHF. Intermediate values (100 to 400 pg/mL) are not specific for CHF and should spur a search for other potential causes for increased BNP and dyspnea (e.g., PE, cor pulmonale). It must be emphasized that clinical judgment should always prevail in the interpretation of plasma BNP levels.

An echocardiogram is essential and allows for the accurate determination of biventricular systolic and diastolic function. With systolic HF, echocardiography demonstrates a depressed LVEF. With pure diastolic HF, echocardiography usually demonstrates LVH, a normal LVEF, and evidence of abnormal diastolic ventricular filling on Doppler evaluation. Echocardiography can also identify valvular abnormalities that may have caused the HF or may reveal evidence of underlying CAD.

In situations when the diagnosis is in doubt or when volume status is uncertain, catheterization (Swan-Ganz catheter) of the PA can be performed, allowing for the direct measurement of intracardiac pressures. This information can be used to guide subsequent therapy. If the cause of the CHF is thought to be CAD, coronary angiography is indicated and will define the extent of the coronary disease and the feasibility of revascularization.

Treatment

General Approach

All patients with HF should limit their ingestion of salt by eating low-salt foods and not adding extra salt to prepared foods. Patients with more severe HF may need to limit their salt intake to <2 g of sodium per day. Restriction of fluid intake is usually not necessary except in the most severe cases. Patients with HF should be encouraged to exercise regularly, and all potentially modifiable risk factors for atherosclerosis should be addressed, including smoking cessation, lipid control, and weight loss. Avoidance of alcohol and illicit drugs should also be encouraged.

The management of individual patients with HF depends in part on the etiology of their disease and the acuity of their symptoms. Potentially reversible causes should be sought and specific treatment initiated. Treatment of the patient with acutely decompensated HF is aimed at improving systemic perfusion, decreasing congestion, and establishing a stable hemodynamic state. The goals of long-term therapy of the compensated HF patient are the control of symptoms, prevention of decompensation, and reduction of mortality.

The choice of specific therapy for the decompensated patient should be directed by the clinical presentation; that is, whether the patient presents with signs of congestion, hypoperfusion, or both. The hemodynamic status of these patients and the most appropriate regimen for their treatment can often be determined by answering two simple questions (see Figure 17-1):

- Is the patient wet (i.e., volume-overloaded with pulmonary and peripheral congestion) or dry?
- Is the patient adequately or inadequately perfused (i.e., normal mentation, adequate urine output, warm extremities)?

Invasive hemodynamic monitoring with a PA catheter is occasionally required and allows for a more precise determination of the severity of HF. The PA catheter can also be used to guide therapy in an effort to normalize a patient's hemodynamics ("tailored therapy"). Ideal hemodynamic parameters in patients with chronic HF include a PCWP of ~15 to 18 mm Hg, right atrial pressure $\leq$8 mm Hg, cardiac index $\geq$2.2 L/min/m^2, and an SVR of 1,000 to 1,200 dynes-sec-cm^{-5}.

Systolic Heart Failure

Pharmacologic Therapies

The pharmacologic therapy of systolic HF centers around the control of excess body water, reduction of afterload, and augmentation of contractility. These hemodynamic changes help to normalize cardiac pressure-volume relationships (see Figure 17-2). Acutely decompensated patients frequently require intravenous medications (Table 17-2), whereas compensated patients can be managed with oral therapy (Table 17-3).

In patients with pulmonary congestion or signs of volume overload, diuretics will usually improve symptoms. Furosemide, which acts in the loop of Henle, is the most common diuretic used for treating HF but has not been shown to decrease mortality. Thiazide diuretics, which act in the distal convoluted tubule, are less frequently used; however, the addition of a thiazide (i.e., metolazone) to furosemide can be remarkably effective for inducing diuresis. This combination may also result in renal potassium and magnesium wasting; electrolyte levels need to be checked regularly when these medications are being used. Spironolactone, an aldosterone inhibitor, is a relatively weak diuretic but has recently been shown to

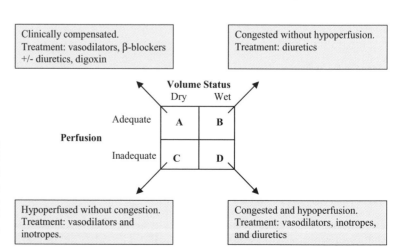

Figure 17-1 • Hemodynamic profiles based on clinical signs in patients with decompensated HF and the associated therapies. Adequate perfusion is indicated by normal mentation, adequate urine output, and warm extremities. Inadequate perfusion is indicated by decreased urine output with worsening renal function, mental status changes, and cool extremities.

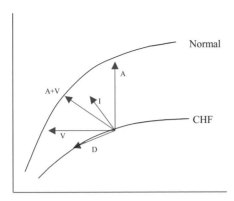

Figure 17-2 • Frank-Starling curve in HF and the effects of specific agents on SV and preload. In the normal setting, as filling pressure (preload) increases, stroke (SV) increases. In HF, the SV is decreased, and an increased preload is required to maintain the same SV. Diuretics (D) and venodilators (V) decrease filling pressures without significantly improving SV. Arterial vasodilators (A) and inotropes (I) improve SV without significantly affecting filling pressures. Combination therapy with venodilators and arterial vasodilators (A + V) both improves cardiac performance and lowers filling pressures.

decrease symptoms as well as improve mortality in patients with NYHA class III to IV HF.

In patients with either asymptomatic left ventricular systolic dysfunction or symptomatic systolic HF, vasodilators are clearly beneficial. These agents decrease systemic vascular resistance, thereby decreasing afterload and improving cardiac output. ACE inhibitors and angiotensin receptor blockers (ARBs) are the most effective oral vasodilators. ACE inhibitors decrease the progression of HF, improve symptoms, and decrease mortality in patients with HF. ARBs may be equally effective but are less well studied. Hydralazine is a less effective vasodilator; however, when combined with an oral nitrate (e.g., isosorbide mononitrate), it is a useful agent for patients who cannot take ACE inhibitors or ARBs because of renal dysfunction or medication intolerance. Additionally, in African Americans, the addition of a hydralazine-nitrate combination to standard HF therapy improves mortality and reduces hospital admissions for HF. In patients with acutely decompensated HF, afterload reduction can be accomplished rapidly with intravenous nitroprusside or nitroglycerin.

TABLE 17-2

Intravenous Agents Used in the Treatment of Patients With Decompensated Heart Failure

Drug	Hemodynamic Effect	Mechanism of Action	Side Effects
Dobutamine	↑CO, ↓SVR, ↓PCWP	α- and β-adrenergic agonist properties	Tachycardia, ventricular arrhythmias
Dopamine	↓SVR, ↔CO, ↔PCWP	Renal and splanchnic vasodilation	Higher doses result in adrenergic stimulation and vasoconstriction
Milrinone	↑↑CO, ↓↓SVR, ↓↓PCWP	Phosphodiesterase inhibitor increases cAMP levels	Hypotension, tachyarrhythmias
Nitroprusside	↓↓SVR, ↑CO, ↓↓PCWP	NO donor, potent arterial and venous vasodilation	Coronary "steal" Cyanide, thiocyanate toxicity
Nitroglycerin	↓SVR, ↔CO, ↓PCWP	Decreases ventricular filling pressures and MVO$_2$, arterial and venous vasodilation	Headache
Furosemide	↓PCWP	Loop diuretic; stimulates salt (and water) loss	Volume depletion, hypotension, electrolyte abnormalities
Nesiritide	↓PCWP, ↓SVR	Recombinant human BNP promotes arterial and venous vasodilation	Hypotension

■ TABLE 17-3

The Beneficial Effects of Oral Agents Used in the Management of Heart Failure			
Drug	Improve Symptoms	Decrease Mortality	Prevent Recurrent CHF
Diuretics	Yes	No	No
Digoxin	Yes	No	+/−
Inotropes	Yes	↑Mortality	No
Direct vasodilators	Yes	Yes	No
Spironolactone	Yes	Yes	No
ACE inhibitors	Yes	Yes	Yes
Beta blockers	Yes	Yes	Yes
Hydralazine/nitrates	Yes	Yes	Yes

Digoxin is a cardiac glycoside that inhibits the Na^+,K^+-ATPase, resulting in higher intracellular calcium levels and thereby augmenting contractility. Digoxin improves symptoms in patients with HF and decreases their need for hospitalization; however, it does not improve mortality. This medication should be used cautiously in patients with renal insufficiency and/or who are elderly, as they are at higher risk for digoxin toxicity. Many other oral inotropic agents have been studied and all have shown either no benefit or increased mortality in HF patients. Dobutamine and dopamine are beta agonists and are effective intravenous inotropic agents; they are especially useful for patients with decompensated HF. These agents augment cardiac output, improve tissue perfusion, and may result in brisk diuresis.

Nitrates are venodilators; as such, they result in decreased preload. When used alone, they are useful for the control of congestive symptoms and angina in patients with concurrent CAD; however, they do not improve mortality.

Beta-blocking agents were long thought to be contraindicated in patients with systolic HF owing to their negative inotropic effects. However, they are now known to be both safe and effective in the treatment of HF; they improve symptoms and substantially decrease mortality. Nonetheless, these agents can lead to an initial worsening of congestive symptoms. Therefore it is important to start these agents at low doses (e.g., carvedilol 3.125 mg twice daily, metoprolol 25 mg daily), increase slowly (titrate upward every 2 to 4 weeks as tolerated), and use diuretics for control of congestive symptoms. A general approach to the outpatient management of chronic HF is summarized in Figure 17-3.

Nesiritide is a recombinant form of human B-type natriuretic peptide (hBNP), which is approved for the intravenous treatment of patients with acutely decompensated CHF. This agent binds to guanylate cyclase receptors and thereby increases levels of cyclic guanosine monophosphate (cGMP). This promotes the relaxation of smooth muscle cells, resulting in arterial and venous vasodilation. The consequent hemodynamic effects are a decrease in PCWP as well as a decrease in SVR. The major side effect is hypotension. Hence this agent is contraindicated in patients with cardiogenic shock, those with an SBP <90 mm Hg, and in patients who are intravascularly volume-depleted.

Device Therapies—Synchronized Biventricular Pacing

Some 30 to 50% of patients with CHF have interventricular conduction defects that are reflected by a prolonged QRS duration on the surface ECG. These conduction abnormalities lead to a delay between the contraction of the right and left sides of the heart (also referred to as dyssynchrony), producing discoordinated contraction of an already failing left ventricle and thereby worsening overall cardiac function. Biventricular pacing resynchronizes the ventricles by electrically activating the right and left ventricles in a synchronized manner. This therapy has been shown to improve ventricular function and reduce the degree of associated MR. CHF patients treated with cardiac resynchronization have demonstrated improvement in symptoms and exercise tolerance.

Surgical Therapies

Coronary artery revascularization, either surgically or percutaneously, should be considered in patients with HF and evidence of ischemic disease. Successful

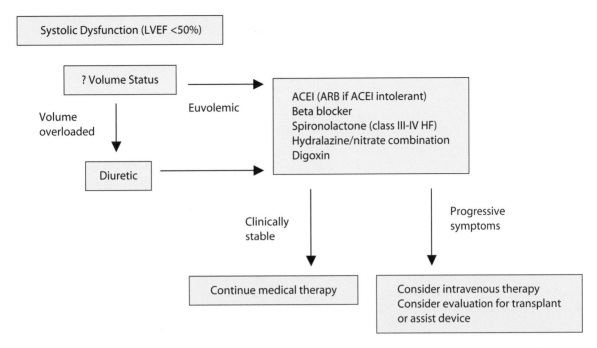

Figure 17-3 • Algorithm for the outpatient management of chronic systolic HF. Initial evaluation of patients with LV dysfunction should include an assessment of volume status. If signs or symptoms of volume overload are present, initial management should include diuresis. In the asymptomatic euvolemic patient, initial therapy should consist of an ACE inhibitor followed by the cautious addition of a beta blocker. Spironolactone should be initiated in patients with moderate to severe symptoms. A hydralazine-nitrate combination should be added in African-American patients and in others with continued symptoms despite the therapy outlined above. Digoxin should be reserved as a second-line agent for those patients who remain symptomatic after treatment with other agents. If symptoms persist despite optimal medical therapy, assist device or transplantation should be considered.

revascularization may improve contractile function, alleviate symptoms, and attenuate the remodeling process.

Patients with cardiogenic shock (persistent HTN, pulmonary congestion, and organ hypoperfusion) may benefit from mechanical devices to assist with ventricular function, as a bridge to either recovery or cardiac transplantation. The most frequently used device is an IABP. This device is placed into the descending thoracic aorta via the femoral artery. It inflates during diastole to improve coronary perfusion and deflates just prior to systole, thereby decreasing afterload and increasing cardiac output. Patients using this device must be closely monitored for complications associated with it, including infection, bleeding, ischemia (limb, renal, spinal, mesenteric), hemolytic anemia with thrombocytopenia (due to shear forces of the balloon), and atherosclerotic plaque embolization. IABPs are contraindicated in patients with aortic dissections, moderate to severe aortic insufficiency, or severe peripheral vascular disease. Ventricular assist devices (VADs) are mechanical pumps that are surgically implanted directly into

the heart and can temporarily sustain a patient's circulation until the heart recovers or the patient receives a heart transplant. Presently, VADs are being used only as temporizing measures; however, these devices may eventually become a more permanent form of therapy.

Cardiac transplantation provides a definite survival advantage over medical therapy in patients with advanced HF and is associated with a 1-year survival rate approaching 80% and a 5-year survival rate of ~65%. Unfortunately, because of a shortage of donor hearts, most patients die while waiting for a transplant. Approximately 40,000 people die each year from chronic HF, while only 2,500 donor hearts become available. As a result of this shortage, attempts have been made to develop a totally artificial heart. These self-contained mechanical devices have been implanted in just a few patients in the course of experimental trials and have had short-term success. With further technical advances, these devices may offer long-term support for patients with severe HF. Currently, the only absolute contraindications to cardiac transplantation are other medical conditions independent of the patient's HF that would limit his or her life expectancy.

Diastolic Heart Failure

The management of pure diastolic dysfunction is problematic, as much less is known about the treatment of diastolic HF than of systolic HF. Management is aimed at treating the underlying cause, alleviating congestive symptoms, and attempting to improve diastolic function with the use of negatively inotropic agents. Both beta blockers and calcium channel blockers appear to be equally effective in this regard, but they may have to be used at high dosages. ACE inhibitors may also yield symptomatic benefit. Diuretics are frequently required to control pulmonary or systemic congestion, but they should be used cautiously as patients with diastolic dysfunction are very preload-dependent. In such patients, overdiuresis may result in hypotension, tachycardia, and worsened diastolic function.

KEY POINTS

1. HF is an increasingly prevalent disease that accounts for the expenditure of billions of health care dollars.
2. Initial management of patients with decompensated HF should be aimed at normalizing volume status and improving systemic perfusion.
3. Therapies that have been shown to decrease mortality in all patients with systolic HF include ACE inhibitors and beta blockers. Spironolactone improves mortality in patients with class III to IV symptoms. Treatment with the combination of hydralazine and nitrates has particular benefit in African Americans.
4. Digoxin, nitrates, and diuretics are used primarily for symptom control.
5. Patients with progressive symptoms despite optimal medical therapy should be considered for cardiac replacement therapy (VAD or transplant).
6. The management of diastolic HF consists primarily of treatment with negative inotropes and limited diuresis. These therapies are, however, of unproven benefit.

18 Myocarditis

Myocarditis is an inflammatory disease of the myocardium that results from a variety of underlying disorders. Its manifestations range from asymptomatic LV dysfunction to fulminant CHF.

Epidemiology

The true incidence of myocarditis is uncertain owing to the high frequency of asymptomatic cases. It is estimated that the myocardium becomes involved in 1 to 5% of patients presenting with an acute viral illness.

Etiology

Causes of myocarditis include:

- Viral infections (e.g., Coxsackie B, adenovirus, influenza, HIV)
- Acute rheumatic fever
- Lyme disease (*Borrelia burgdorferi*)
- Chagas disease (*Trypanosoma cruzi*)
- Toxins (e.g., cocaine, anthracyclines, catecholamines)
- Systemic diseases (collagen vascular, autoimmune, or granulomatous diseases)
- Hypersensitivity reactions to a variety of antibiotics, antihypertensives, and anticonvulsants

The vast majority of cases are the result of viral infections.

Pathogenesis

The offending agent or toxin may cause direct myocyte damage or necrosis. More importantly, an immune response is stimulated in which macrophages and T lymphocytes infiltrate the myocardium and release proinflammatory cytokines such as tumor necrosis factor and interleukin-1. This reaction may proceed for months and eventually result in LV dysfunction.

Clinical Manifestations

History

The typical patient with acute myocarditis is an otherwise healthy young adult. The clinical presentation varies widely. Most cases are probably minimally symptomatic and never come to medical attention. Symptomatic patients usually present with HF of recent onset. Other presenting symptoms include palpitations, chest pain, syncope, and sudden cardiac death. Patients may recall a preceding viral syndrome.

Physical Examination

The physical examination is similar to that of other patients with HF. Most patients are tachycardic and moderately dyspneic. A pericardial friction rub may be present if the pericardium is also inflamed. Signs of systemic disease should be sought, including lymphadenopathy (suggests sarcoidosis), rash (suggests hypersensitivity reaction), and features of acute rheumatic fever (see Chapter 26).

Diagnostic Evaluation

Abnormal laboratory findings in acute myocarditis include:

- Elevated CK and troponin (elevated only in the acute phase)
- Elevated ESR
- Abnormal ECG that may show transient STE, diffuse T-wave inversions, atrial and ventricular arrhythmias
- Elevated acute viral titers

Echocardiography typically demonstrates ventricular systolic dysfunction, which may be either global or regional. Intracardiac thrombi, valvular regurgitation, and pericardial effusions may also be seen. Nuclear scanning and contrast-enhanced MRI can detect the degree and extent of inflammation in myocarditis, but they are of uncertain utility.

Endomyocardial biopsy can definitively establish the diagnosis of myocarditis; demonstration of an inflammatory myocardial infiltrate with associated myocyte damage confirms the diagnosis. However, a negative biopsy does not exclude the diagnosis, because the histologic changes may be short-lived and the involvement of the myocardium may be heterogeneous. Biopsy should be considered if the clinical evaluation suggests a specific disorder for which treatment is available; however, its routine use remains controversial.

Differential Diagnosis

Acute myocarditis can mimic AMI (chest pain, ST-T-wave changes, myocardial enzyme elevation, and regional wall-motion abnormalities). A careful history must be obtained to distinguish between the two entities. One distinguishing feature is the pattern of cardiac enzyme elevation. Following an AMI, the CK-MB rises within hours, peaks within the first day, and slowly returns to normal over the next several days. With myocarditis, the CK-MB may remain persistently elevated for days to weeks.

Prognosis

Given the variability in the etiology and presentation of this disease, prognostication is difficult. In general, approximately one-third of patients presenting with acute myocarditis and LV dysfunction will regain normal cardiac function; one-third will have persistent mild LV dysfunction; and one-third will develop progressive symptomatic LV dysfunction.

Treatment

The treatment of acute myocarditis is largely supportive, including restricted activity, monitoring for arrhythmias, and institution of routine therapy for HF (see Chapter 17). In certain forms of myocarditis (e.g., Lyme disease, Chagas disease, acute rheumatic fever), specific therapy may be available; however, in most forms of myocarditis (i.e., viral myocarditis)

immunosuppressive and immunologic therapy is of no proven benefit. NSAIDs have been shown to increase myocyte damage in animal models and are contraindicated in the early phase of myocarditis.

Patients with fulminant myocarditis may develop cardiogenic shock and require inotropic support or mechanical assist devices (see Chapter 17). Although many of these patients improve with aggressive medical therapy, patients with severe, progressive myocardial dysfunction should be considered for heart transplantation.

KEY POINTS

1. Viral infections are the most common cause of myocarditis.
2. Myocarditis can result in diffuse or patchy involvement of the myocardium.
3. The clinical presentation of myocarditis varies from asymptomatic LV dysfunction to fulminant ventricular failure with cardiogenic shock.
4. Anti-inflammatory and immunosuppressive therapy does not have proven benefit for the treatment of acute myocarditis.

19 The Cardiomyopathies

The CMPs are primary diseases of the myocardium. They may result from a variety of conditions but can largely be classified into dilated, hypertrophic, and restrictive forms.

■ CLASSIFICATION

These three classes of CMP may be distinguished by their morphologic appearance and LV function.

- **Dilated cardiomyopathy (DCM)** is characterized by LV dilation and systolic dysfunction. Often, four-chamber dilation is present. Regional wall-motion abnormalities may be present even in the absence of significant CAD.
- **Hypertrophic cardiomyopathy (HCM)** is characterized by marked thickening of the ventricular myocardium, small LV cavity size, and hyperdynamic systolic function.
- **Restrictive cardiomyopathy (RCM)** is characterized by normal LV size and systolic function and impaired diastolic function. Mild ventricular thickening may be present.

There is significant overlap among classes, and features of more than one type may be present in the same individual. Diastolic dysfunction is a prominent feature of all three.

■ DILATED CARDIOMYOPATHY

Epidemiology

The reported incidence of DCM is 5 to 8 cases per 100,000 people per year. It is more common in males than in females and in African Americans than in their Caucasian counterparts.

Etiology

A wide variety of disorders can result in DCM, including:

- Viral infections (e.g., adenovirus, enterovirus, HIV)
- Immunologic/inflammatory diseases [e.g., systemic lupus erythematosus (SLE), rheumatoid arthritis, scleroderma]
- Toxins (e.g., alcohol, anthracyclines)
- Metabolic disorders (hyper- or hypothyroidism, beri-beri, selenium deficiency)
- Pregnancy (postpartum CMP)
- Tachycardia (AF, atrial flutter)

In addition, genetic factors may also play a role. In approximately one-quarter of cases of DCM, the cause remains unknown; most of these "idiopathic" cases are likely the result of prior viral myocarditis.

Clinical Manifestations

History and Physical Examination (See Also Chapter 17)

Most patients with DCM present between 20 and 50 years of age. Symptoms of left-sided HF predominate, although arrhythmias (atrial and ventricular tachyarrhythmias), thromboembolic events (from atrial or ventricular thrombi), syncope, and SCD are not uncommon. The physical examination of patients with DCM is indistinguishable from that of patients with other forms of systolic HF.

Diagnostic Evaluation

Echocardiography is the main diagnostic modality in DCM and usually reveals four-chamber dilation with depressed LV systolic function. Other routine diagnostic studies in a patient with CMP should include electrolytes, complete blood count (CBC), thyroid function tests, and iron studies. The ECG often demonstrates an intraventricular conduction delay and left axis deviation. The CXR reveals cardiomegaly and may demonstrate pulmonary congestion.

Patients should be questioned about occupational exposures, alcohol consumption, illicit drug use, and family history of CMP. Stress testing and coronary angiography are useful in patients in whom the history suggests underlying CAD. Myocardial biopsy is not routinely performed.

Treatment

The treatment of DCM is the same as that of other forms of systolic dysfunction (see Chapter 17).

■ HYPERTROPHIC CARDIOMYOPATHY

HCM, an inherited disorder of the cardiac sarcomere, is characterized by marked ventricular hypertrophy. It is a heterogeneous disease with varied morphologic, clinical, and hemodynamic manifestations resulting in a variety of descriptive subtypes, including hypertrophic obstructive cardiomyopathy (HOCM), idiopathic hypertrophic subaortic stenosis (IHSS), and asymmetric septal hypertrophy (ASH).

Epidemiology

Patients with HCM typically present in adolescence or early adulthood. There is an increased risk of SCD (1 to 6% per year), the following factors being associated with the highest risk:

- Younger age at diagnosis (≤14 years)
- History of syncope or nonsustained ventricular tachycardia
- Family history of SCD

HCM is the leading cause of sudden death in athletes below 35 years of age. 10 to 15% of patients with HCM progress to LV dilation and systolic dysfunction.

Etiology

At least 50% of cases of HCM are familial, usually with autosomal dominant inheritance. Over 70 genetic alterations of at least 9 different genes on 4 chromosomes (1, 11, 14, 15) have been identified in familial forms of HCM. These genes encode various proteins of the cardiac sarcomere, including myosin heavy and light chains, troponin T and I, tropomyosin, and myosin-binding protein C. The etiology of sporadic cases of HCM remains unknown.

Pathogenesis

Marked ventricular hypertrophy (wall thickness >15 mm, with normal being <11 mm) is the hallmark of HCM; most patients demonstrate asymmetric septal involvement. On myocardial biopsy, myocyte hypertrophy, myofibrillar disarray, and fibrosis are characteristic findings.

Asymmetric septal hypertrophy causes a narrowing of the left ventricular outflow tract (LVOT), which worsens during systole. The resulting increase in flow velocity in the LVOT pulls the anterior mitral leaflet toward the interventricular septum (Venturi effect); this results in further obstruction to LV outflow by the mitral valve leaflet and can also result in MR.

Diastolic dysfunction, MR, and myocardial ischemia also contribute to the symptoms of HCM. Myocardial ischemia may occur despite normal epicardial coronary arteries as a result of increased muscle mass, elevated diastolic filling pressure, increased wall stress, and decreased capillary density. The increased LV pressure and MR result in increased LA pressure and predispose to AF.

Death from HCM is most often the result of SCD (usually caused by ventricular tachyarrhythmias and less commonly resulting from the LVOT obstruction). Other common causes of morbidity and mortality in this condition include CHF and stroke, the latter resulting from AF.

Clinical Manifestations

Physical Examination

Patients with HCM often have a prominent fourth heart sound and a hyperdynamic precordial impulse. The dynamic LV obstruction often found in this disorder produces a coarse, crescendo-decrescendo, systolic murmur over the left sternal border that increases during expiration or during the strain phase of Valsalva (see Table 2-2). This feature and the lack of radiation to the carotids distinguish the murmur of HCM from that of AS.

Diagnostic Evaluation

ECG usually reveals marked LVH, LA enlargement, and LAD. Echocardiography is the diagnostic test of choice and demonstrates marked LV (and frequently RV) thickening; other characteristic features include systolic anterior motion of the mitral apparatus, MR, and a dynamic intraventricular gradient.

Cardiac catheterization may also aid in the diagnosis of HCM by demonstrating a pressure gradient within the ventricle. This gradient may be quite labile and not apparent at rest, but it may be brought out by the Valsalva maneuver.

Treatment

High-dose beta blockers and calcium antagonists (primarily verapamil) are the mainstays of medical therapy. These drugs are negatively inotropic, resulting in decreased LV contractile force and thereby reducing the LVOT obstruction. They frequently improve both symptoms and exercise tolerance. Disopyramide may also be effective if these agents fail. Diuretics, if clinically indicated, should be used cautiously, as the cardiac output in HCM is dependent on adequate preload.

Septal myomectomy (with or without mitral valve replacement) should be considered for patients with severe HCM (LVOT gradient > 50 mm Hg) who do not respond to medical therapy. This procedure significantly reduces the LVOT gradient in over 90% of patients and results in clinical improvement. Alcohol infusion into the septal arteries is an alternative to myomectomy and produces an infarction of the septum with resultant thinning of the septal myocardium and relief of the LVOT obstruction.

The role of dual-chamber pacing (may reduce the LVOT obstruction) and implantable defibrillators (for prevention of SCD) is unclear in HCM. Atrial arrhythmias are common in HCM. Loss of organized atrial contraction owing to AF can result in significant hemodynamic compromise. Thus attempts should be made to restore and maintain sinus rhythm in these patients.

▆ RESTRICTIVE CARDIOMYOPATHY

Pure RCM is characterized by diastolic dysfunction in the absence of a dilated or hypertrophic LV.

Etiology

RCM may be a primary disorder (idiopathic) or secondary to another disease. Its causes are as follows:

• Idiopathic (endomyocardial fibrosis, hypereosinophilic syndrome)

• Infiltrative (amyloidosis, sarcoidosis, hemochromatosis, glycogen storage disease)
• Scleroderma
• Carcinoid heart disease

Clinical Manifestations

The presentation of RCM is similar to that of severe constrictive pericarditis (see Chapter 33). Evidence of biventricular failure is usually present, although signs and symptoms of right HF predominate. The jugular venous pulsations classically demonstrate rapid x and y descents (see Figure 2-1).

Differential Diagnosis

RCM may mimic other forms of HF; however, the main differential lies in the distinction between RCM and constrictive pericarditis (see below).

Diagnostic Evaluation

In primary RCM, echocardiography demonstrates normal ventricular size and systolic function and abnormal diastolic function. In secondary RCM, myocardial thickening and/or LV and RV systolic dysfunction are often present.

The distinction between constrictive pericarditis and RCM is often aided by their hemodynamic profiles. Both RCM and constrictive pericarditis demonstrate elevated venous pressures and a rapid rise and then plateau of diastolic ventricular pressure (square-root sign) (Figure 19-1). However, in constriction, the restraining effect of the pericardium affects both ventricles equally; therefore, the RV and LV diastolic pressures remain equal throughout the respiratory cycle, even after volume loading. Most restrictive diseases affect the LV in excess of the RV and the diastolic pressures dissociate with inspiration or volume loading. The presence of pericardial calcification on CXR, CT, or MRI also suggests constrictive disease.

Treatment

The treatment of primary RCM does not differ dramatically from that of other forms of diastolic HF (see Chapter 17). In secondary forms of RCM, specific therapy (when available) should be directed at the underlying cause. Venous congestion should be managed with cautious diuresis, as ventricular underfilling can result in decreased cardiac output, hypotension, and hypoperfusion. AF is a common occurrence,

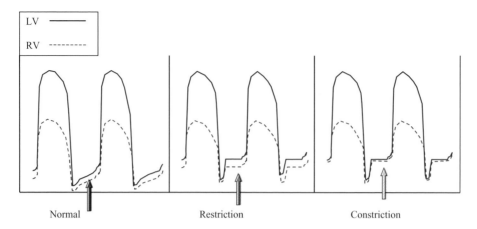

Figure 19-1 • Left (LV) and right (RV) ventricular pressure tracings in a normal heart, in restrictive cardiomyopathy, and in constric-tive pericarditis. In the normal setting, diastolic pressure in the LV exceeds that in the RV; both rise gradually during diastole (black arrow). In restriction, the ventricles are poorly compliant, diastolic pressures are elevated, and ventricular filling results in a rapid rise in pressure followed by diastasis (the **dip**-and-**plateau pattern**, or **square-root sign**). Pressure in the LV still exceeds that in the RV owing to a greater effect of the restrictive process on the LV (medium blue arrow). In constriction, a similar pattern is seen, but the LV and RV pressures are identical secondary to the equal effect of the constricting pericardium on both ventricles (light blue arrow).

and restoration and maintenance of sinus rhythm should be the goal. Malignant ventricular arrhythmias can be seen in certain restrictive cardiomyopathies, particularly sarcoidosis, and may require the place-ment of an implantable defibrillator. Cardiac trans-plantation should be considered for patients with refractory symptoms.

■ DIFFERENTIAL DIAGNOSIS OF THE CARDIOMYOPATHIES

Other cardiovascular diseases may result in depressed LV systolic function, abnormal diastolic function, and/or myocardial thickening and can thereby mimic the CMPs. These conditions include valvular heart disease, hypertensive heart disease, and ischemic heart disease. It is important to identify these under-lying causes, as correction of the primary abnormality may restore cardiac function.

KEY POINTS

1. DCM, HCM, and RCM all result in congestive HF but do so through different mechanisms.
2. DCM is characterized by LV (and frequently four-chamber) dilation, resulting in predominantly systolic dysfunction.
3. HCM is characterized by severe LV and RV thicken-ing, resulting in predominantly diastolic dysfunc-tion. LV systolic function is usually preserved.
4. RCM is characterized by impairment of diastolic function; it frequently results from infiltrative disease.
5. DCM is treated with afterload reduction, diuretics, and beta blockers.
6. HCM is treated with negatively inotropic medica-tions (calcium channel blockers, beta blockers). Treatment with dual-chamber pacing and septal myomectomy should be considered in patients with HCM and LVOT obstruction who fail medical therapy.

Part Five

Arrhythmias

Mechanisms of Arrhythmogenesis

Before approaching specific arrhythmias, a discussion of the mechanisms of their production is in order. Specialized cells in the RA, known collectively as the sinoatrial (SA) node, rhythmically generate electrical impulses and thereby function as the pacemaker of the heart. These electrical impulses are propagated through specialized conduction pathways known as the His-Purkinje system, resulting in the orderly and sequential depolarization of the atria and then the ventricles (see Figure 3-1). Abnormal production or propagation of these electrical impulses produces arrhythmias, whereas abnormal conduction of the electrical impulses results in HB (see Table 20-1).

◼ PHYSIOLOGY OF THE ACTION POTENTIAL

Although a comprehensive review of the cardiac action potential (AP) is beyond the scope of this text, some

◼ TABLE 20-1

Mechanism of Various Types of Arrhythmias		
	Mechanism of Arrhythmia	**Examples**
Tachyarrhythmias	Increased automaticity	Atrial, junctional, and ventricular premature complexes Accelerated junctional rhythm Accelerated idioventricular rhythm Ectopic atrial rhythm Some forms of ventricular tachycardia
	Triggered activity	Some forms of VT, torsades de pointes, bradycardia-dependent VT, long-QT syndrome (early afterdepolarizations) Digoxin toxicity (late afterdepolarizations)
	Reentry	AV-nodal reentrant tachycardia AV-reentrant tachycardia (i.e., WPW) Atrial fibrillation Atrial flutter Most forms of VT
Bradyarrhythmias	Disorders of impulse formation	Sinus bradycardia Sinus-node dysfunction (sick sinus syndrome) Junctional and ventricular escape rhythms
	Disorders of impulse conduction (HB)	Sinus nodal exit block First-, second-, and third-degree AV block Infranodal (His-Purkinje) block

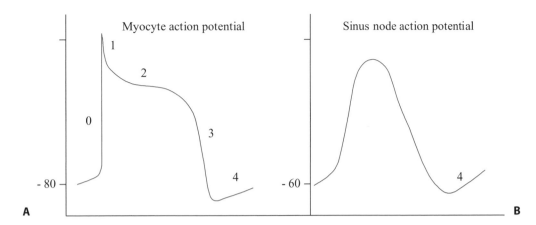

Figure 20-1 • The AP of ventricular myocardium and sinus nodal tissue. The slope of phase 4 repolarization is steeper in SA nodal tissue and accounts for its faster rate of spontaneous depolarization. See text for details.

basic knowledge of cardiac electrophysiology is necessary to understand the mechanisms of arrhythmias. The AP is the summation of the electrical activity of a cardiac myocyte (Figure 20-1). In the resting state, the transmembrane potential of the myocyte is maintained at approximately −80 mV (intracellular relative to extracellular) by the active accumulation of potassium ions (K^+) in the cell and the active expulsion of sodium ions (Na^+) from the cell. When the myocyte is depolarized to −60 mV (threshold potential), it becomes highly permeable to Na^+ and calcium (Ca^{2+}). The subsequent ion fluxes result in rapid cellular depolarization (phase 0 of the AP), which is represented by the QRS complex on the surface ECG. Phases 1, 2, and 3 of the AP represent stages in cellular repolarization and are represented on the surface ECG by the ST segment and T wave. During these later phases, the myocyte gradually returns to its resting membrane potential, primarily as a result of K^+ efflux from the cell (Figure 20-1A). During phase 4 of the AP, the membrane potential gradually and spontaneously depolarizes toward threshold potential, at which time a new AP is generated. This property is known as automaticity. The slope of phase 4 in SA nodal tissue is steeper that that of other cardiac tissue (Figure 20-1B); hence, the SA node reaches threshold potential more quickly than the rest of the myocardium and thereby determines the rate of depolarization of the heart (the HR).

▨ MECHANISMS OF TACHYARRHYTHMIAS

A tachyarrhythmia is a cardiac rhythm that produces an HR greater than 100 beats per minute (bpm). Most tachyarrhythmias are produced by one of three mechanisms: increased automaticity, triggered activity, or reentry. Almost all cardiac tissue demonstrates automaticity. The SA node's automaticity results in an inherent heart rate of 60 to 100 bpm. Other cardiac tissue has slower automaticity and thus is suppressed by the SA node's activity. Occasionally an area of the myocardium develops abnormally increased automaticity (steeper slope in phase 4 of AP) and thereby stimulates a tachyarrhythmia. The abnormal focus of depolarization may arise in the atrial tissue (e.g., atrial premature complexes, ectopic atrial tachycardia), the AV node (e.g., junctional tachycardia), or the ventricular myocardium (e.g., ventricular premature complexes, idioventricular rhythm).

In normal cardiac tissue, low-amplitude oscillations of the transmembrane potential occur during or at the end of electrical repolarization (early or delayed afterdepolarizations respectively; see Figure 20-2). In abnormal myocardium, higher-amplitude oscillations may develop and cause the membrane potential to reach threshold prematurely, thereby "triggering" another AP. Examples of triggered automaticity include digitalis-induced arrhythmias and some forms of VT (e.g., torsades de pointes).

Reentry is a common mechanism of arrhythmogenesis and reflects the formation of an abnormal electrical circuit in the heart. Two distinct electrical pathways in the myocardium, each with differing electrical properties, form this circuit. One pathway conducts rapidly but repolarizes slowly, whereas the other conducts slowly and repolarizes rapidly (Figure 20-3). These characteristics allow an electrical loop to be formed and an impulse to reenter the loop in a continuous fashion. The reentrant circuit can occur in a small focus

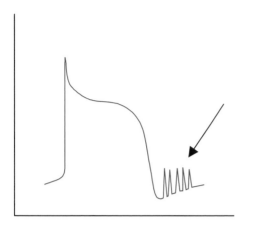

Figure 20-2 • Delayed afterdepolarizations. Oscillations of the membrane potential (arrow) may reach threshold potential and trigger recurrent depolarization.

of myocardium (a microreentrant circuit) or can involve anatomically distinct pathways (a macroreentrant circuit). Examples of reentrant arrhythmias include atrioventricular nodal reentrant tachycardia (AVNRT); atrioventricular reentrant tachycardia (AVRT), which uses a bypass tract (i.e., WPW syndrome); atrial flutter; AF; and most VTs.

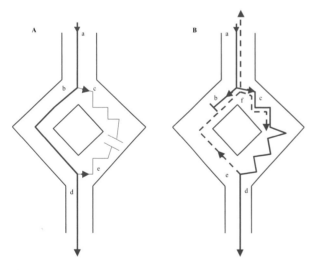

Figure 20-3 • The mechanism of reentry. (A) In the normal setting, the atrial impulse enters the superior aspect of the reentrant loop (a) and then travels down both the fast (b) and slow (c) pathways. On reaching the inferior aspect of the loop, the impulse travels distally (d) and retrograde up the slow pathway (e), where it is extinguished. (B) A premature impulse enters the loop (a) and finds the fast path refractory (b). It then proceeds down the slow path (c) and continues distally (d) as well as retrograde up the fast pathway (e), where it then reenters the loop (f).

■ MECHANISMS OF BRADYARRHYTHMIAS

A bradyarrhythmia is a rhythm that produces an HR of less than 60 bpm. Bradyarrhythmias may arise due to abnormally slow impulse formation by the sinus node or as a result of impaired conduction of an impulse to the remainder of the myocardium. When the sinus node slows its rate of depolarization (sinus bradycardia) or fails to depolarize altogether (sinus arrest), the area of the heart with the next fastest inherent depolarization rate (usually the AV node) will take over as the pacemaker of the heart. The AV node will then beat at a rate of 40 to 60 bpm (junctional rhythm). If the AV node fails, the ventricular myocardium will beat at a rate of 20 to 30 bpm (idioventricular rhythm). Rhythms such as these, which are unmasked by failure of a faster pacemaker site, are referred to as **escape rhythms**.

Bradycardia may also result from failure of a normal impulse to be propagated through the conduction system. This is termed **heart block (HB)**. HB can occur anywhere along the conduction system, although it most commonly occurs at the AV node. The block can be partial (first- or second-degree block) or complete (third-degree block), and it can be intermittent or persistent.

KEY POINTS

1. Tachyarrhythmias produce heart rates of >100 bpm; bradyarrhythmias produce rates of <60 bpm.
2. Specific ion fluxes result in depolarization and repolarization of the myocyte and generate the cellular electrical activity known as the AP.
3. *Automaticity* refers to the inherent ability of cardiac tissue to produce spontaneous APs.
4. The SA node normally has the fastest automaticity and thus functions as the pacemaker of the heart.
5. The three main mechanisms that produce tachyarrhythmias are increased automaticity, triggered activity, and reentry.
6. Mechanisms of bradycardia include delayed or abnormal impulse formation and impaired impulse conduction.

21 Tachyarrhythmias

Tachycardias are defined as arrhythmias that produce heart rates of greater than 100 bpm. The three primary mechanisms that produce tachyarrhythmias are enhanced automaticity, triggered activity, and reentry. These are discussed in detail in Chapter 20 and are referred to here in the context of specific arrhythmias.

Etiology

Tachyarrhythmias are more likely to occur in patients with underlying structural heart disease, including:

- Prior MI
- LV aneurysm
- Cardiomyopathy
- Valvular disease
- Hypertrophic heart disease
- Arrhythmogenic RV dysplasia

However, even patients with structurally normal hearts may develop tachyarrhythmias under certain circumstances, such as:

- Increased catecholamines (e.g., fear, pain, anxiety)
- Metabolic abnormalities (e.g., hyper- or hypokalemia, hypomagnesemia, hypocalcemia, hyperthyroidism)
- Drugs (e.g., caffeine, cocaine, ethanol)
- Medications (e.g., beta agonists, theophylline, antiarrhythmic agents, thyroid hormone replacement).

Clinical Manifestations

History

Patients with tachycardias may be asymptomatic, mildly symptomatic, or have fulminant hemodynamic collapse. Furthermore, the same type of tachyarrhythmia occurring at the same rate can produce vastly different symptoms in different patients.

The symptoms of tachyarrhythmias may be intermittent or persistent and may include:

- Palpitations
- Light-headedness or dizziness
- Syncope
- Chest pain
- Dyspnea

Many of these symptoms are secondary to a reduction in CO resulting from decreased ventricular filling time during the tachycardia. Other important historic information that should be reviewed includes the patient's medical history (specifically a prior history of cardiac disease), family history (of SCD), and medication regimen (identify cardiac and vasoactive medications).

Physical Examination

It is essential to measure the BP of a patient with tachycardia in order to assess the hemodynamic significance of the arrhythmia. Arrhythmias that result in hypotension (systolic blood pressure <90 mm Hg) require urgent treatment. Palpation of the carotid arterial pulse will reveal the regularity and rate of the rhythm and examination of the JVP may demonstrate cannon A waves, suggesting AV dissociation (see below), a sign that is highly suggestive of VT. Variability of the S_1 and an intermittent S_3 and S_4 also suggest AV dissociation. Auscultation of the lung fields may reveal evidence of pulmonary vascular congestion, reflecting LV dysfunction, which may be preexisting or a result of the arrhythmia itself.

Differential Diagnosis

Tachycardias can arise from any part of the heart, including the sinus node, atria, AV node, His-Purkinje

■ **TABLE 21-1**

Differential Diagnosis of Tachyarrhythmias

QRS Morphology	Pattern	Examples
Narrow complex	Regular	Sinus tachycardia Ectopic atrial tachycardia Atrial flutter Junctional tachycardia AVNRT Orthodromic AVRT
	Irregular	AF (P waves absent) Multifocal atrial tachycardia (≥ three different P waves present) Atrial flutter with variable conduction (flutter waves present)
Wide complex	Regular	VT SVT with aberrancy, including antidromic AVRT
	Irregular	AF with aberrancy

system, or ventricles. The most frequently encountered tachyarrhythmias are outlined in Table 21-1.

Diagnostic Evaluation

The ECG is the primary tool for differentiating among various tachyarrhythmias. Determining the exact type of tachyarrhythmia is essential for selecting appropriate therapy. The most important aspect of diagnosing a tachyarrhythmia is determining whether it is a SVT, which arises from the atria or AV node, or a VT, which arises from the ventricular myocardium. The QRS morphology helps to distinguish these arrhythmias; those with a narrow QRS complex (<0.120 seconds) are almost always SVTs, whereas those with a wide QRS complex (>0.120 seconds) may be VTs or SVTs with aberrant conduction. Two other diagnostically helpful features on the ECG are the regularity of the rhythm and the presence or absence of P waves (see Table 21-1).

When narrow-complex tachycardias occur at very fast HRs, it is often difficult to determine the exact type of SVT present. Adenosine (or other AV-nodal blocking agents) can be very helpful in this setting by causing a transient block of the AV node and resultant slowing of the ventricular rate. For SVTs that are independent of the AV node, the slower ventricular rate allows the underlying atrial activity to become evident. Additionally, for SVTs that use the AV node as part of a reentrant loop (AVNRT, AVRT), the transient blockade of the AV node frequently aborts the arrhythmia. Importantly, adenosine should not be used for the diagnosis of wide-complex tachycardias as it can cause hemodynamic deterioration when given to patients with VT.

Treatment

In general, the goals of therapy of SVT are to control the ventricular rate, terminate the arrhythmia, and prevent its recurrence. The following methods are available:

- Vagal maneuvers [e.g., carotid sinus massage (CSM), Valsalva maneuver] and intravenous adenosine transiently block AV nodal conduction and may abort SVTs that are dependent on the AV node for part of a reentrant circuit (i.e., AVNRT, AVRT).
- Drugs that block the AV node (e.g., calcium channel blockers, beta blockers, digitalis) are useful for controlling the rate of SVTs, as they slow the conduction of the arrhythmia to the ventricles.
- Antiarrhythmic medications can restore and maintain normal sinus rhythm in patients with atrial flutter or AF.
- Synchronized electrical countershock (cardioversion) can restore normal sinus rhythm in patients with AF or atrial flutter.
- Catheter-guided radiofrequency ablation (RFA) can be used to modify or destroy reentrant circuits (AVNRT, AVRT, atrial flutter) and thereby terminate the arrhythmia and prevent its recurrence.

The treatment of VT differs from that for SVT. Ventricular arrhythmias are frequently hemodynamically unstable rhythms that require urgent or emergent therapy. Vagal maneuvers and AV node–blocking drugs are not effective in this setting because the AV node is not involved in the propagation of the tachycardia. The mainstays of treatment are electrical defibrillation to emergently convert unstable rhythms and antiarrhythmic medications (e.g., amiodarone, lidocaine, procainamide) to convert hemodynamically stable VT back to sinus rhythm and prevent its recurrence. Placement of an ICD may be indicated to prevent SCD when these ventricular tachyarrhythmias recur (see Chapter 25).

FEATURES OF SPECIFIC TACHYCARDIAS

SINUS TACHYCARDIA

Sinus tachycardia almost always occurs as a response to some physiologic stimulus (e.g., fever, exercise, volume depletion, thyrotoxicosis, hypotension). The ECG demonstrates normal-appearing P waves (inverted in lead aVR, upright in lead II), and the rate rarely exceeds 200 bpm. If the increased HR is causing symptoms, it can be slowed with the AV nodal–blocking drugs mentioned above; however, the treatment of sinus tachycardia should be directed toward correcting the underlying cause.

ECTOPIC ATRIAL TACHYCARDIA

Atrial tachycardias originate from an area of the atria distinct from the SA node, have similar triggers as does sinus tachycardia, but may also occur in the absence of an identifiable precipitant. Frequently the ECG demonstrates P waves that are inverted in the inferior leads (leads II, III, aVF) and upright in lead aVR, reflecting the origin of this arrhythmia from the inferior aspect of the atria. Treatment is similar to the treatment

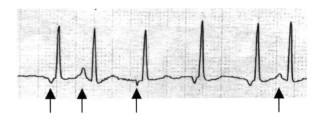

Figure 21-1 • Multifocal atrial tachycardia. Note the irregular rhythm and various p wave morphologies (arrows).

of sinus tachycardia. Chronic treatment with beta blockers or calcium channel blockers may be required to prevent recurrences.

MULTIFOCAL ATRIAL TACHYCARDIA (MAT) (FIGURE 21-1)

MAT is a form of atrial tachycardia in which multiple areas of the atria generate impulses. It is most commonly seen in patients with severe lung disease. The ECG demonstrates an irregularly irregular rhythm with three or more different P-wave morphologies and three or more different PR intervals. The heart rate is usually difficult to control, although verapamil may be effective. The mainstay of therapy is treatment of the underlying lung disease.

ATRIAL FIBRILLATION (FIGURE 21-2)

AF is one of the most common types of SVT. The risk factors for developing AF include RHD, HTN, CHF, and advanced age. During AF, the atria fibrillate at ~400 to 600 bpm but produce no effective atrial contraction. This predisposes to the formation and subsequent embolization of atrial clots and accounts for the almost fivefold increase in stroke risk in patients with AF compared with those in normal sinus rhythm. Atrial systole contributes ~20% of diastolic LV filling; the loss of atrial contraction during AF can significantly reduce CO, especially in patients with reduced LV systolic function. The ECG

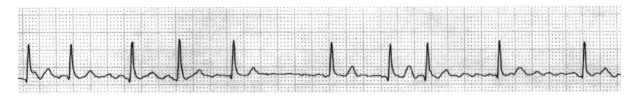

Figure 21-2 • Atrial fibrillation. Note the irregularly irregular rhythm without discernable P waves.

in AF demonstrates no P waves and an irregularly irregular ventricular rhythm, usually at a rate of 100 to 170 bpm.

There are three goals of treatment for AF:

- Control of HR
- Prevention of stroke
- Restoration and maintenance of sinus rhythm (rhythm control)

The ventricular rate can usually be controlled with AV nodal–blocking medications (ideal heart rate: <80 bpm). Beta blockers or calcium channel blockers are usually used; digoxin is rarely effective on its own. The risk of stroke in patients with chronic or paroxysmal AF can be decreased with the use of warfarin to maintain an INR of ~2 to 3. Patients under age 60 without a history of stroke, preexisting heart disease, diabetes mellitus, or hypertension (so-called **lone atrial fibrillation**) may be treated with aspirin instead of warfarin, as their risk of embolic events is quite low. AF may be converted to normal sinus rhythm electrically or with certain antiarrhythmic agents (e.g., propafenone, quinidine, amiodarone). Unless required because of hemodynamic compromise, cardioversion should be avoided until the patient has been therapeutically anticoagulated for at least 3 weeks or has been shown to be free of atrial thrombi by TEE. In the past, attempts were made at restoring sinus rhythm in most patients with AF and then stopping their anticoagulation. However, recent studies have shown that rhythm control is associated with an increased embolic risk (due to cessation of anticoagulation) without clinical benefit. Therefore rhythm control is likely unnecessary except in patients in whom rate control has proven difficult or who continue to have symptoms associated with the arrhythmia.

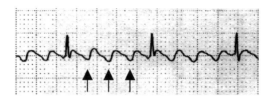

Figure 21-3 • Atrial flutter. Note the regular, "sawtooth" flutter waves (arrows).

■ ATRIAL FLUTTER (FIGURE 21-3)

Atrial flutter is caused by a macroreentrant circuit in the atrium. It tends to be an unstable rhythm and frequently either reverts spontaneously to sinus rhythm or degenerates to AF. The ECG demonstrates "flutter waves," which have a "sawtooth" appearance in leads II, III, and aVF and occur at a rate of 250 to 350 bpm. However, the usual ventricular rate is one-half of this (2:1 block) because of the inability of the AV node to conduct at such rapid rates—a property known as decremental conduction. Predisposing factors and treatment are the same as for AF. In addition, RFA (see Chapter 7) may cure this rhythm.

■ AV-NODAL REENTRANT TACHYCARDIA (FIGURE 21-4)

AVNRT results from a small reentrant loop (microreentrant circuit) within the AV node itself. AVNRT is usually initiated by a premature atrial beat and propagates at a rate of 170 to 220 bpm. The ECG demonstrates a regular tachycardia, either without discernible P waves, or with P waves occurring after the QRS complex ("retrograde P waves"). AV nodal–blocking drugs are the treatment of choice and stop the arrhythmia

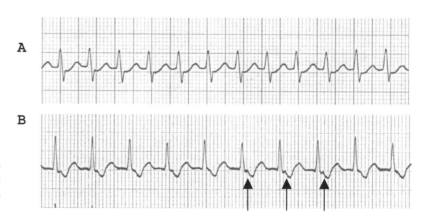

Figure 21-4 • Two different AV-nodal reentrant tachycardias. (a) No P wave is seen (hidden in QRS). (b) Retrograde P waves are seen in the ST segment (arrows).

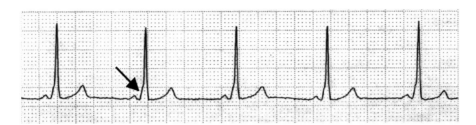

Figure 21-5 • WPW syndrome. Note the slurred upstroke of the QRS (delta wave) and the short PR interval.

by slowing conduction through the reentrant circuit. Adenosine is effective for acutely terminating AVNRT, while beta blockers or calcium channel blockers are often effective at preventing its recurrence. RFA may be curative.

ATRIOVENTRICULAR REENTRANT TACHYCARDIA

AVRT involves a large reentrant loop (macroreentrant circuit), with one limb of the circuit including the AV node and the other being an abnormal connection between the atria and ventricles (an accessory bypass tract). The most common type of bypass tract occurs in the WPW syndrome. The ECG in this syndrome demonstrates a delta wave in normal sinus rhythm owing to partial preexcitation of the ventricles via rapid conduction of the atrial impulse through the bypass tract (Figure 21-5). AVRT is usually initiated by a premature beat and may be associated with a narrow QRS complex if the circuit proceeds down the AV node and up the bypass tract (orthodromic AVRT). If the circuit proceeds in the opposite direction (antidromic AVRT), a wide QRS complex occurs. Treatment is the same as for AVNRT, but with a lower threshold to proceed to RFA in patients with symptomatic AVRT. Care must be taken when patients with bypass tracts develop atrial arrhythmias (e.g., AF or atrial flutter). If AV-nodal blocking agents are given in this situation, the impulses will be preferentially shunted rapidly down the bypass tract and can precipitate hemodynamic collapse.

VENTRICULAR TACHYCARDIA (FIGURE 21-6)

VT is usually associated with symptoms and may cause SCD if it is sustained or if it degenerates into VF. It is usually produced by a reentrant circuit located in either ventricle and is seen most often in the following circumstances:

- Acute cardiac ischemia resulting from CAD
- Prior MI
- Cardiomyopathy (ischemic or nonischemic)
- Electrolyte abnormalities (e.g., hypokalemia, hypomagnesemia)
- Drug toxicity (e.g., digitalis)
- Congenital abnormalities (e.g., RV dysplasia)

The ECG in VT manifests a regular wide-QRS-complex tachycardia. Occasional P waves may be seen, but they have no relation to the QRS complexes. This lack of association between the electrical activity of the atria and ventricles, referred to as **AV dissociation**, is a hallmark of VT.

Torsades de pointes is a specific form of VT in which the axis of the QRS complex constantly changes, causing a waxing and waning QRS amplitude on ECG (Figure 21-7). This type of VT is frequently

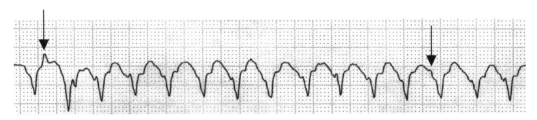

Figure 21-6 • Ventricular tachycardia. Note the wide QRS and evidence of AV dissociation (P waves marked by arrows).

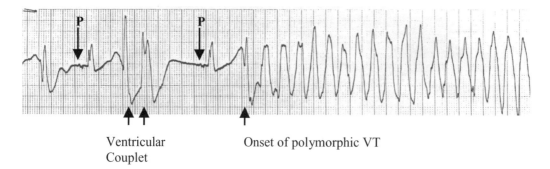

Ventricular Couplet   Onset of polymorphic VT

Figure 21-7 • Polymorphic ventricular tachycardia (**torsades de pointes**). The underlying rhythm is sinus (note P waves) with a long QT. Multiple premature ventricular complexes are present and induce a ventricular couplet and then polymorphic VT.

the result of myocardial ischemia or drug toxicity and can also be seen in patients with an abnormally prolonged QT interval (congenital long-QT syndrome). Treatment of VT includes direct-current countershock if it is hemodynamically unstable and pharmacologic therapy with antiarrhythmic drugs including lidocaine and amiodarone. Recurrences of VT may be prevented by antiarrhythmic medications (e.g., amiodarone, sotalol, propafenone) or treated with an ICD. Torsades de pointes may be treated with magnesium or by pacing the ventricle at a faster rate (overdrive pacing).

Differentiation of Wide-Complex Tachycardias

Most wide-complex tachycardias (duration of QRS complex >0.12 second) are ventricular in origin (i.e., VT). However, at times, SVT may present as a wide-complex tachycardia due to aberrant electrical conduction through the His-Purkinje system. Distinguishing VT from SVT with aberrancy is critical for determining the most appropriate therapy. The following features of the history, physical, and ECG favor VT as the diagnosis:

- History of CAD and/or recent or prior MI
- ECG or physical evidence of AV dissociation
- Shift in QRS axis from baseline ECG
- QRS duration >0.160 second

Although these signs are not conclusive for VT, they can aid in the diagnosis if they are noted.

KEY POINTS

1. The most important aspect of arrhythmia management is identifying the particular arrhythmia present. The presence of P waves, the morphology of the QRS complex, and the regularity of the rhythm are key features in this regard.
2. The main goals of treating supraventricular tachyarrhythmias are control of the ventricular rate, restoration of sinus rhythm, and prevention of recurrences.
3. Ventricular tachyarrhythmias are frequently hemodynamically unstable rhythms that require urgent/emergent cardioversion to restore sinus rhythm.
4. Wide-complex tachyarrhythmias may be ventricular in origin or may originate in the atria but conduct aberrantly to the ventricles. Features that favor VT over SVT in this setting include a history of CAD or CMP, QRS duration >160 milliseconds, evidence of AV dissociation, and a shift in the QRS axis from baseline.

Bradyarrhythmias (Bradycardia and Heart Block)

Bradycardia is defined as an HR of less than 60 bpm. When the normal conduction from the atria to the ventricles is delayed or interrupted, heart block (HB) is present. Bradycardia may occur with or without HB, and HB may occur with or without bradycardia. In general, bradycardia is a benign rhythm unless it produces symptoms, whereas HB is usually more ominous.

Etiology

Although the causes of bradyarrhythmias are varied, it is useful to think of them in terms of functional or structural abnormalities (see Table 22-1). Functional abnormalities produce bradycardia by depressing impulse generation and can result in HB by slowing or preventing conduction through the AV node and His-Purkinje system. In general, functional abnormalities are the result of autonomic (predominantly increased vagal tone) or pharmacologic influences and are reversible upon treating the precipitating cause. Structural abnormalities, on the other hand, reflect inherent conduction system disease, are frequently progressive, and require definitive treatment.

■ TABLE 22-1			
Causes of Bradycardia and Heart Block			
Category		**Examples**	**Treatment**
Functional	Autonomic influences	Increased vagal tone (fear, GI disorders, acute IMI, increased ICP, CSS, highly trained athletes)	Atropine for vagal episodes
		Decreased sympathetic tone (hypothyroidism)	Thyroid replacement
	Medications	Beta blockers Calcium channel blockers Digoxin Antiarrhythmic agents	Stop medications Specific antidotes for overdose*
Structural		Fibrosis of SA and/or AV node Infiltration of SA and/or AV node (amyloidosis, sarcoidosis, hemochromatosis) Ischemia or infarction Infection (Lyme disease, Chagas disease, endocarditis) Congenital complete HB	Pacemaker is usually indicated, especially if symptomatic

*Glucagon for beta-blocker overdose, intravenous calcium for calcium channel blocker overdose, digoxin antibodies for digoxin overdose.

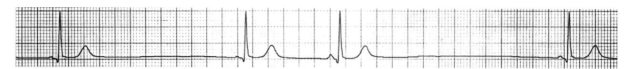

Figure 22-1 • A prolonged sinus pause.

Clinical Manifestations

History

The clinical importance of bradycardia rests almost entirely on the symptoms it produces; nonetheless, many individuals are asymptomatic despite very slow heart rates. If symptoms do develop, they usually reflect decreased cardiac output and/or hypotension and include:

- Syncope or near-syncope
- Angina pectoris
- Dizziness and light-headedness
- Congestive heart failure
- Confusion
- Fatigue

Patients may also experience palpitations, the pattern of which depends on the type of arrhythmia present.

It is essential to obtain a thorough medication history to exclude possible medication-induced bradyarrhythmias and to perform a review of systems to identify underlying disorders or precipitating causes (e.g., headaches, nausea, pain, and so on that could result in increased vagal tone).

Physical Examination

Aside from revealing a slow heart rate, the examination of patients with bradyarrhythmias may be unremarkable. It is essential to measure the BP to exclude hypotension (SBP <90 mm Hg) and determine the hemodynamic significance of the rhythm and the urgency of therapy. In patients with AV dissociation (e.g., complete HB), intermittent prominent pulsations may be seen in the jugular venous waveform. These "cannon A waves" reflects atrial contraction against the closed tricuspid valve during ventricular

systole. Cardiac auscultation may demonstrate a variable intensity of S_1 and an intermittent S_3 or S_4. In patients with carotid sinus hypersensitivity, palpation of the carotid arteries may provoke marked bradycardia or transient ventricular asystole.

Differential Diagnosis

The term *bradyarrhythmias* encompasses a variety of rhythm abnormalities. In general, these rhythms can be distinguished by close inspection of the surface ECG.

Sinus Bradycardia

Sinus bradycardia is marked by an HR < 60 bpm and a normal-appearing P wave preceding each QRS complex. It is generally a benign rhythm caused by medications or increased vagal tone. The latter mechanism accounts for the sometimes marked bradycardia (HR < 50 bpm) that occurs during sleep and is seen in many athletes. Other conditions associated with sinus bradycardia include hypothyroidism, hypothermia, obstructive jaundice, and intrinsic disease of the SA node (see below).

Sinus Node Dysfunction (SND)

This condition may be due to infiltration (e.g., amyloid, sarcoid, hemochromatosis) or fibrosis (e.g., normal aging) of the SA node and can result in sinus bradycardia, intermittent prolonged sinus pauses (Figure 22-1), or complete sinus arrest. It reflects failure of the SA node to generate an electrical impulse (sinus pause or arrest) or failure of the impulse to propagate beyond the region of the node (sinus exit block). If the SA node slows or pauses long enough, junctional or ventricular escape rhythms will supervene. **Sick sinus syndrome** (SSS) refers to the association of SND with

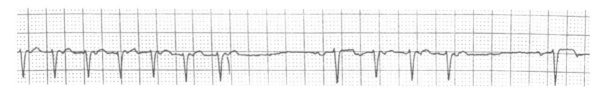

Figure 22-2 • Tachy-brady syndrome. There is a run of supraventricular tachycardia followed by a moderate pause.

symptomatic bradycardia. In a subset of patients with SSS, intermittent tachyarrhythmias such as atrial fibrillation alternate with bradyarrhythmias (tachycardia-bradycardia syndrome) (Figure 22-2).

AV Node Conduction Disorders (Heart Block)

Even in the presence of normal SA node function and a normal rate of impulse formation, bradycardia can still develop if the impulse cannot propagate through the AV node (i.e., is "blocked"). This may occur as a result of functional or structural influences (see Table 22-1). Varying degrees of HB can occur and can be intermittent or persistent. The degree of block can be diagnosed on a 12-lead ECG by observing the relationship between depolarization of the atria (the P wave) and ventricles (the QRS complex). In first-degree AV block, there is fixed prolongation of the PR interval (>200 milliseconds), representing slowed conduction through the AV node (Figure 22-3).

Higher degrees of AV block (second- and third-degree AV block) are associated with the failure of atrial impulses to conduct to the ventricles (a P wave occurs without a resultant QRS complex). In second-degree HB, the failure of AV conduction is intermittent and may occur in two different patterns:

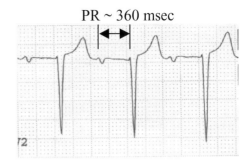

Figure 22-3 • First-degree AV block.

- Mobitz I (Wenckebach)
- Mobitz II

In the Wenckebach type, the PR interval progressively prolongs until a P wave fails to conduct and the subsequent QRS complex is "dropped" (Figure 22-4). This may occur sporadically or in a fixed pattern (e.g., every third or fourth beat), is usually the result of increased vagal tone, and is a relatively benign rhythm. In Mobitz II HB, the PR interval remains constant for all conducted beats; however, occasionally one or more P waves fail to conduct to the ventricles (Figure 22-5). This form of second-degree HB is usually the result of

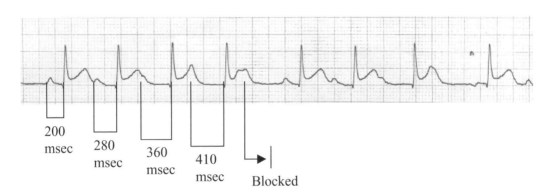

Figure 22-4 • Mobitz I second-degree HB (Wenckebach). Note the progressive prolongation of the PR interval preceding the nonconducted P wave.

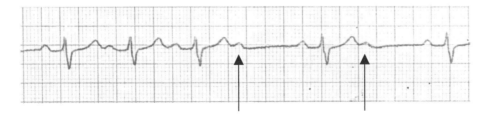

Figure 22-5 • Mobitz II second-degree HB. Note the nonconducted P waves (arrows) in the absence of progressive PR prolongation.

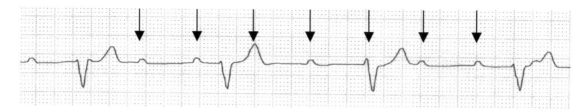

Figure 22-6 • Complete HB. Note that the P waves (arrows) march out faster than the QRS complexes and independent of them.

structural disease, is frequently associated with symptoms, and may progress to higher-degree HB.

The most severe form of AV-nodal block is third-degree HB (complete HB). This is characterized by complete inability of any atrial impulse to pass through the AV node. Thus, the ECG demonstrates normal P waves without associated QRS complexes (AV dissociation) (Figure 22-6). When complete HB occurs, the AV node or ventricular myocardium takes over as the heart's pacemaker (an escape rhythm). These tissues possess a slower intrinsic rate than the sinus node and therefore bradycardia ensues.

Diagnostic Evaluation

The most important diagnostic test in the evaluation of bradyarrhythmias is the 12-lead ECG. The pattern of P waves and their relationship to the QRS complexes will usually allow identification of the specific bradyarrhythmia present. Owing to the intermittent nature of conduction disturbances, prolonged monitoring with a 24-hour Holter monitor or a 30-day event recorder (see Chapter 7) is sometimes required to identify these arrhythmias in patients with suggestive symptoms. Rarely, the mechanism of bradycardia or HB cannot be determined on ECG and electrophysiologic study is required. An evaluation of thyroid function is warranted in patients with bradycardia, and a thorough review of medications is necessary.

It is important to distinguish HB from AV dissociation. With AV dissociation, the atria and ventricles beat independently of each other. As such, complete HB is a form of AV dissociation. However, the presence of AV dissociation does not necessarily imply HB, as AV conduction may be completely normal but dissociation occurs because the ventricles are beating faster than the atria (e.g., VT, accelerated idioventricular rhythm). With true HB, AV dissociation is present and the ventricles beat at a slower rate than the atria owing to the development of an escape rhythm.

Treatment

In the absence of symptoms, sinus bradycardia itself does not generally require treatment. Similarly, first-degree HB and Mobitz I second-degree HB (Wenckebach) are generally benign rhythms with few clinical implications. In many instances, correcting the underlying cause (e.g., hypothyroidism, hypothermia) may restore a normal HR. Drugs that slow conduction should be discontinued and ischemia or infarction should obviously be treated. In patients with symptomatic bradycardia and in most patients with higher degrees of HB (second-degree Mobitz type II and third-degree), treatment is warranted. Atropine may increase the HR acutely when the cause of the arrhythmia is functional, but it can worsen HB that occurs on a structural basis. Patients with persistent symptomatic bradycardia despite removal of aggravating causes and those with SND or higher degrees of HB generally require implantation of a permanent pacemaker.

KEY POINTS

1. Sinus bradycardia is usually a benign rhythm caused by medication or increased vagal tone.
2. Sick sinus syndrome involves the association of sinus node dysfunction with symptomatic bradycardia.
3. Second-degree HB type I (Wenckebach) is associated with progressive prolongation of the PR interval until a nonconducted P wave occurs. Second-degree HB type II is associated with a nonconducted P wave in the absence of preceding progressive PR prolongation.
4. Sinus bradycardia and Wenckebach are generally benign rhythms that do not require treatment.
5. Mobitz II second- and third-degree HB is often associated with structural heart disease and may require placement of a permanent pacemaker.

Syncope

Syncope is the sudden transient loss of consciousness and postural tone followed by spontaneous recovery. Presyncope is the sensation of impending syncope without loss of consciousness.

Epidemiology

Syncope is a common clinical entity, accounting for approximately 3% of ED visits and 6% of all hospital admissions. The incidence of syncope increases with advancing age, and approximately one-third of the population will suffer an episode of syncope at some point in their lives.

Pathogenesis

Syncope can result from a variety of cardiovascular or noncardiovascular causes. The common physiologic link among all cardiovascular causes of syncope is a transient decrease in cerebral blood flow. This usually results from a sudden fall in BP, producing bilateral cortical or brainstem hypoperfusion; unilateral carotid artery disease is unlikely to cause syncope. Noncardiovascular causes of syncope produce loss of consciousness by inducing diffuse brain dysfunction via electrical or metabolic derangement.

Differential Diagnosis

The cardiovascular causes of syncope can be separated into those that are reflex-mediated and those resulting from a structural cardiac problem (Box 23-1). The most common type of reflex-mediated syncope is vasovagal syncope, also known as neurocardiogenic syncope, in which various stimuli trigger the sudden development of vasodilation ("vaso") and bradycardia ("vagal"), resulting in hypotension. Vasovagal syncope precipitated by a specific trigger (such as coughing or micturition) is referred to as situational syncope. A similar reflex can be provoked in some people by applying gentle pressure over the carotid artery (carotid sinus hypersensitivity). This may result in vasodilation (vasodepressor response), bradycardia (cardioinhibitor response), or both. Orthostatic hypotension resulting from volume depletion or antihypertensive medication is another frequent cause of syncope.

Structural cardiac disease and arrhythmias account for approximately 15 to 20% of all syncope. Common mechanical causes include aortic stenosis and HOCM; MS, pulmonary HTN, and cardiac tamponade are less common causes. Both bradyarrhythmias (sick sinus syndrome, AV-nodal blockade, etc.) and tachyarrhythmias (VT or SVT) can result in a fall in CO, thereby precipitating syncope. Of note, SVT rarely causes syncope in the absence of underlying structural heart disease or a bypass tract.

Noncardiovascular causes of syncope include neurologic (seizure, vertebrobasilar insufficiency) and metabolic (hypoglycemia) causes. Psychiatric causes (anxiety, pseudoseizure) are uncommon.

Clinical Manifestations

History

The history is the most important aspect of evaluating a patient with syncope and frequently gives clues to the underlying cause. It is important to obtain the history not only from the patient, but also from any witnesses and to ask the following questions:

1. What was the patient doing at the time of the syncopal episode?
2. Were there any symptoms (e.g., chest pain, palpitations) preceding the event?

BOX 23-1 CARDIOVASCULAR CAUSES OF SYNCOPE

Reflex-mediated (neurocardiogenic)
Situational (vasovagal)
  Micturition
  Tussive
  Valsalva
  Postprandial
  Adverse stimulus
Orthostatic
  Volume depletion
  Medications
  Carotid sinus hypersensitivity

Structural
Cardiac
  AS
  MS
  HCM
  Atrial myxoma
  MI
  Pericardial tamponade
Vascular
  PE
  Pulmonary HTN
  Vertebrobasilar insufficiency

Arrhythmic
SVT
VT
Sinus node dysfunction
AV-nodal block

- Exertional syncope
- Syncope without warning or aura

Table 23-1 outlines important historic features of syncope and the diagnoses they suggest.

Physical Examination

On physical examination it is important to evaluate the patient for orthostatic changes in BP and for signs

TABLE 23-1

Historic Features of Syncope and Suggested Etiologies

Historical Feature of Syncopal Episode	Suggested Cause(s)
Exertional	AS or MS, HCM, pulmonary HTN
Associated with chest pain	Myocardial ischemia, PE, aortic dissection
Associated with palpitations	Tachy- or bradyarrhythmias
Patient with history of CAD or CMP	Ventricular tachyarrhythmia
Family history of syncope or SCD	Hereditary long-QT syndrome, HCM
Associated with emotional stress, pain, unpleasant auditory or visual stimuli	Vasovagal episode
Following cough, micturition, or defecation	Situational syncope (form of vasovagal syncope)
After arising from lying or sitting position	Orthostatic hypotension, hypovolemia
After turning head; during shaving	Carotid sinus sensitivity
Associated with certain body position	Atrial myxoma or "ball valve" thrombus
Diuretic medication use	Hypovolemia
Antiarrhythmic or antipsychotic medication use	Ventricular tachyarrhythmias
Parkinson disease, DM	Autonomic insufficiency
Premonitory aura, tonic-clonic movements, incontinence, tongue-biting, or postictal state	Seizure
History of stroke or head trauma	Seizure

3. Is the patient on any medications?
4. Does the patient have a history of heart disease?
5. Was there any sign of seizure activity? Any incontinence or tongue biting?
6. How long did the patient remain unconscious?
7. When the patient awoke, was he or she confused?

It is important to identify patients who have a cardiac cause of their syncope, as their prognosis is much worse than with a noncardiac cause. Cardiac syncope is always sudden in onset, may be preceded by chest pain or palpitations, and resolves spontaneously (usually in less than 5 minutes). The following findings on history suggest true cardiac syncope:

- Syncope following chest pain
- Syncope preceded by palpitations

TABLE 23-2

Diagnostic Modalities in the Evaluation of Syncope

Diagnostic Procedure	Syncope Types in Which It May Be Helpful
ECG	Arrhythmias, heart block, conduction disease
Tilt-table testing	Neurocardiogenic syncope (vasovagal)
Electrophysiologic testing	VT, some SVT, some bradycardias
24-hour Holter monitor	Arrhythmias that occur frequently
Event monitor	Infrequent arrhythmias (can monitor for ~1 month)
Implantable loop monitor	Very infrequent arrhythmias (can monitor up to 18 months)
EEG, CT scan	Seizure disorder
CSM	Carotid sinus hypersensitivity

of volume depletion as well as to listen for the murmurs of AS, MS, or HOCM. CSM should be carefully performed if the history is suggestive; however, carotid vascular disease should first be excluded by inquiring about a history of TIA or stroke and listening for carotid bruits.

Diagnostic Evaluation

Many procedures are available to aid in determining the etiology of syncope (Table 23-2); however, the use of these ancillary tests should be guided by results of the history and physical examination. In at least one-third of cases of syncope, a specific diagnosis cannot be determined, and in approximately one-half of cases in which a diagnosis is made, it is suggested by the initial history or physical examination.

A 12-lead ECG should be obtained in all patients with syncope unless the history clearly suggests a noncardiac cause. The ECG may reveal the actual cause (i.e., HB, tachyarrhythmias) or suggest potential causes (i.e., evidence of ischemic heart disease, bypass tracts, etc.). In patients in whom an arrhythmia is suspected but not documented on ECG, prolonged monitoring with a 24-hour Holter monitor, event recorder, or implantable recorder may be helpful. An echocardiogram is indicated in patients suspected of having underlying structural heart disease and may reveal the cause of the syncope (e.g., AS or MS), or

demonstrate evidence of prior infarction, thereby raising the suspicion of an arrhythmic cause. If the history, physical examination, or initial diagnostic tests suggest an arrhythmic cause for syncope, an EPS may be indicated, especially if the patient is also suspected of having CAD (see Chapter 7). During EPS, the arrhythmia that caused the syncope can frequently be reproduced or HB identified. In patients without underlying heart disease, EPS rarely identifies the cause of syncope.

Most patients without structural heart disease or clinical evidence of arrhythmias have a reflex cause of syncope (usually vasovagal), and further invasive diagnostic studies are usually not indicated. In such patients who have recurrent syncope, the diagnosis of neurocardiogenic syncope can be confirmed with tilt-table testing (see Chapter 7). Patients who are suspected of having seizures or a psychiatric cause of syncope warrant neurologic or psychiatric evaluation, respectively.

Prognosis

Young patients (age < 60) with syncope but without underlying heart disease have an excellent prognosis. Patients with a normal ECG have a low probability of an arrhythmic cause of syncope and a low risk of SCD. Patients who have a cardiac cause of syncope have an annual mortality rate as high as 30%.

TABLE 23-3

Treatment for Some Specific Causes of Syncope

Type of Syncope	Possible Therapies
Vasovagal/ neurocardiogenic	Avoid provoking stimuli; consider beta blockers; volume repletion
Orthostasis	Volume repletion, avoid antihypertensive drugs; mineralocorticoid supplementation for primary autonomic insufficiency
VT	Implantable defibrillator, antiarrhythmic drugs
SVT	Rate-controlling medications, antiarrhythmic drugs, RFA
Bradycardia	Pacemaker
AS or MS	Valve replacement
HCM	Myomectomy, ICD
Situational	Avoid precipitating factor

Treatment

The treatment of syncope depends entirely on its cause (Table 23-3). Most types of situational or vasovagal syncope require no specific therapy. Recurrent reflex-mediated syncope in the absence of triggering factors (i.e., neurocardiogenic syncope) may respond to treatment with beta blockers. Arrhythmias require specific therapy based on the type of arrhythmia present (see Chapters 21 and 22). In general, SVTs can be treated with rate-lowering medications (e.g., beta blockers, calcium channel blockers, digoxin), antiarrhythmic drugs, or occasionally RFA, whereas VT almost always requires treatment with antiarrhythmic drugs and/or implantation of an ICD. Syncope resulting from bradyarrhythmias requires placement of a pacemaker unless a reversible cause is identified (e.g., medications, metabolic abnormalities).

Syncope resulting from underlying heart disease requires correction of the structural abnormality. For example, AS and MS require valve replacement, and ischemic heart disease (ischemia or infarction) requires coronary revascularization with percutaneous balloon angioplasty or CABG.

KEY POINTS

1. Syncope is the sudden transient loss of consciousness and can arise as a result of cardiac or noncardiac disorders.
2. Cardiac syncope is always sudden in onset, may be preceded by chest pain or palpitations, is short-lived, and resolves spontaneously.
3. The most common type of syncope is vasovagal (i.e., neurocardiogenic syncope).
4. Structural heart disease and arrhythmias account for approximately 15 to 20% of syncopal episodes.
5. A thorough history is the most important aspect of the evaluation of a patient with syncope.

24 Sudden Cardiac Death

The term *sudden cardiac death* (SCD) refers to unexpected natural death from a cardiac cause occurring within 1 hour of the onset of symptoms in a patient without a preexisting fatal condition. The term *SCD survivor* refers to a patient who suffered SCD but was successfully resuscitated.

Epidemiology and Risk Factors

In the United States, sudden cardiac death leads to 400,000 to 600,000 deaths annually, accounting for almost half of all death from cardiac causes. Approximately 70% of cases of SCD occur in patients with CAD; therefore the risk factors for SCD closely parallel those for CAD. These include:

- Tobacco use
- High cholesterol
- Advanced age
- Male gender
- HTN

Other noted risk factors for SCD include:

- LVH
- Intraventricular conduction block
- Depressed LV systolic function

In patients with a prior MI, the strongest predictor of SCD is an LVEF of ≤30%. Frequent ventricular ectopy, especially NSVT, is also a strong predictor of SCD in these patients.

The incidence of SCD is highest from birth until 6 months of age, due to sudden infant death syndrome (SIDS) and some congenital cardiac anomalies. The incidence declines during adolescence and young adulthood and then rises sharply during middle and advanced age owing to the development of CAD. Approximately 75% of all cases of SCD occur in males. This gender predisposition is even more marked with advancing age; the male:female ratio is approximately 7:1 in the middle-aged and elderly population.

Etiology and Pathogenesis

Most cases of SCD result from cardiac disorders, predominantly CAD. Over 75% of patients who suffer SCD have pathologic evidence of a prior MI; in as many as 25% of patients with CAD, SCD is the first manifestation of their disease. Other cardiac causes of SCD are outlined in Table 24-1 and include structural abnormalities of the heart and conditions other than CAD that predispose to arrhythmia.

Although the specific mode of death in SCD may be difficult to ascertain, many cases are attributed to malignant arrhythmias such as VT and VF. Bradyarrhythmias are a much less common mechanism of SCD. The mechanisms that produce VT and VF in SCD include reentry, increased automaticity, and triggered activity and may depend on factors such as autonomic tone (see Chapter 20).

Patients with long-QT syndrome as noted on the surface ECG, defined as a corrected QT interval >0.44 second, may develop a type of polymorphic VT known as torsades de pointes (see Chapter 21), which can cause death by degenerating to VF. Although long-QT syndrome may be a congenital condition, it is more commonly the result of various drugs or metabolic disturbances such as:

- Class Ia, Ic, and some class III antiarrhythmics
- Antihistamines (e.g., terfenadine)
- Antimicrobials (mostly antifungals)
- Tricyclic antidepressants
- Phenothiazines
- Electrolyte abnormalities (hypokalemia, hypomagnesemia, hypocalcemia)

TABLE 24-1

Cardiac Causes of Sudden Death

Cause	Examples
I. Coronary artery disease	Atherosclerosis, congenital anomalies, coronary aneurysms, coronary embolism, coronary spasm
II. Structural heart disease (other than CAD)	
Valvular heart disease	AS
Hypertrophic heart disease	HCM, hypertensive heart disease
DCM	Ischemia, idiopathic, postviral, alcohol-associated, myocarditis, arrhythmogenic RV dysplasia
Infiltrative heart disease	Amyloidosis, hemochromatosis, Chagas disease
Congenital heart disease	AS, Eisenmenger syndrome
III. Arrhythmogenic disorders	
Prolonged-QT syndrome	Congenital, drug effect (antiarrhythmics, phenothiazines), electrolyte abnormalities (hyper- or hypokalemia, hypocalcemia, hypomagnesemia)
Preexcitation syndromes	WPW syndrome
Brugada syndrome	
Bradyarrhythmias	Complete HB, asystole
IV. Other	
Cardiac tumors	Atrial myxoma
Pericardial tamponade	
PE	
Aortic dissection	

The congenital forms of QT prolongation have recently been attributed to genetic defects that lead to abnormal myocyte potassium and sodium channels. The resultant alterations in ionic fluxes result in abnormal ventricular repolarization, thereby predisposing to the development of **torsades de pointes**, possibly through the generation of abnormal after depolarizations.

Several factors may predispose to the development of SCD in patients with underlying cardiac disease. These include:

- Electrolyte imbalances (potassium, magnesium, calcium)
- Transient myocardial ischemia
- Hypoxia

Prognosis

The vast majority of patients (>80%) who suffer an episode of SCD do not survive, and the incidence of recurrent SCD among initial survivors is as high as 30% in the first year following the event. The most common causes of death in survivors of SCD relate to neurologic injury at the time of the event or infectious complications as a result of prolonged intubation. Among survivors of SCD who survive to hospital discharge, over one-third suffer persistent neurologic deficits.

Clinical Manifestations

History

The history obtained form survivors of SCD should be directed toward identifying potential causes and should include a review of:

- Prior cardiac disease
- Concomitant medical conditions
- Medication usage

If available, the patient's activities and symptoms immediately preceding the event should be reviewed, as they may offer insight into the etiology.

Physical Examination

The physical examination of survivors of SCD should similarly be geared toward identifying potential causes. Evidence of cardiomyopathy (e.g., S_3, displaced PMI) or valvular heart disease (e.g., murmur of AS) should be noted. In addition, a thorough neurologic examination should be performed to identify neurologic deficits that may have occurred during the prolonged period of cerebral hypoxemia that often accompanies SCD.

Diagnostic Evaluation

The initial evaluation in SCD survivors includes an ECG and basic laboratory tests. The ECG may reveal evidence of CAD (old or evolving MI, active ischemia), electrical predisposition to ventricular tachyarrhythmias (preexcitation, long QT), ventricular irritability (frequent ventricular premature complexes, NSVT), or evidence of HB. Initial laboratory tests should include an electrolyte panel and tests for myocardial injury (creatine kinase, troponin). If the initial ECG suggests an AMI, cardiac catheterization to define the coronary anatomy and feasibility of revascularization should be considered.

Once stabilized, all survivors of SCD should undergo echocardiography to seek evidence of CAD or valvular heart disease and to determine the LVEF. Patients with normal LV function but with risk factors for CAD should undergo diagnostic exercise stress testing. In patients with a depressed EF, cardiac catheterization may be warranted to exclude significant underlying CAD, and EPS may be indicated for risk stratification and guidance of therapy.

Treatment

The initial management of survivors of SCD is in large part supportive, with most requiring intubation and mechanical ventilation for several days. Hemodynamic lability is common, as are CHF, recurrent arrhythmias, and infection (especially aspiration pneumonia). Most survivors are neurologically impaired following the event but have neurologic recovery (albeit often incomplete recovery) over the course of several days. Hypothermic therapy has been shown to improve overall neurologic outcome following SCD and should be instituted in patients who remain unresponsive after resuscitation. Hypothermia is achieved via cooling blankets or intravascular cooling devices. The patient's temperature should be reduced to 32 to 34°C for 24 hours, after which passive warming is allowed. Patients must be sedated, and pharmacologic paralysis is required during hypothermia to prevent shivering.

The specific treatment of survivors of SCD depends on the etiology of the event. If a reversible cause is identified (e.g., medication toxicity or electrolyte abnormality), treatment involves correcting the underlying problem. However, if the patient is thought to have suffered an acute ischemic event as the basis for SCD, cardiac catheterization should be performed and percutaneous or surgical revascularization undertaken if possible. Implantation of an ICD should be strongly considered in all SCD survivors who have had a previous MI or have an underlying cardiomyopathy and who are felt to have had an arrhythmic event as the cause of SCD (see Chapter 25). These devices will monitor for and treat recurrent arrhythmias and reduce mortality in this setting. A formal EPS may be warranted in SCD survivors for

whom an arrhythmic cause is not certain in order to determine the inducibility of ventricular tachyarrhythmias. Many of these patients will require treatment with an antiarrhythmic agent (such as amiodarone) and most will require implantation of an ICD. Patients with long-QT syndrome require removal of offending medications, correction of metabolic abnormalities, and frequently ICD placement.

The primary prevention of SCD is difficult because many patients do not manifest signs or symptoms that may indicate their high risk of SCD. Since most cases of SCD are due to CAD or underlying structural heart disease, screening for disease in at-risk individuals may reduce the incidence of SCD by identifying patients with predisposing conditions and allowing for adequate therapy before SCD occurs. In general, correcting, or at least improving, cardiac function in those diseases known to cause SCD can reduce its incidence.

Patients with a depressed LVEF who also have nonsustained VT (especially those with underlying CAD) have a significantly increased risk of developing SCD. These patients may warrant ICD placement.

KEY POINTS

1. SCD is a major cause of death in the United States.
2. CAD is the leading cause of SCD and accounts for over 70% of cases.
3. SCD is most often the result of ventricular tachyarrhythmias; bradyarrhythmias are a less common cause.
4. The initial evaluation of SCD survivors should include an ECG, electrolyte panel, cardiac enzymes, and an echocardiogram.
5. If SCD results from CAD, cardiac catheterization and revascularization are indicated. Hypothermic therapy should be considered for survivors of SCD who remain unresponsive after initial resuscitation.
6. Treatment depends in large part on the underlying cause and the LV function. Antiarrhythmic agents may be necessary to prevent recurrences, whereas ICD placement is usually indicated to treat recurrences.

Pacemakers and Implantable Cardioverter-Defibrillators

With the major advances in microprocessor technology of the last two decades, patients who have symptomatic bradycardias and malignant tachycardias can be treated effectively with permanent pacemakers and ICDs, respectively. This chapter outlines the basic components, function, and indications for implantation of these devices.

▣ PACEMAKERS

A cardiac pacemaker consists of a battery-powered pulse generator connected to a system of electrical leads. With a permanent pacemaker, the pulse genera-

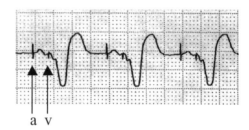

Figure 25-2 • Rhythm strip of patient with a dual-chamber pacemaker. Note the atrial (a) and ventricular (v) pacemaker spikes that precede the P wave and QRS complex. Also note the wide QRS complex that results from direct activation of the ventricular myocardium.

tor is implanted subcutaneously in the chest wall, usually below the left clavicle. The leads pass from the pulse generator through the cephalic or subclavian veins and are anchored into the RA and/or RV (Figure 25-1). The device can be programmed to sense intrinsic cardiac electrical activity. If the intrinsic heart rate falls below a predetermined rate, the device delivers an electrical impulse to the myocardium, causing it to depolarize. Temporary pacemakers are also available and can be inserted transvenously or can deliver the electrical impulse directly through the chest wall (transcutaneously). The electrical impulse from the pacemaker can be seen on an ECG as an electrical spike immediately preceding the P wave or QRS complex (Figure 25-2).

Indications for Pacemaker Implantation

The most common indications for placement of a pacemaker are outlined in Box 25-1. In general, pacemakers are implanted as treatment for symptomatic bradyarrhythmias (see Chapter 22). Asymptomatic bradyarrhythmias are usually benign but occasionally

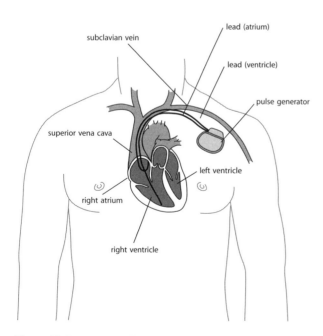

Figure 25-1 • Diagram of pacemaker placement.

BOX 25-1 — COMMON INDICATIONS FOR IMPLANTATION OF A PERMANENT PACEMAKER

Heart block
Symptomatic third-degree AV block
Asystole > 3 seconds
Symptomatic second-degree HB regardless of Mobitz
  type
Asymptomatic third-degree HB with escape rate
  < 40 bpm
Mobitz II second-degree HB

Sinus node dysfunction (sick sinus syndrome)
Sick sinus syndrome with symptomatic bradycardia
Symptomatic chronotropic incompetence
Tachycardia-bradycardia syndrome with symptomatic
  bradycardia

Syncope
Recurrent syncope caused by carotid sinus stimulation
Cardioinhibitory response (asystole > 3 seconds) with
  minimal CSM

Dilated cardiomyopathy (biventricular pacemaker)
Symptomatic HF with wide QRS on ECG and LVEF < 35%

---

require pacemaker placement owing to a high likelihood of progression to symptomatic bradycardia in some settings. Temporary pacemakers are used to treat transient bradyarrhythmias that result from reversible causes, whereas permanent pacemakers are used to treat irreversible disorders.

Pacemaker Modes

Single-chamber pacemakers have a lead in the RA or RV, whereas dual-chamber pacemakers have a lead in both chambers. These leads allow the device both to sense the electrical activity in the atrium and/or ventricle and to pace the chambers at a preset rate.

Pacemakers can be programmed to various modes of activity described by a standardized three- or four-letter code. The first letter refers to the chamber being paced and the second to the chamber being sensed [A = atrium; V = ventricle; D = dual (both atrium and ventricle); O = neither]. The third letter refers to the response of the pacemaker to a sensed native heartbeat. The sensed beat may inhibit (I) the pacemaker from pacing; may trigger (T) the pacemaker to

pace; or may have a dual effect (D) whereby it inhibits atrial pacing while triggering subsequent ventricular pacing. The fourth letter refers to special functions of the pacemaker. Some pacemakers can sense an increase in a person's activity level and respond by increasing the pacing rate (denoted by R for "rate-responsive").

Choice of Pacemaker Mode

The choice of pacing mode depends mainly on the underlying arrhythmia. For patients with bradycardia but with an underlying sinus rhythm (sick sinus syndrome, HB, etc.), dual-chamber pacing (usually DDD mode) is preferred because it maintains AV synchrony. For patients with AF and bradycardia, single-chamber ventricular pacing is used (usually VVI mode) because the fibrillating atrium cannot be paced. Other pacing modes are used less frequently.

Biventricular Pacing

An important advance in pacemaker technology is the biventricular pacemaker, which provides the ability to simultaneously pace the RV and LV via leads placed in the RV and the coronary sinus. This mode of pacing has been shown to increase cardiac output and improve quality of life in patients with advanced systolic HF and a widened QRS on ECG. In general,

---

BOX 25-2 — INDICATIONS FOR IMPLANTATION OF A CARDIOVERTER-DEFIBRILLATOR

1. Nonsustained VT in the setting of CAD, LV systolic dysfunction, and prior MI, with inducible VT on EPS*
2. Spontaneous, sustained VT in the absence of a reversible cause and/or in the setting of structural heart disease
3. Survivors of cardiac arrest resulting from VT or VF without reversible cause
4. Syncope of undetermined etiology with inducible VT on EPS (when drug therapy is ineffective or not tolerated)

* Many physicians agree that an ICD is indicated in patients with history of MI at least 1 month prior and an LVEF of <30%, even without documented NSVT or inducible VT at EPS.

a QRS duration of >130 milliseconds signifies delayed depolarization of the LV and dysynchronous ventricular contraction. Resynchronization therapy with a biventricular pacemaker should be considered in patients with a wide QRS and an EF < 35% who remain highly symptomatic from their HF despite maximal medical therapy.

■ IMPLANTABLE CARDIOVERTER-DEFIBRILLATORS

An ICD is similar to a pacemaker in that it consists of an endocardial lead in the RV apex connected to a pulse generator implanted in the chest wall. However, although ICDs have pacing capability, their primary role is in treating ventricular tachyarrhythmias (VT or VF). When the device detects one of these arrhythmias, it attempts to terminate it either by transiently pacing the heart faster than the rate of the arrhythmia (overdrive pacing), or by delivering a high-energy shock to the myocardium (cardioversion/defibrillation).

Indications for ICD Implantation

ICDs are highly effective at terminating ventricular tachyarrhythmias and decrease the risk of SCD in certain patient populations. The patients who benefit the most from ICDs include those with CAD, depressed LV systolic function, and documented runs of nonsustained VT as well as those who have survived an episode of SCD. Recent evidence suggests that all patients with a cardiomyopathy (LVEF <30%) may benefit from ICD placement even in the absence of symptoms or a documented arrhythmia. Other patients who are felt to be at increased risk of SCD may be further stratified as to risk by EPS (see Chapter 7). Some of these patients who have inducible VT may benefit from ICD implantation. Box 25-2 outlines the currently accepted indications for ICD placement.

KEY POINTS

1. Pacemakers are generally used for the treatment of symptomatic bradyarrhythmias.
2. Dual-chamber pacing maintains AV synchrony. Biventricular pacing may be indicated in patients with symptomatic systolic HF and a wide QRS.
3. ICDs are used for the treatment of ventricular tachyarrhythmias and decrease mortality in certain patient populations.

Part Six

Valvular Heart Disease

26 Rheumatic Fever

Acute rheumatic fever (RF) is an immune-mediated inflammatory disease resulting from untreated group A beta-hemolytic streptococcal pharyngitis. The chronic sequela of this disease is progressive cardiac valvular dysfunction with resulting HF.

Epidemiology

Acute RF is an uncommon illness in developed nations. It is rare in infancy (<5 years of age), uncommon in adulthood, and usually seen in the 5- to 15-year-old age group. Males and females are equally affected. Its incidence is directly related to the prevalence of streptococcal pharyngitis in the community. During prior epidemics of streptococcal pharyngitis, approximately 3% of those affected developed acute RF. Patients with a prior history of acute RF have a high risk of recurrence (5 to 50%) with subsequent untreated streptococcal pharyngitis. Most cases in the United States are sporadic, although clusters have been reported in dormitories, military barracks, closed institutions, and densely populated poor urban neighborhoods.

Etiology and Pathogenesis

Several epidemiologic and prospective studies have established the association of RF with antecedent streptococcal pharyngitis. Group A streptococci with M-protein serotypes 1, 3, 5, 6, 18, 19, and 24 are the most rheumatogenic strains. Streptococcal skin infections (e.g., cellulitis, impetigo), even when caused by the above serotypes, are not associated with RF. The exact mechanism whereby the disease process is initiated remains uncertain but likely involves molecular mimicry. Neither streptococci nor streptococcal antigens can be demonstrated in the pathologic lesions of RF.

The principal organs involved in RF are the heart, large joints, brain, skin, and subcutaneous tissues. The pathognomonic lesion of rheumatic carditis is the Aschoff body, which consists of interstitial edema, fragmentation of collagen fibers, and mononuclear cell infiltration. Valvulitis, as a result of rheumatic endocarditis, can result in acute valvular regurgitation. More commonly, as the valvulitis heals, scarring, thickening, and adhesion of valve cusps and chordae occur and lead to valvular stenosis and/or regurgitation.

Clinical Manifestations

All patients with RF have had preceding streptococcal pharyngitis; this may have been asymptomatic in as many as 50% of cases. The symptoms and signs of RF typically begin 3 weeks after the incident pharyngitis.

Major Manifestations

The major manifestations can be remembered by using the mnemonic J♥NES—where "J" stands for *joints* (arthritis), the "♥" stands for *carditis*, "N" stands for subcutaneous *nodules*, "E" stands for *erythema marginatum*, and "S" stands for *Sydenham chorea*.

Carditis

Rheumatic carditis is present in at least 50% of patients with acute RF. Acute rheumatic carditis varies in severity, is often asymptomatic, and affects all three layers of the heart. Endocarditis most commonly involves the MV, followed by the AV, and rarely the TV and PV. Acute valvular regurgitation can occur and may result in HF. Most patients with acute rheumatic carditis have a systolic murmur of MR and may have a low-pitched apical middiastolic murmur (Carey-Coombs murmur) resulting from flow across the inflamed valve. Rheumatic myocarditis usually manifests as sinus tachycardia disproportionate to the degree of fever, with or without other symptoms or signs of HF. Rheumatic pericarditis may result in chest pain, an audible friction rub, and pericardial effusion, although pericardial tamponade is rare. Myocarditis or pericarditis in the absence of endocarditis is not likely to be secondary to RF.

Arthritis

An asymmetric, nonerosive, migratory polyarthritis with a predilection for large joints of the extremities (knees, ankles, elbows, wrists) is the most common symptom of RF. Effusions are common, but there is no residual joint deformity.

Erythema Marginatum

This transient, erythematous, migratory, nonpruritic rash is characteristic of RF but is seen in only 5% of affected patients. The rash may vary in size with serpiginous, slightly raised margins and a pale center. It is usually localized to the trunk and proximal extremities.

Subcutaneous Nodules

Pea-sized, firm, painless, freely mobile nodules on the extensor surface of the elbows, knees, and wrists and over the scapulae, vertebrae, and occipital scalp are seen in 3% of patients with RF (usually in patients with carditis).

Chorea

Also known as Sydenham chorea and St. Vitus dance, chorea is seen in 20% of RF patients and reflects inflammation of the basal ganglia and caudate nucleus. It is characterized by purposeless, involuntary movements of the face and extremities, nervousness, explosive speech, and emotional lability. Symptoms are absent during sleep and resolve spontaneously in 1 to 2 weeks. Unlike the other symptoms, chorea appears 3 to 6 months after the initial pharyngitis.

Minor Manifestations

Fever, arthralgia (without arthritis), epistaxis, abdominal pain, and tachycardia (without other features of carditis) may all be present in acute RF.

Late Manifestations

Approximately 50% of patients who have carditis during an episode of acute RF will eventually develop chronic rheumatic valvular disease. Aortic and mitral regurgitation may occur during the acute phase or develop years later. Valvular stenosis is a late sequela, usually occurring decades after the acute illness. The MR is most commonly affected, followed by the AV and the TV. The PV is rarely if ever involved.

Combined MV and AV disease is more common than isolated rheumatic AV disease; TV disease is invariably accompanied by MV disease.

Diagnostic Evaluation

There is no definitive diagnostic test for acute RF; the Jones criteria (Box 26-1) serve as the standard diagnostic modality. The presence of either two major criteria or one major and two minor criteria, with supporting evidence of antecedent streptococcal infection, indicates a high probability of RF. The absence of positive cultures or serologic evidence of recent streptococcal infection makes the diagnosis of RF doubtful except when the presenting symptom is chorea. Diagnostic workup should include a pharyngeal swab, blood cultures, blood tests for acute-phase reactants, and serum analysis for antistreptococcal antibodies. An ECG and echocardiogram should be performed to evaluate for evidence of conduction disturbance and carditis, respectively.

BOX 26-1	CLINICAL CRITERIA FOR THE DIAGNOSIS OF ACUTE RHEUMATIC FEVER

Modified Duckett Jones Criteria (AHA 1992)
Major criteria
Carditis
Polyarthritis
Erythema marginatum
Subcutaneous nodules
Chorea

Minor criteria
Clinical findings
  Fever
  Arthralgia
Laboratory findings
  Elevated acute-phase reactants (ESR or CRP)
  Prolonged PR interval

Evidence of antecedent streptococcal infection
Positive pharyngeal culture or rapid streptococcal antigen test
Elevated or rising titers of antistreptococcal antibodies (anti–streptolysin O, anti–DNase B, antihyaluronidase, Antistreptozyme)

Differential Diagnosis

Several illnesses can mimic acute RF, including infective endocarditis and various arthritides. However, with infective endocarditis, blood cultures are usually positive, vegetations are seen on echocardiography, and the associated arthritis is nonmigratory. Hepatosplenomegaly and lymphadenopathy are prominent features of juvenile rheumatoid arthritis but not of RF. Rheumatoid arthritis is not related to RF and is typically a disease of adults characterized by erosive, nonmigratory polyarthritis.

Treatment

Most patients with acute RF should be admitted to the hospital for observation; those with arthritis and/or carditis should be placed on bed rest until their joint inflammation has subsided and the acute-phase reactants have returned to normal. Even if pharyngeal swabs are negative for streptococci, all patients should receive a 10-day course of penicillin VK, 250–500 mg four times daily (erythromycin if penicillin-allergic) to eradicate residual infection. Arthritis usually responds well to high-dose salicylates (100 mg/kg/day in four to five divided doses); treatment duration depends on disease severity and clinical response. Patients with significant carditis and those who do not respond to an adequate dose of aspirin are treated with steroids (usually prednisone 1–2 mg/kg/day). Most patients require 4 to 12 weeks of therapy, followed by gradual tapering of the dose. As many as 5% of patients may have attacks that last 6 months or longer. Occasionally, symptoms recur when salicylates or steroids are tapered. Chorea usually responds to benzodiazepines; phenothiazines may also help ameliorate this symptom.

Prevention

Primary Prevention

Prompt treatment of streptococcal pharyngitis will prevent RF. Oral penicillin VK (250–500 mg four times daily for 10 days) or a single IM injection of benzathine penicillin (0.6–1.2 million units) is an acceptable regimen. Erythromycin may be used in penicillin-allergic patients. Sulfa drugs are not acceptable because they do not eradicate streptococci.

Secondary Prevention

All patients with an established diagnosis of RF, Sydenham chorea, or RHD should receive secondary prophylaxis to prevent recurrent acute RF. Intramuscular benzathine penicillin (1.2 million units every 3–4 weeks) or oral penicillin VK (250 mg twice daily) are the preferred antibiotic regimens. For those patients who are allergic to penicillin, oral sulfadiazine (0.5–1 g once daily) or oral erythromycin (250 mg twice daily) are acceptable alternatives. Prophylaxis is recommended for at least 10 years after the most recent episode of acute RF and generally until age 40. Lifelong prophylaxis is advisable for those patients with established RHD, especially if they are living in an endemic area, as well as for those patients who have had their affected valves replaced.

Patients with rheumatic valvular disease will also require additional antibiotic prophylaxis to prevent bacterial endocarditis. Patients with a history of acute RF without evidence of valvular involvement do not require endocarditis prophylaxis.

KEY POINTS

1. RF follows untreated group A beta-hemolytic streptococcal pharyngitis.
2. Carditis, arthritis, erythema marginatum, chorea, and subcutaneous nodules are the cardinal manifestations of acute RF.
3. Carditis can lead to both acute and chronic valvular disease. The MV is most commonly involved, followed by the AV. TV or PV involvement is unusual.
4. Prompt treatment of streptococcal pharyngitis is essential to prevent RF.
5. Following an episode of acute RF, all patients should receive long-term antibiotic prophylaxis.

27 Disorders of the Aortic Valve

Valvular heart disease encompasses a wide array of disorders ranging from asymptomatic murmurs to life-threatening disease. In general, diseases of the AV and MV are far more common and clinically important than diseases of the TV or PV. This chapter and the next are, therefore, limited to a discussion of AV and MV disorders.

■ AORTIC STENOSIS

Etiology

AS may be congenital (bicuspid or unicuspid valve) but is more commonly acquired. Acquired AS is three times more common in men than in women and is most often the result of senile degenerative changes ("wear and tear") or RHD.

Pathogenesis

AS is a disease of pressure overload, which produces progressive obstruction to LV outflow. As the obstruction worsens, the pressure required to pump blood across the valve increases and a transvalvular pressure gradient results (Figure 27-1). As compensatory hypertrophy develops, the LV becomes poorly compliant, resulting in elevated ventricular diastolic pressure. This pressure is transmitted to the LA and pulmonary system, resulting in pulmonary congestion and dyspnea. The noncompliant LV is dependent on the "atrial kick" to maintain adequate filling during diastole; thus, the onset of AF in a patient with AS may precipitate rapid decompensation. Over time, the ventricle weakens and systolic failure occurs.

In congenital AS, the valve leaflets are fused at the commissures, resulting in an orifice of reduced effectiveness. In acquired cases, there is thickening, calcification, fibrosis, and fusion of the leaflets, resulting in reduced leaflet excursion. Most patients with rheumatic AS have associated aortic insufficiency and rheumatic MV disease.

Clinical Manifestations

History

The cardinal symptoms of AS are dyspnea (CHF), chest pain (angina), and syncope. CHF may result from systolic or diastolic dysfunction. Angina may reflect concomitant CAD but may also result from myocardial oxygen supply/demand mismatch as a result of increased LV mass and LV diastolic pressure

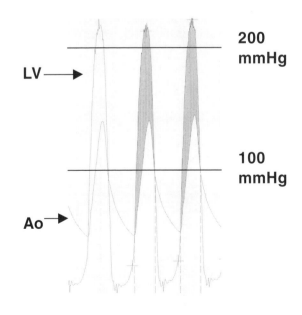

Figure 27-1 • Hemodynamic tracing in a patient with critical AS. Note that the LV pressure exceeds the Ao pressure. The shaded area represents the pressure gradient. The AV area was 0.3 cm².

in the face of decreased CO and diminished coronary perfusion pressure. Exertional syncope occurs as a result of peripheral vasodilation and consequent hypotension in the presence of a fixed CO. Syncope at rest is usually secondary to an arrhythmia.

Symptoms usually develop in the third to fourth decades of life in patients with bicuspid AS, in the fourth to fifth decades with rheumatic AS, and in the sixth or later decades with degenerative AS. Symptoms are of prognostic importance—once angina, syncope, or HF develops, the average survival without surgery is 5, 3, and 1½ years, respectively.

Physical Examination

Characteristic physical findings of AS include:

- Pulsus parvus et tardus (diminished upstroke and a delayed peak of the carotid pulse)
- Sustained and displaced (inferiorly and laterally) LV apical impulse; often bifid as a result of a palpable S_4
- A low-pitched, harsh, crescendo-decrescendo, systolic murmur, loudest at the second right intercostal space and radiating to the carotid arteries (Table 2-2)
- Soft or absent AV closure sound (A_2)
- Paradoxical splitting of the second heart sound (which suggests associated ventricular dysfunction)
- A systolic thrill over the upper sternal border

The peak intensity of the murmur helps to estimate the severity of AS. An early-peaking murmur is associated with mild disease, whereas a late-peaking murmur is heard with severe stenosis. The murmur may also radiate to the LV apex (Gallavardin phenomenon). An S_4 is often heard. In patients with bicuspid AS, an aortic ejection sound may be heard immediately after S_1.

Diagnostic Evaluation

The ECG usually demonstrates LVH if significant AS is present, and CXR may demonstrate AV calcification and LV enlargement. However, the key component of the evaluation is measurement of the transvalvular pressure gradient and calculation of the valve area. The normal aortic valve area is 3.5 cm^2. An area of 1.5 to 2.0 cm^2 is considered mild stenosis, 1.0 to 1.5 cm^2 moderate stenosis, and <1.0 cm^2 (or a mean gradient of >50 mm Hg) severe stenosis. "Critical" stenosis involves an aortic valve area of <0.75 cm^2. The valve area can usually be estimated accurately by echocardiography. Once valve replacement is warranted, cardiac catheterization is usually performed to assess for concomitant CAD. Although in the past

catheterization has been the "gold standard" for determining the severity of AS, it is not required if a good-quality echocardiogram demonstrates severe disease.

Treatment

There is no effective medical management for symptomatic AS. In fact, many medications may cause adverse effects by decreasing preload or afterload and precipitating hemodynamic collapse.

Patients with asymptomatic moderate AS should be followed with clinical examinations every 6 to 12 months and serial echocardiograms every 1 to 2 years. Patients with asymptomatic severe AS should be followed with clinical examinations at least every 6 months and serial echocardiograms every year. Such patients should avoid strenuous exertion.

Symptomatic AS, asymptomatic critical AS, and severe AS with LV dysfunction, even if asymptomatic, are indications for surgical valve replacement. The decision to operate is usually based on symptoms and not on an absolute valve area or pressure gradient. Percutaneous balloon valvuloplasty is associated with an unacceptably high restenosis rate in patients with AS but may be attempted in critically ill patients as a bridge to surgery or in those who are not surgical candidates owing to significant comorbid disease.

■ AORTIC INSUFFICIENCY

Etiology

Aortic insufficiency may be caused by a variety of valvular disorders, including:

- Rheumatic fever (usually with concomitant AS)
- Bicuspid AV (secondary to incomplete valve closure and/or prolapse)
- Infective endocarditis
- Trauma
- Connective tissue disease (SLE, rheumatoid arthritis)

It may also result from disorders that primarily cause dilation of the ascending aorta and aortic root, including Marfan syndrome, aortic dissection, syphilitic aortitis, and the seronegative spondyloarthropathies.

Epidemiology

AI is more common in men than in women. When associated with RHD, AI is usually accompanied by some degree of AS and MV disease.

Pathogenesis

AI is a disease of volume overload and may be acute or chronic. In acute AI, the abrupt increase in blood volume entering the small, noncompliant LV during diastole results in a sudden rise in LV diastolic pressure. This is transmitted to the pulmonary system and results in pulmonary edema and dyspnea.

In chronic AI, the excess volume initially results in LVH. This is followed by ventricular dilation and increased end-diastolic volume, thereby augmenting contractility by the Frank-Starling mechanism. The increased stroke volume results in bounding pulses with an increased systolic pressure. Peripheral vasodilation and the regurgitation of blood back into the LV results in a lower diastolic pressure and a widened pulse pressure. Such patients are often well compensated and asymptomatic. However, with continued enlargement, the LV systolic function declines and HF ensues.

Clinical Manifestations

History

Patients with acute AI often present with pulmonary edema and hemodynamic instability. The symptoms of the underlying disease (i.e., aortic dissection, endocarditis) may predominate. Patients with chronic AI usually present with exertional dyspnea and may complain of a pounding sensation in the neck, resulting from the increased LV stroke volume. Angina may result from the combination of increased oxygen demand from LVH and low diastolic pressures, causing reduced coronary perfusion.

Physical Examination

Chronic AI is associated with a variety of physical findings, all of which relate to the increased stroke volume and widened pulse pressure (Table 27-1).

Severe AI may be associated with a double peaking bisferious pulse. The apical impulse is usually hyperdynamic and displaced downward and laterally, signifying LV dilation and hypertrophy. The characteristic murmur of AI is a high-pitched, decrescendo, diastolic murmur (see Table 2-2) that is best heard at the second right or third left intercostal space. The longer the murmur, the more chronic and severe the AI. A systolic aortic flow murmur is usually present and is the result of increased flow across the valve. The S_1 may be soft, owing to premature MV closure, and a mitral middiastolic murmur (Austin-Flint murmur) may be audible at the apex.

Patients with acute AI frequently have hemodynamic instability and signs of pulmonary edema, but the murmur may be inaudible and peripheral manifestations are frequently absent.

Diagnostic Evaluation

The ECG usually reveals LVH. Echocardiography is the initial test of choice to confirm the diagnosis, assess the severity of AI, and assess LV dimensions and function. Cardiac catheterization and aortography can also assess the severity of AI and identify associated aortic pathology. MRI is a useful tool for anatomic assessment of the thoracic aorta, especially in the presence of aneurysms.

Treatment

Acute severe AI is an indication for early surgical intervention. Death from pulmonary edema, ventricular arrhythmias, or circulatory collapse is common in these patients even with aggressive medical management.

Most patients with chronic mild to moderate AI are asymptomatic and require no specific therapy aside from antibiotic prophylaxis for procedures and close monitoring for the development of symptoms. Many patients with chronic severe AI are also asymptomatic. If such patients have normal LV size and function, surgery can be deferred. They should be closely monitored for symptoms, with exercise testing if necessary, and with periodic echocardiography to assess LV systolic function and dimensions. Chronic

■ TABLE 27-1

Peripheral Signs of Aortic Insufficiency

Sign	Eponym
Systolic head bobbing	De Musset sign
Visible pulsations in the nail beds	Quincke pulses
Rapid-rising and rapid-collapsing carotid pulse	Corrigan pulse
Pistol-shot sounds over the radial or femoral artery	Traube sign
To-and-fro bruit over the femoral artery	Duroziez sign
Systolic bobbing of the uvula	Müller sign
SBP in leg >20 mm Hg higher than in arm	Hill sign

administration of long-acting nifedipine or ACE inhibitors may delay the development of symptoms and the need for surgery in these patients.

Indications for surgery include:

- Onset of symptoms attributable to AI
- Progressive LV dysfunction (LVEF <55%)
- Progressive LV dilation (end-systolic dimension >55 mm)

Valve replacement is usually necessary for primary valvular disorders. When AI is secondary to a dilated aortic root, root repair alone may be adequate.

KEY POINTS

1. The cardinal symptoms of AS are chest pain, syncope, and shortness of breath.
2. Patients with symptoms of AS and a valve area <1.0 cm^2 should undergo valve replacement. Valvuloplasty is not an effective long-term therapy for AS.
3. Patients with severe AI should undergo valve replacement if they have symptoms of CHF, if their LVEF falls below 55%, or if their end-systolic LV dimension increases to >55 mm.

Chapter 28

Disorders of the Mitral Valve

Disorders of the MV are the most common types of valvular heart disease and may occur as either the sequela of a primary valve disorder or the secondary result of other cardiac disease. These disorders may be categorized as those that result in valvular stenosis and those that result in valvular regurgitation.

▓ MITRAL STENOSIS

Etiology

MS is predominantly a sequela of RF (see Chapter 26). Rarely it may be congenital, iatrogenic (following MV repair or replacement), or secondary to systemic diseases such as rheumatoid arthritis, SLE, or carcinoid heart disease. It is more common in women than in men.

Pathogenesis

The normal MV area (MVA) is 4.0 to 6.0 cm^2. The stenosis is considered mild if the MVA is 1.5 to 2.5 cm^2, moderate if it is 1.0 to 1.5 cm^2, and severe if it is <1.0 cm^2. With rheumatic MS, fibrosis of the valve occurs, producing commissural fusion, and the narrowed orifice takes on the classic "fish mouth" appearance. As the valve narrows, the pressure gradient across it increases (see Figure 28-1). During tachycardia, there is less time available for transmitral flow, and the transvalvar gradient increases even further. The increased pressure gradient results in elevated left atrial (LA) pressure, LA enlargement, pulmonary venous congestion, and pulmonary HTN. Eventually, RV dilation, tricuspid regurgitation, and RV failure ensue. In MS, the LV is relatively protected and does not dilate or hypertrophy in the absence of other cardiovascular disease.

Clinical Manifestations

History

The most common symptoms of patients with MS include:

- Left HF (dyspnea on exertion, paroxysmal nocturnal dyspnea, orthopnea)
- Hemoptysis (from rupture of small bronchial veins owing to elevated LA pressure)
- Cerebral or systemic emboli (result from AF or stasis in a dilated LA)
- Chest pain (from pulmonary HTN)
- Right HF (fatigue, ascites, edema)
- Palpitations (AF)

Patients generally have a gradual onset of symptoms, usually by age 28. Severe enlargement of the LA may occasionally compress the left recurrent

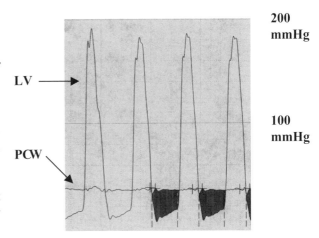

Figure 28-1 • Hemodynamic tracing in MS. The MV impairs the flow of blood from the LA (measured as PCW) to the LV. Thus, during diastole, there is a continuous pressure gradient (shaded region) between these two chambers.

laryngeal nerve, resulting in hoarseness (Ortner syndrome) or compress the esophagus, causing dysphagia.

Physical Examination

Patients with MS frequently demonstrate signs of chronic left and/or right HF and pulmonary HTN. Classic physical findings of MS include:

- Loud S_1
- Loud P_2 (pulmonary HTN)
- OS (crisp sound after S_2 heard best with the diaphragm of the stethoscope; most characteristic auscultatory finding of MS)
- Diastolic "rumble" (with presystolic accentuation if in sinus rhythm; see Table 2-2)
- Right parasternal heave (RV enlargement)

Diagnostic Evaluation

The ECG often demonstrates sinus tachycardia, LA enlargement, and RV hypertrophy. AF is frequently present. CXR may reveal straightening of the left heart border (LA and RV dilation), dilated pulmonary arteries, and pulmonary vascular congestion.

Echocardiography is the test of choice by which to confirm the diagnosis of MS and assess its severity (see Figure 28-2). The size of the MV orifice can be measured, the extent of valvular thickening and calcification assessed, the severity of pulmonary HTN estimated, and associated valvular abnormalities identified. Cardiac catheterization can also quantify MS severity and mea-

sure PA pressure. It is often performed in conjunction with coronary angiography prior to valve surgery.

Treatment

Endocarditis prophylaxis is essential for any patient with MS. Asymptomatic patients should be closely monitored for the development of symptoms, atrial arrhythmias, and silent systemic embolism. Serial echocardiograms (every 6 to 12 months, depending on valve severity) should be performed to evaluate the progression of valvular stenosis.

Symptomatic patients with MS may initially be managed with beta blockers (calcium channel blockers or digoxin are alternatives) to control the ventricular HR, thereby prolonging diastole and minimizing the transvalvar pressure gradient. Diuretics are used to reduce pulmonary congestion. Arterial vasodilators should be avoided. When AF accompanies MS, it is associated with ~12% per year risk of stroke, compared with ~4 to 6% in AF that is not valvular-related. Every effort must be made to maintain sinus rhythm, including electrical cardioversion and administration of antiarrhythmic agents (see Chapter 21). If AF is chronic, patients should be anticoagulated to prevent systemic embolization and the ventricular rate controlled with beta blockers, calcium channel blockers, or digoxin.

Patients with symptomatic severe or moderately severe MS, worsening pulmonary HTN, or recurrent systemic embolization should undergo mitral val-

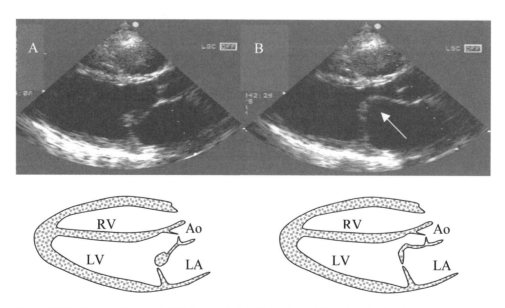

Figure 28-2 • Echocardiogram in MS. In systole (a), thickening of the mitral leaflets is seen. In diastole (b), the anterior mitral leaflet is seen "doming" into the LV cavity (arrow).

votomy or valve replacement. Valvotomy may be performed percutaneously by balloon dilation or surgical commissurotomy. Balloon valvuloplasty is the procedure of choice in young patients with pliable valves, minimal valvular calcification, and no significant associated MR. Patients who undergo valvotomy usually require a second procedure in 5 to 15 years. Patients with heavily calcified valves and/or associated significant MR require valve replacement (see Chapter 30).

■ MITRAL REGURGITATION

Etiology and Epidemiology

MR may result from a variety of conditions and may be acute or chronic (Box 28-1). Mitral valve prolapse (MVP) is the most common cause of isolated MR; the posterior leaflet is more frequently involved than the anterior leaflet. MVP affects 3 to 5% of the population and is slightly more common in women. It is often an isolated condition but may be associated with congenital heart disease (e.g., ASD, bicuspid AV) and connective tissue disorders. Rheumatic MR is more common in men than in women and may occur in isolation or in association with MS.

Pathogenesis

The significance of MR depends in part on its acuity and the compliance of the LA. In acute MR, the LA is normal in size and poorly compliant. The acute regurgitation of blood into the atrium results in marked elevation of LA and pulmonary venous pressures, resulting in pulmonary edema. In chronic MR, the regurgitation progresses over time, allowing the LA to dilate gradually and become compliant. In this setting, patients are able to tolerate moderate to severe MR for several years with only a slight increase in LA and PA pressures.

Initially with MR, the augmented LV preload results in increased contractility (Starling mechanism), resulting in hyperdynamic LV function. Over time, the LV hypertrophies and dilates, stretching the mitral annulus and worsening the MR severity. Eventually, LV systolic function deteriorates and HF ensues.

Clinical Manifestations

History

Patients with acute MR have an abrupt onset of symptoms and often present with acute pulmonary

BOX 28-1	CAUSES OF MITRAL REGURGITATION

Acute MR
Valve leaflet perforation (endocarditis)
Ruptured chord (endocarditis, trauma, myxomatous degeneration)
Papillary muscle dysfunction or rupture (ischemia, blunt chest trauma)
Acute mechanical failure of prosthetic valve (strut fracture, cusp perforation, or degeneration)

Chronic MR
MV prolapse
RHD
Annular dilation (CMPs)
Rheumatologic diseases (SLE, scleroderma)
Connective tissue disorders (Marfan, Ehlers-Danlos, pseudoxanthoma elasticum)
Congenital (parachute mitral valve, cleft mitral valve, endocardial cushion defects)
Hypertrophic CMP
Mitral annular calcification
Anorexigenic drugs (e.g., Fen-Phen)
Any cause of acute MR

edema or cardiogenic shock. Patients with chronic MR may be asymptomatic for years; eventually progressive exertional dyspnea develops. A history of anginal chest pain (ischemic MR), recent dental work (endocarditis), or distant rheumatic fever should be noted. Most patients with MVP are asymptomatic, although many report nonspecific symptoms such as vague chest discomfort, palpitations, presyncope, and fatigue (Barlow syndrome).

Physical Examination

Patients with MR frequently demonstrate signs of chronic left and/or right HF and pulmonary HTN. Patients with acute MR are often hypotensive and tachycardic and may be in acute respiratory distress. Classic findings of MR include:

- Holosystolic murmur (may be late systolic with MVP)
- Apical systolic thrill (with severe MR)
- Soft S_1 (incomplete coaptation of the mitral leaflets)
- Loud P_2 and RV heave (pulmonary HTN)
- Midsystolic click (with MVP)

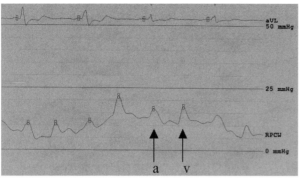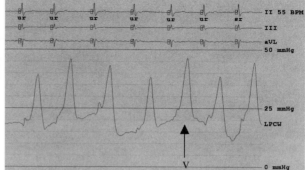

Figure 28-3 • Hemodynamic tracing in severe MR. (a) Normal a and v waves in a PCW pressure tracing. (b) PCW tracing in severe MR. Note the prominent v wave reflecting direct transmission of the LV pressure to the pulmonary system.

Diagnostic Evaluation

The ECG often demonstrates LA enlargement and LVH. AF is often present. CXR may reveal straightening of the left heart border (LA dilation), a dilated LV, and pulmonary vascular congestion.

Echocardiography is the test of choice for the assessment of MR. The severity of MR is graded from 1 to 4, based on the volume of regurgitant flow seen by color Doppler. In addition, the atrial and ventricular chamber sizes can be measured, LV systolic function quantified, pulmonary HTN assessed, and associated valvular abnormalities identified. Echocardiographic findings may suggest the etiology of MR by revealing rheumatic changes, MVP, ruptured chordae, vegetations (endocarditis), or LV dilation. Cardiac catheterization has been the "gold standard" for the quantification of MR and can also directly measure PA pressure. In severe MR, the LV pressure is transmitted to the pulmonary system and produces a prominent v wave in the PCWP tracing (see Figure 28-3). Cardiac catheterization is usually performed prior to valve surgery to confirm the severity of MR and assess for concomitant CAD.

Treatment

There is no specific medical management of asymptomatic or minimally symptomatic patients with mild or moderate MR aside from endocarditis prophylaxis. Empiric use of afterload-reducing agents (e.g., ACE inhibitors) has not been shown to be of benefit and may mask the symptoms of progressive LV dysfunction. Serial echocardiograms should be performed every 6 to 12 months (depending on MR severity) to evaluate progression of regurgitation and assess LV size and systolic function.

Surgery is indicated in patients with moderate to severe symptomatic MR. Valve repair is desirable if possible, as it avoids the risks of anticoagulation and prosthetic valve dysfunction. If the valve is replaced, the papillary muscles and chordae are often preserved and help to maintain LV geometry and function.

The ideal timing of surgery for the asymptomatic or mildly symptomatic patient with severe MR remains controversial. Nonetheless, there is general consensus that a decrease in the LVEF to ≤60% and/or an increase in end-systolic LV dimension to >45 mm are indications for surgery.

Patients with acute, severe MR require urgent therapy. Hypotensive patients should have an IABP inserted, followed by emergent valve repair or replacement. Patients who are not hypotensive should be managed with diuretics and vasodilators such as nitroprusside or ACE inhibitors while arrangements are made for surgery.

KEY POINTS

1. MS is predominantly a sequela of rheumatic fever.
2. The most common etiology of MR and most common indication for MV replacement is MV prolapse.
3. The classic physical findings of MS include a loud S$_1$, an OS, and a diastolic rumble. The classic physical finding of MR is a holosystolic murmur associated with a midsystolic click in the presence of MVP.
4. Patients with moderate to severe MS or MR who have symptoms despite medical therapy should undergo valve surgery.

29 Infective Endocarditis

IE is an infection of the endocardial surface of the heart. The structures most commonly affected are the valves; however, valvular chordae and the atrial and ventricular walls may also be involved. IE is associated with significant morbidity and mortality; early diagnosis, appropriate treatment, and prompt recognition of complications are essential for the management of these patients.

Epidemiology

The incidence of IE in the United States is 15,000 to 20,000 new cases per year. Males are affected twice as often as females. The average age of those affected is 54 years; however, the median age of those affected changes continuously as a consequence of changes in the population at risk. For instance, IE in IV drug users favors younger patients with an average age of 32.5 years. The MV is most commonly affected, followed in order by the AV, TV, and PV. IE in IV drug users has a predilection for the TV. IE can be divided into three general categories: native valve endocarditis (NVE), prosthetic valve endocarditis (PVE), and endocarditis in IV drug users. The causative organisms, symptoms, treatment, and prognosis differ significantly among these groups.

Risk Factors

Predisposing factors for IE include:

- Acquired valvular heart disease (RHD, MVP, degenerative valve disease)
- Prosthetic heart valves
- Congenital heart disease (VSD, bicuspid aortic valve, PDA)
- HCM
- Indwelling central venous catheters or temporary pacing catheters
- IV drug use
- Prior endocarditis

In the past, the most common predisposition for IE was RHD; however, RHD now accounts for only 7 to 10% of cases. MVP and degenerative valvular disease are now the most common antecedent conditions. In 20 to 40% of adults with IE, no obvious risk factor is identified.

Pathogenesis

The normal cardiac endothelium is resistant to infection. However, endothelial injury may occur as a result of turbulent blood flow across a valve or valvular trauma from intravascular catheters. This results in the deposition of platelets and fibrin on the valve surface (nonbacterial thrombotic endocarditis). During subsequent bacteremia, microorganisms adhere to the fibrinous material, colonize it, and proliferate. This bacteremia may occur during dental, gastrointestinal, genitourinary, or gynecologic procedures; dental procedures are associated with the highest incidence. Transient bacteremia also frequently occurs after tooth brushing, eating, and bowel movements. Bacteria that produce dextran and those that have surface receptors for fibronectin are especially likely to adhere to these vegetations. PVE occurring in the first year after surgery is usually the result of contamination at the time of surgery, whereas that occurring later results from transient bacteremia.

Causative Organisms

The microbiology of IE depends on the underlying predisposing factors (Box 29-1). NVE in non-IV drug

BOX 29-1   MICROORGANISMS CAUSING ENDOCARDITIS

Prosthetic valve: <1 year after implant
Staphylococcus epidermidis
Staphylococcus aureus
Gram-negative bacilli
Candida
Diphtheroids
Enterococci
Streptococci
Atypical mycobacteria, *Mycoplasma*

Prosthetic valve: >1 year after implant
Viridans streptococci
Staphylococcus epidermidis
Staphylococcus aureus
Enterococci
HACEK organisms

Native valve endocarditis
Viridans streptococci
Group A streptococci
Enterococci
Staphylococcus aureus
Staphylococcus epidermidis
HACEK organisms

Intravenous drug use
Staphylococcus aureus
Streptococci
Enterocci
Gram-negative bacilli
Candida

NVE develop symptoms within 2 weeks of the presumed initiating bacteremia. Patients may present with constitutional symptoms resulting from activation of the immune system or with symptoms of acute valvular dysfunction or embolic events. Common constitutional symptoms include:

- Fever (present in 80 to 85% of affected individuals)
- Rigors
- Night sweats
- Fatigue, malaise
- Anorexia, weight loss
- Myalgias, arthralgias

Patients with SBE tend to present with constitutional symptoms, whereas those with ABE tend to present with CHF from valvular dysfunction. Occasionally the initial symptom is the result of an embolic event, which may manifest as stroke (CNS embolism), limb ischemia (vascular embolism), flank pain and hematuria (renal embolism), left-upper-quadrant or left shoulder pain (splenic embolism), diffuse abdominal pain and hematochezia (mesenteric embolism), or MI (coronary artery embolism). IV drug users with TV or PV endocarditis may present with cough, hemoptysis, and pleuritic chest pain resulting from septic PE. In obtaining the history from a patient with suspected IE, it is important to ask about predisposing conditions and recent procedures.

Physical Examination

Most patients (80 to 85%) with IE have a murmur, although the murmur is often faint or inaudible in patients with isolated tricuspid valve involvement. In patients with preexisting valvular disease, a new or changing murmur may occasionally be noted. A significant proportion of patients with IE and a new regurgitant murmur will develop signs of CHF. Cutaneous manifestations may be present and reflect peripheral embolic phenomena and immunologic vascular injury (see Table 29-1). Cutaneous manifestations as well as digital clubbing and splenomegaly are much more common in the subacute forms of endocarditis.

Differential Diagnosis

The differential diagnosis of IE includes other forms of intravascular infection (septic thromboembolism, infected indwelling vascular catheters). IE may mimic other chronic inflammatory diseases and must be considered in the differential diagnosis of patients with fever of unknown etiology or persistent bacteremia.

users is usually caused by streptococci and less commonly by staphylococci. The reverse is true of NVE in IV drug users. PVE occurring within the first year after surgery is predominantly caused by coagulase-negative staphylococci (*Staphylococcus epidermidis*), whereas that occurring after the first year is usually caused by streptococci. IE caused by enterococci usually follows genitourinary tract procedures; patients with *Streptococcus bovis* endocarditis often have colonic neoplasms and should be evaluated with colonoscopy.

Clinical Manifestations

History

IE may be an indolent disease (SBE) or have a dramatic clinical course (ABE). More than 80% of patients with

■ TABLE 29-1

Cutaneous Manifestations of Infective Endocarditis

Cutaneous Finding	Etiology	Description
Petechiae	Immunologic	Tiny hemorrhagic lesions in the conjunctiva, oral mucosa, and extremities
Splinter hemorrhages	Immunologic	Linear hemorrhages in the proximal two-thirds of the nail beds
Osler nodes	Immunologic	Small, raised, painful lesions in the finger pads
Janeway lesions	Embolic	Erythematous, painless lesions on the palms and soles
Roth spots	Immunologic	Whitish, oval retinal lesions with surrounding hemorrhage

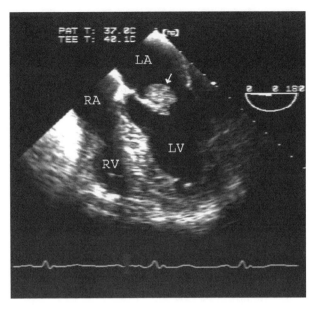

Figure 29-1 • TEE in a patient with MV endocarditis. There is a large rounded vegetation (arrow) on the atrial surface of the anterior MV leaflet.

Diagnostic Evaluation

The diagnosis of IE is usually suspected on the basis of clinical findings and confirmed by blood cultures and echocardiography. When IE is suspected, at least three sets of blood cultures should be drawn over 24 hours from different venipuncture sites, ideally before antibiotics are administered. Blood cultures may be negative in ≤5% of patients with IE, usually as a result of inadequate microbiologic techniques, infection with highly fastidious bacteria or nonbacterial microorganisms, or from the administration of antimicrobial agents before blood for culture is drawn. Infection with organisms such as *Coxiella burnetti, Bartonella* spp., *Brucella abortus,* and *Chlamydia pneumoniae* may only be identifiable by serologic tests or polymerase chain reaction.

TTE is the initial test of choice to visualize valvular vegetations and quantitate valvular dysfunction. However, TEE is more sensitive (>80%) for the detection of vegetations (see Figure 29-1) and for assessing local complications such as valve-ring or aortic-root abscesses and valvular destruction or perforation. A negative TEE does not exclude IE and may occur when the vegetation is very small, the vegetation has embolized, or inadequate images are obtained. When the clinical

suspicion of IE is high, a repeat study in 7 to 10 days may demonstrate previously undetected vegetations.

Laboratory evaluation in patients with IE frequently reveals:

- Normocytic anemia (~75% of cases)
- Leukocytosis (~30% of cases)
- Elevated ESR (~75% of cases)
- Proteinuria (~50% of cases)
- Microscopic hematuria (~50% of cases)

A positive rheumatoid factor and false-positive VDRL and Lyme titers may also be noted.

The CXR may show consolidation or evidence of parenchymal abscesses as a result of septic emboli from right-sided endocarditis. The ECG is of limited diagnostic value but may show conduction abnormalities (progressive AV block) when a perivalvular abscess burrows into the conduction system.

The diagnosis of IE is relatively obvious in patients with the classic features of bacteremia, vegetations, and embolic phenomena. In those without such features, the Duke criteria may aid in the diagnosis (see Box 29-2).

Treatment

Once IE is suspected, empiric antibiotic therapy should be started until the diagnosis is confirmed and an

BOX 29-2 CLINICAL CRITERIA FOR DIAGNOSING INFECTIVE ENDOCARDITIS

The clinical diagnosis of IE can be made if a patient has:
  2 major criteria, OR
  1 major and 3 minor criteria, OR
  5 minor criteria

Major criteria
Positive blood culture (≥2 positive cultures drawn
  >12 hours apart OR all 3 cultures positive if drawn
  at least 1 hour apart OR a majority positive if 4 or
  more cultures are drawn)
Echocardiographic evidence of endocardial involvement

Minor criteria
Predisposing cardiac condition or IV drug use
Fever (temperature ≥38.0°C)
Vascular phenomena: major arterial emboli, septic pul-
  monary infarcts, mycotic aneurysm, intracranial
  hemorrhage, conjunctival hemorrhages, and
  Janeway lesions
Immunologic phenomena: glomerulonephritis, Osler
  nodes, Roth spots, and elevated rheumatoid factor
Microbiologic evidence: positive blood culture but
  does not meet a major criterion as noted above
Echocardiographic findings: consistent with IE but do
  not meet a major criterion as noted above

organism identified. It is important that bactericidal antibiotics be used in order to effectively eradicate the infection. High-dose penicillin G (12 million units daily) is the usual initial regimen in patients with suspected streptococcal infections, whereas nafcillin (2 g every 4 hours) should be used in patients with suspected staphyloccal infections. Vancomycin may be substituted in penicillin-allergic patients. The addition of an aminoglycoside during the first week of therapy has been shown to hasten sterilization of the blood but does not improve the cure rate. Once the infecting organism has been identified, antibiotic treatment should be guided by sensitivity studies. Almost 75% of patients will defervesce within a week of starting antibiotic therapy and 90% will be afebrile by the second week. In general, however, 4 to 6 weeks of IV antibiotic therapy is required to treat IE adequately.

Patients should be closely observed for response to treatment and the development of complications, including:

- Emboli to major organs resulting in ischemia, infarction, or abscess
- CHF from valvular destruction
- Perivalvular abscess formation
- Intracranial hemorrhage from ruptured mycotic aneurysms
- Immune complex–mediated glomerulonephritis resulting in renal insufficiency

Patients at a higher risk of complications include those with prosthetic heart valves, cyanotic CHD, systemic-to-pulmonary shunts, left-sided IE, *S. aureus* or fungal IE, recurrent IE, symptoms of >3 months duration, and poor response to antimicrobial therapy. Serial clinical examinations in association with echocardiography will identify most mechanical complications. Recurrence of fever may indicate treatment failure but can also result from hypersensitivity reactions to antibiotics. "Surveillance" blood cultures are recommended during antibiotic therapy, especially in staphylococcal IE, in order to detect persistent bacteremia. Cultures should also be drawn in the first 8 weeks following completion of treatment to diagnose relapses.

BOX 29-3 INDICATIONS FOR SURGERY IN INFECTIVE ENDOCARDITIS

Native valve endocarditis
Acute AI or MR with heart failure
Fungal endocarditis
Annular or aortic abscess or aneurysm
Persistent infection with valve dysfunction
Recurrent emboli despite therapy
IE with gram-negative organisms or organisms with
  poor response to antibiotics
Large mobile vegetations (>10 mm)

Prosthetic valve endocarditis
Early IE (within 2 months of surgery)
HF with valve dysfunction
Fungal endocarditis
Evidence of significant paravalvular regurgitation
Annular or aortic abscess or aneurysm
IE with gram-negative organisms or organisms with
  poor response to antibiotics
Persistent bacteremia despite 7 to 10 days of antibiotic
  therapy
Recurrent emboli despite therapy
Relapse after optimal therapy

■ TABLE 29-2

Cardiac Conditions Associated with Infective Endocarditis

IE Prophylaxis Recommended		IE Prophylaxis Not Recommended
High risk category	**Moderate risk category**	**Low or negligible risk**
Prosthetic heart valves	Most other congenital cardiac malformations	Isolated secundum ASD
Previous IE	Acquired valvular dysfunction (e.g., senile	Successfully repaired ASD, VSD,
Congenital cyanotic	degenerative valve disease, RHD)	or ductus
heart disease	Hypertrophic CMP	Previous CABG
Surgically constructed	MVP with regurgitation and/or	MVP without regurgitation
systemic pulmonary	thickened leaflets	Previous rheumatic fever without
shunts or conduits		valve dysfunction
		Cardiac pacemakers, ICD

Despite appropriate antibiotic therapy, many patients with IE will require surgery to replace or repair an infected valve. Box 29-3 summarizes the currently accepted indications for surgery in the setting of IE.

Prognosis

The overall mortality rate in NVE is ~15%. Markers of increased mortality include advanced age (>65 years old), AV infection, CHF, CNS involvement, and persistence or recurrence of fever more than 7 to 10 days after the initiation of antibiotics. The overall mortality rate for PVE is 20 to 25%.

Prevention

In those patients at risk for IE (see Table 29-2) who are undergoing dental, genitourinary, or GI procedures, antibiotic prophylaxis is essential to minimize the risk. In general, amoxicillin 2 g, or clindamycin 600 g (if penicillin-allergic) given 1 hour before the procedure is the recommended prophylactic regimen. In high-risk patients undergoing genitourinary or GI procedures, the addition of gentamicin (1.5 mg/kg IV) is suggested.

KEY POINTS

1. Risk factors for IE include acquired valvular heart disease, CHD, prosthetic heart valves, IV drug abuse, indwelling central venous catheters, and prior endocarditis.
2. MVP and degenerative valvular disease are the most common antecedent conditions.
3. NVE in non-IV drug users is usually caused by streptococci and less commonly by staphylococci. The reverse is true of NVE in IV drug users.
4. PVE occurring within the first year after surgery is predominantly caused by coagulase-negative staphylococci (*Staphylococcus epidermidis*), whereas that occurring after the first year is usually caused by streptococci.
5. Over 80% of patients with IE present with fever; the vast majority also have a murmur.
6. When IE is suspected, at least three sets of blood cultures should be drawn over 24 hours from different venipuncture sites.
7. IV antibiotic therapy for 4 to 6 weeks is required to adequately treat IE, although most patients will become afebrile within a week of starting treatment.
8. Antibiotic prophylaxis is essential in patients at risk for developing IE.

Valve replacement surgery is the treatment of choice for severe valvular heart disease. A variety of prosthetic valves exist; each has its own benefits and drawbacks. These valves are quite effective at correcting a variety of valvular disorders. Unfortunately, they are also prone to a variety of complications, including infection, thrombosis, and degeneration.

■ TYPES OF PROSTHETIC VALVES (SEE FIGURE 30-1)

Prosthetic valves may be classified as mechanical prosthetic valves (MPVs) or tissue valves (bioprosthetic valves, or BPVs). Mechanical valves are usually composed of metal or carbon alloys and are available in three main types:

- Ball-in-cage (Starr-Edwards)
- Single tilting disc (Björk-Shiley, Medtronic-Hall, or Omniscience)
- Bileaflet tilting disc (St. Jude, Medtronic-Hall)

Mechanical prostheses are very durable, lasting at least 20 years; however, they are thrombogenic and require lifelong anticoagulation. Ball-in-cage valves are the most thrombogenic, followed by single-tilting-disc valves; bileaflet-tilting-disc valves are the least thrombogenic. The thrombotic potential of these valves is also dependent in part on the position in which they are placed—MV prostheses pose a higher risk of thrombosis than do AV prostheses.

Tissue valves may also be of several different types:

- **Heterograft (xenograft):** either an explanted animal valve (usually porcine; i.e., Carpentier-Edwards, Hancock) or a valve created from bovine, porcine, or equine pericardial tissue.

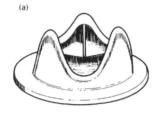
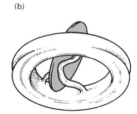
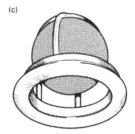
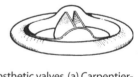

Figure 30-1 • Diagram of various prosthetic valves. (a) Carpentier-Edwards porcine xenograft. (b) Björk-Shiley tilting disc valve. (c) Starr-Edwards ball-in-cage valve. (d) St. Jude Medical bileaflet valve. (Reproduced with permission from Swanton RH. Pocket Consultant: Cardiology. Oxford, UK: Blackwell, 2003.)

- **Homograft:** aortic valves harvested from human cadavers.
- **Autografts:** the patient's own pulmonary valve, which is harvested and placed in the aortic position; a prosthetic valve is then placed in the pulmonary position (see below).

The main advantage of BPVs is that they are less thrombogenic than MPVs and require only short-term anticoagulation (~3 months) after implantation; however, with the exception of the pulmonary autograft, they are not as durable and often have to be replaced 10 to 15 years after implantation.

CLINICAL EVALUATION

Heterografts may produce mildly accentuated heart sounds and, when placed in the aortic or pulmonary position, may produce a short ejection systolic murmur. Frequently, however, tissue valves may be indistinguishable from native valves by auscultation. Mechanical prostheses produce crisp, metallic opening and closing sounds; in some cases these may be audible without a stethoscope. Mechanical prostheses also result in short flow murmurs—systolic in the aortic and pulmonary positions and middiastolic in the mitral and tricuspid positions. All mechanical valves have mild transvalvar regurgitation, which is rarely audible. In general, audible prosthetic valve regurgitation should trigger an evaluation for valve dysfunction.

DIAGNOSTIC EVALUATION

A baseline ECG and an echocardiogram should be obtained postoperatively in all patients who have undergone valve replacement. Patients with mechanical valves require no further echocardiographic follow-up after their baseline study unless there is a clinical change. BPVs pose an increased risk of valve degeneration after 5 years in the mitral position and 8 years in the aortic position. Nevertheless, scheduled echocardiography for these patients is not generally recommended. Rather, as with mechanical valves, the clinical history and physical examination should guide the need for further echocardiographic studies. When regurgitation is detected, echocardiography is indicated every 3 to 6 months. Signs and symptoms of HF, new murmurs, significant changes in the intensity of the prosthetic valve sounds, embolic events, persistent fevers, and bacteremia should also prompt evaluation with a TTE. Frequently, a TEE is also required to evaluate suspected prosthetic valve endocarditis and/or valvular dysfunction. Mechanical valve leaflet mobility and integrity can also be evaluated with fluoroscopy.

FACTORS AFFECTING THE CHOICE OF PROSTHETIC VALVE TYPE (SEE TABLE 30-1)

The major advantage of an MPV is its durability, whereas the major advantage of a BPV is the avoidance of anticoagulation. Factors to consider in selecting a valve for a particular patient include:

- Patient's age
- Risk of bleeding
- Other indications for anticoagulation (e.g., atrial fibrillation)
- Potential for pregnancy
- Medication compliance
- Surgical considerations (size of the aortic root)

The surgeon has a central role in valve selection and must consider such factors as the patient's size, the size of the valvular annulus into which the prosthesis will

TABLE 30-1

Preferred Type of Prosthetic Valve in Specific Clinical Scenarios		
Clinical Scenario	Preferred Valve	Reasons for Choice
Age >70	BPV	Slow valve deterioration in this age group Patient less likely to outlive valve
Patient with bleeding risk	BPV	Avoids need for anticoagulation
Medication noncompliance	BPV	Avoids subtherapeutic anticoagulation of mechanical valve
Women desiring pregnancy	BPV	Avoids need for anticoagulation due to bleeding risk and teratogenicity
Other indication for anticoagulation	MPV	Need for anticoagulation negates advantage of tissue valve
Most patients age <70	MPV	Greater durability; patients likely to outlive tissue valve
Children; adults age <35	MPV	Rapid deterioration of tissue valve in this age group Greater durability
Chronic renal failure	MPV	Rapid deterioration of tissue valve in this group
Young patients (<40) with AV disease	Pulmonary autograft	Avoids long-term anticoagulation risk Excellent durability of autograft in this group

be sewn, and the hemodynamic profile of the specific valve (bileaflet tilting discs or bioprosthetic valves offer a slightly larger orifice than other prosthetic valves).

The pulmonary autograft (the Ross procedure) may be the valve replacement procedure of choice in young patients with AV disease. In this procedure, the patient's own PV is used to replace the diseased AV and a tissue valve (usually a homograft) is placed in the pulmonary position. This is a technically challenging operation, but the autograft provides excellent durability, grows with the adolescent or child, and obviates the need for anticoagulation.

Anticoagulation of Prosthetic Valves

Mechanical valves are predisposed to thromboembolic complications and require lifelong anticoagulation with warfarin. The intensity of anticoagulation depends on the type of valve, its position, and the presence of other risk factors for thrombosis (i.e., AF, LV dysfunction, prior thromboembolism, hypercoagulable state). Ball-in-cage valves are the most thrombogenic, while bileaflet valves are the least thrombogenic. Additionally, these valves are all more thrombogenic in the mitral position than in the aortic position. In general, the goal INR range is 2.5 to 3.5; however, patients who have bileaflet valves in the aortic position may safely be kept at an INR range of 2.0 to 3.0. The addition of aspirin (81 mg daily) to warfarin should be considered in patients with thrombotic risk factors.

■ PROBLEMS ASSOCIATED WITH PROSTHETIC VALVES

Although valve-replacement surgery can be lifesaving and provides significant symptom relief in patients with severe disease, prosthetic valves themselves are associated with several potential problems that carry substantial risks of morbidity and mortality.

Valve Thrombosis and Thromboembolism

With mechanical valves, the risk of valve thrombosis is related to valve type, valve position, and the number of prosthetic valves present. Ball-in-cage valves, older tilting disc valves (Björk-Shiley, Omniscience), TV and MV positions, and multiple-valve prostheses are associated with higher thrombotic risk. Other predisposing factors include LV dysfunction, inadequate anticoagulation, and a prior history of thromboembolism. Valve thrombosis can present as embolic

episodes or valve dysfunction, the latter frequently precipitating HF. Despite anticoagulation of mechanical valves, there is at least a 1 to 2%-per-year risk of thromboembolism, which is associated with a 0.2% rate mortality. Tissue valves do not require long-term anticoagulation, and have a slightly lower thromboembolic complication rate.

Hemorrhagic Complications

Anticoagulation with warfarin carries a 0.2%-per-year risk of fatal intracranial bleeding and 2%-per-year risk of nonfatal but significant bleeding. Predisposing factors include advanced age, gait instability, alcoholism, and the use of medications that potentiate the effect of warfarin.

Valve Degeneration

Valve degeneration is the main complication limiting the use of tissue valves. Degeneration, fibrosis, perforation, and calcification can affect the valve cusps as early as the fifth postoperative year and may result in hemodynamically significant stenosis and/or regurgitation. Usually, the deterioration is insidious; rarely, it is acute, with resultant catastrophic HF. As many as 60% of bioprosthetic valves may need to be replaced within 15 years; reoperation carries a 5 to 15% mortality risk. Valvular degeneration may be particularly rapid in the young and in those with chronic renal failure or hyperparathyroidism.

Arrhythmias

Atrial fibrillation occurs in ~50% of patients after valve replacement surgery. It is typically self-limited in patients with no prior history of arrhythmia. If it persists for >48 hours, anticoagulation should be started and electrical cardioversion considered. Some 2 to 3% of patients who have undergone valve-replacement surgery experience high-degree HB and require implantation of a permanent pacemaker. This occurs as a result of surgical trauma to the conduction system or postoperative edema of the periannular tissue.

Hemodynamic Issues

Prosthetic valves generally have a smaller orifice area than the native valves they replace and are, therefore, intrinsically mildly stenotic. In patients with a small aortic annulus, this degree of obstruction may be hemodynamically significant.

Infective Endocarditis
(See Also Chapter 29)

With the exception of the pulmonary autograft, all prosthetic valves are prone to endocarditis. This complication occurs in 3 to 6% of patients with prosthetic valves. Early endocarditis (<60 days after surgery) principally results from perioperative seeding of bacteria and is most commonly caused by staphylococcal organisms. It is associated with a mortality of 30 to 80%. Late prosthetic valve endocarditis (>60 days postop) is usually caused by streptococci and is associated with a mortality of 20 to 40%. Meticulous attention to dental hygiene, appropriate antibiotic prophylaxis for invasive procedures, and early aggressive treatment of infections elsewhere are essential for the prevention of prosthetic valve endocarditis.

Hemolysis

Mechanical valves usually result in mild intravascular hemolysis owing to traumatic destruction of red blood cells. Perivalvular regurgitation from endocarditis or suture dehiscence may also cause clinically significant hemolysis.

Pregnancy-Related Problems

Anticoagulation during pregnancy increases the risk of fetal loss and peripartum hemorrhage. Pregnancy also increases the risk of thromboembolic complications. In addition, warfarin is teratogenic, and first-trimester fetal exposure results in a 4 to 10% risk of an embryopathy characterized by telecanthus, small nasal bones, choanal hypoplasia, and long-bone epiphyseal dysplasia.

KEY POINTS

1. Prosthetic heart valve recipients require close life-long follow-up.
2. Mechanical valves are durable for the lifetime of the patient but carry a risk of thromboembolism and require lifelong anticoagulation.
3. Tissue valves do not require chronic anticoagulation but are not as durable.
4. Factors to consider in deciding which type of valve should be used in a particular patient include his or her age, risk of bleeding, presence of other indications for anticoagulation, and pregnancy potential.
5. Fatal intracranial hemorrhage, endocarditis, hemolysis, and warfarin-induced teratogenicity are other potential complications.
6. TEE is useful when valvular dysfunction is present or SBE suspected.

Part Seven

Pericardial Diseases

Pericarditis

Acute pericarditis is a syndrome caused by inflammation of the pericardium; it is characterized by chest pain, distinctive ECG changes, and a pericardial friction rub on physical examination.

Epidemiology

The incidence of pericardial inflammation noted at autopsy ranges from 2 to 6%; however, pericarditis is diagnosed in only 1 in 1,000 hospital admissions, suggesting that this process is often clinically inapparent. Pericarditis is generally more common in men than in women and is fairly uncommon in children.

Pathogenesis

The normal pericardium is a smooth, double-layered structure. The inner serous visceral pericardium constitutes the epicardial surface of the heart and is separated from the outer fibrous parietal pericardium by the pericardial space. This space usually contains less than 50 mL of fluid, which lubricates the pericardium and prevents friction between the layers during cardiac contraction. Pericarditis is marked by infiltration of the pericardium by polymorphonuclear leukocytes, with eventual deposition of fibrin in the pericardial space. The inflamed pericardial layers rub against each other during each cardiac contraction, often resulting in pain and an audible friction rub. Inflammatory fluid may collect in the pericardium, producing a pericardial effusion; large effusions may result in pericardial tamponade (see Chapter 32). Chronically, the inflammatory process may produce pericardial thickening and reduced pericardial compliance, resulting in pericardial constriction (see Chapter 33).

Etiology

Acute pericarditis is most commonly viral or idiopathic in origin; infections of the latter type are usually presumed to be viral. A variety of other causes have been identified, including other infections and systemic diseases (Table 31-1).

Clinical Manifestations

History

The clinical history may provide clues to the cause of pericarditis. For example, a preceding upper respiratory tract infection suggests viral pericarditis, whereas a prior history of SLE or rheumatoid arthritis suggests autoimmune pericarditis. Regardless of the cause, most patients with acute pericarditis complain of chest pain. This pain is usually sudden in onset, retrosternal in location, variable in intensity, and may be confused with angina. Several characteristic features of pericardial pain include:

- It is pleuritic in nature, exacerbated by deep breathing or coughing.
- It is alleviated by sitting upright and leaning forward and is aggravated in the supine position.
- It may radiate to the trapezius ridge and neck.
- It may become worse with swallowing.

Patients with pericarditis will often complain of systemic symptoms, including fevers, myalgias, and generalized fatigue.

Physical Examination

The classic physical examination finding for acute pericarditis is a pericardial friction rub. This is a scratching, high-pitched, superficial sound noted on

TABLE 31-1

Selected Causes of Pericarditis

Category	Examples
Idiopathic	Unknown, by definition
Viral	Coxsackie A and B virus, HIV, adenovirus, EBV
Autoimmune	SLE, scleroderma, rheumatoid arthritis, Wegener granulomatosis
Radiation	Mantle radiation for chest malignancies
Bacterial	Pneumococcus, streptococcus, *Neisseria* spp., TB
MI	Dressler syndrome, acute regional pericarditis
Medications	Procainamide, hydralazine
Trauma	Cardiac surgery (postpericardiotomy syndrome), cardiac contusion
Renal	Uremia, hemodialysis-associated
Neoplastic	Lung and breast cancer, lymphoma, melanoma
Miscellaneous	Amyloidosis, sarcoidosis, dissecting aortic aneurysm

cardiac auscultation; it may be localized over the left lower sternal border or heard across the precordium. A rub is best appreciated with the diaphragm of the stethoscope, with the patient leaning forward or in the left lateral decubitus position. Classically, the rub consists of three components corresponding to atrial systole, ventricular systole, and ventricular diastole. In many instances, only one or two components may be heard, and they are often mistaken for murmurs. A rub may be intermittent and may change in quality from one examination to the next; its presence is diagnostic for acute pericarditis but its absence does not exclude the diagnosis. The clinician should always examine the patient for any signs of underlying disorders that may cause pericarditis.

Diagnostic Evaluation

ECG abnormalities during acute pericarditis reflect inflammation of the myocardium underlying the visceral pericardium. They may develop within hours of the onset of chest pain and may persist for days. The typical ECG abnormalities include (see Figure 31-1):

- Diffuse STE
- PR-segment depression

Over a period of days, a typical evolution of ECG abnormalities occurs (see Table 31-2). Although some ECG abnormality is seen in 90% of cases, the absence of these findings does not exclude pericarditis. Once pericarditis has been diagnosed, a search for the underlying cause is warranted. Serum markers of inflammation (e.g., ESR) are invariably elevated. Specific testing for human immunodeficiency virus (HIV) or other viral antigens, blood cultures, ASO (antistreptolysin O) titer, autoimmune antibodies, and tuberculin skin testing should be considered. An echocardiogram is not necessary in uncomplicated cases of pericarditis but can be useful if associated myocarditis is suspected and to assess for associated pericardial effusion.

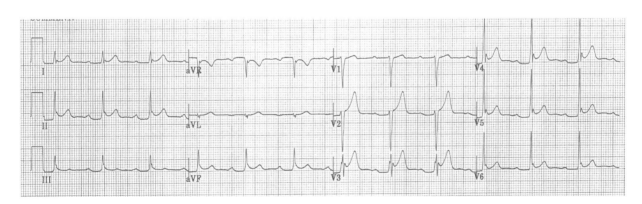

Figure 31-1 • ECG of stage I pericarditis. Note the diffuse STE and the PR depression in lead II. A first-degree AV block is also present (unrelated).

■ TABLE 31-2

Electrocardiographic Stages of Pericarditis

Stage	ST Segment	PR Interval	T Waves
I	Elevated	Depressed or normal	Upright
II	Normal	Depressed or normal	Upright
III	Normal	Normal	Inverted
IV	Normal	Normal	Upright

Treatment

The cornerstone of therapy for acute pericarditis is treatment of the underlying disorder. The inflammatory process and the associated pericardial pain usually respond to treatment with NSAIDs (e.g., ibuprofen or indomethacin); systemic steroids and/or colchicine may be required for severe unremitting pain. Anticoagulant drugs should be avoided in the early stages of pericarditis owing to the risk of intrapericardial hemorrhage. The first-line treatment for post-MI pericarditis is aspirin, not any of the other NSAIDs, as the latter can cause coronary vasoconstriction. Steroids also should be avoided, as they are associated with an increased risk of myocardial rupture in this setting. Viral pericarditis is usually self-limited and resolves spontaneously over a period of days without significant sequelae. Occasionally recurrent pericarditis may develop weeks or months after the initial event. Acute bacterial pericarditis is a life-threatening disease and requires emergent drainage of purulent pericardial fluid and administration of IV antibiotics. Some forms of pericarditis (especially malignancy-associated cases) may result in cardiac tamponade and require emergent percutaneous or surgical drainage. Chronically, pericarditis can result in pericardial scarring and constriction.

KEY POINTS

1. Pericarditis is an inflammatory disease of the pericardium.
2. The most common causes of pericarditis are viral and idiopathic.
3. Pericarditis is a clinical diagnosis whose classic features include pleuritic chest pain, a pericardial friction rub, and diffuse STE and PR-segment depression on ECG.
4. Therapy involves treating the underlying cause and administering anti-inflammatory agents.

Chapter 32

Cardiac Tamponade

Cardiac tamponade is a characteristic hemodynamic syndrome resulting from the accumulation of fluid in the pericardial space, with resultant compression of the cardiac chambers.

Etiology

Cardiac tamponade may result from any disease process that can produce pericarditis or a pericardial effusion (see Table 31-1). The most common causes of cardiac tamponade include:

- Neoplasm (50% of cases)
- Idiopathic/viral pericarditis (15% of cases)
- Uremia (10% of cases)

Other causes include bacterial and tuberculous pericarditis, blunt or penetrating chest trauma, myxedema, SLE, aortic dissection with rupture into the pericardial space, and MI with LV free-wall rupture.

Pathogenesis

Normally, the pericardial space contains approximately 50 mL of fluid and the intrapericardial pressure is similar to intrathoracic pressure (i.e., lower than RV and LV diastolic pressures). When additional fluid enters the pericardial space, intrapericardial pressure rises. If the fluid accumulation is rapid, intrapericardial pressure will rise significantly after only 80 to 100 mL. If the fluid accumulates gradually, the pericardium may be able to accommodate several liters of fluid with only a small rise in pressure.

During diastole, the increased intrapericardial pressure is transmitted to the heart, resulting in the simultaneous elevation of diastolic pressure in all cardiac chambers (equilibration of diastolic pressures). The increased ventricular diastolic pressures impair ventricular filling and result in decreased CO and elevated JVP. Tachycardia and peripheral vasoconstriction occur as a compensatory mechanism. Once the intrapericardial pressure exceeds intracardiac pressure, cardiac compression occurs, CO falls precipitously, and hypotension ensues, resulting in cardiogenic shock.

Clinical Manifestations

History

Patients with tamponade often present with shortness of breath, light-headedness, presyncope, or hemodynamic collapse. Palpitations or chest pain may also be present, as may symptoms of poor peripheral perfusion such as confusion and agitation. Patients with slowly developing tamponade may present with symptoms of progressive right HF (edema, fatigue) or symptoms relating to compression of adjacent structures by the enlarging pericardial sac, including dysphagia (esophageal compression), hiccups (phrenic nerve compression), and dyspnea (lung compression).

Physical Examination

The classic features of cardiac tamponade are described by the Beck triad:

- Elevated JVP
- Systemic hypotension
- "Quiet" heart sounds (blunted transmission of sound across the precordium due to the presence of pericardial fluid)

Other physical findings include:

- Pulsus paradoxus
- Tachypnea

- Tachycardia
- Pericardial friction rub (often absent or evanescent)

The jugular venous pulsations in tamponade classically demonstrate a rapid x descent (rapid atrial filling after atrial contraction) and an absent y descent (no passive filling of the ventricle owing to increased ventricular diastolic pressure) (see Figure 2-1). Pulsus paradoxus is the inspiratory fall in systolic arterial BP. Normally, the increased venous return during inspiration causes the right heart to expand, pushing the interventricular septum slightly to the left. This impairs LV stroke volume and accounts for the normal pulsus paradoxus of <10 mm Hg. In tamponade, the pericardial effusion limits the total blood volume of the heart. Consequently, during inspiration, as augmented RV filling occurs, the interventricular septum is pushed further to the left and LV filling is compromised, resulting in a marked fall in LV stroke volume and a pulsus paradoxus of >10 mm Hg. Other causes of an increased pulsus paradoxus include severe COPD, acute PE, and constrictive pericarditis.

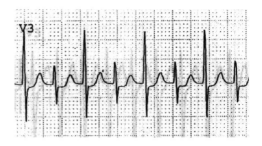

Figure 32-2 • ECG demonstrating electrical alternans. The QRS axis alternates with each beat as the heart swings within a large effusion.

Diagnostic Evaluation

The diagnosis of cardiac tamponade is made on the basis of historic features and physical findings. Ancillary testing should be used to confirm the clinically suspected diagnosis. Helpful diagnostic modalities include:

- Echocardiography—demonstrates pericardial fluid, compression of cardiac chambers, and impaired ventricular diastolic filling (Figure 32-1).
- CXR—cardiac silhouette may appear as a "water bottle" due to a large pericardial effusion.
- ECG—usually demonstrates tachycardia; low QRS amplitude may be present with large effusions; electrical alternans may occur as the heart swings back and forth within the pericardial fluid (Figure 32-2).
- Right cardiac catheterization—demonstrates elevated intracardiac filling pressures and equalization of diastolic pressures.

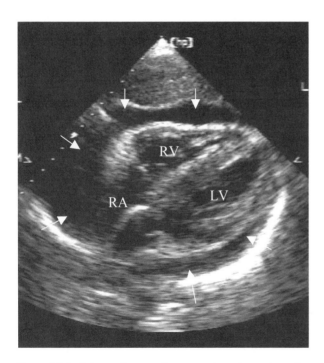

Figure 32-1 • Echocardiogram demonstrating a large circumferential pericardial effusion (arrows) in a patient with pericardial tamponade. The RA is compressed by the fluid and is poorly visualized.

Treatment

Cardiac tamponade is a medical emergency requiring rapid diagnosis and treatment. The cornerstone of therapy is immediate drainage of the pericardial fluid. This may be performed percutaneously via a hollow-bore needle inserted into the pericardium from the subxiphoid region (pericardiocentesis). Hemodynamically unstable patients should be supported with volume expansion and vasopressors (i.e., dopamine) while preparations for pericardiocentesis are being made. Both vasodilators such as nitrates and diuretics should be avoided as they may precipitate hypotension in this setting. Following pericardial drainage, rapid recovery of BP and normalization of HR is the rule. The pericardial fluid should be sent for chemical analysis, culture, and cytology. Often, a catheter is left in the pericardial space for 1 to 2 days after pericardiocentesis to allow for continued drainage. In patients in whom percutaneous drainage is unsuccessful or rapid reaccumulation of the fluid occurs, surgical resection of a portion of the pericardium (pericardiectomy or the creation of a "pericardial window") can be performed. This allows for chronic drainage of the fluid from the pericardial space into the left thorax, thereby preventing recurrent tamponade.

KEY POINTS

1. Cardiac tamponade is caused by the accumulation of excessive pericardial fluid.
2. The most common causes of pericardial tamponade include malignancies, viral pericarditis, and uremia.
3. The hemodynamic hallmarks of tamponade include increased intrapericardial pressure, elevated and equilibrated intracardiac diastolic pressures, reduced diastolic filling of the ventricles, and reduced CO.
4. Classic features of tamponade include hypotension, elevated JVP, and muffled heart sounds (the Beck triad).
5. Other physical findings characteristic of tamponade include tachycardia, prominent x descent and absent y descent in the jugular venous waveform, and elevated pulsus paradoxus.
6. Definitive therapy for tamponade is emergent pericardiocentesis (acutely) and surgical pericardiotomy (for recurrent effusions).

Chapter

33 Constrictive Pericarditis

Constrictive pericarditis, one of the sequelae of acute pericarditis, is characterized by a thickened, noncompliant pericardium that impairs filling of the cardiac chambers and thereby results in HF.

Etiology

Most cases of constrictive pericarditis evolve following an initial episode of acute pericarditis; therefore the etiologies are similar (Table 33-1). Worldwide, TB is the leading cause of constrictive pericarditis; however, in developed countries, idiopathic constrictive pericarditis predominates.

Pathogenesis

The hallmark of constrictive pericarditis is impairment of diastole without impairment of systole. Normally, the pericardium is compliant and allows the ventricles to fill freely during diastole. After an episode of acute pericarditis, fibrosis may develop and can severely

reduce pericardial elasticity. When this occurs, intracardiac pressures begin to rise. Early in diastole, the ventricles fill rapidly, owing to unimpeded ventricular relaxation and increased atrial pressure. However, once the cardiac volume has reached the limits of the constrictive pericardium, further diastolic filling is severely reduced. Throughout diastole, as a result of equivalent effects of the constrictive pericardium on the RV and LV, the ventricular pressures are elevated and equal (Figure 33-1). This is to be distinguished from the

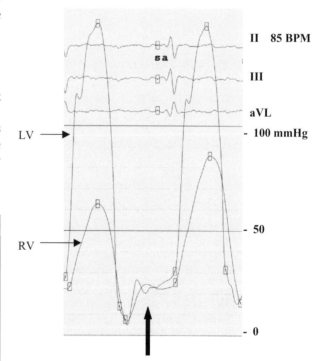

Figure 33-1 • Intraventricular pressure tracings in a patient with pericardial constriction. The ventricular diastolic pressures are equal and elevated, demonstrating the "square-root sign" (block arrow) characteristic of this condition.

■ TABLE 33-1

Common Causes of Constrictive Pericarditis

Category	Examples
Infectious	TB, viral and bacterial causes
Connective tissue disorders	SLE, rheumatoid arthritis
Neoplasms	Lung and breast cancer, mesothelioma, lymphoma, melanoma
Radiation-induced	Following mantle radiation
Trauma	Postcardiac surgery
Idiopathic	Nonspecific

■ TABLE 33-2

Comparative Features of Pericardial Constriction, Pericardial Tamponade, and Restrictive Cardiomyopathy

	Pericardial Constriction	Pericardial Tamponade	Restrictive Cardiomyopathy
Pulsus paradoxus	Usually absent	Present	Absent
JVP waveform	Prominent x and y descents	Prominent x descent, absent y descent	Prominent x and y descents
Kussmaul sign	Usually present	Absent	May be present
Hemodynamic pattern	LV and RV diastolic pressures equal and have "dip-and-plateau" pattern	Equalization of all cardiac diastolic pressures	LV diastolic pressure >5 mm Hg higher than RV, both have "dip-and-plateau" pattern

hemodynamic pattern of restrictive cardiac disease, which predominantly affects the LV, resulting in elevated but unequal RV and LV diastolic pressures (see Figure 19-1). The elevated diastolic pressure produces many of the clinical features of this syndrome. Systolic cardiac function, however, remains intact.

Clinical Manifestations

History

Elevated RV and LV end-diastolic pressure may manifest as right and left HF, respectively. However, in most patients with pericardial constriction, right-sided symptoms predominate and include:

- Peripheral edema
- Abdominal fullness, nausea (resulting from intestinal edema and ascites)
- Right-upper-quadrant tenderness (owing to liver congestion)
- Fullness in the neck [resulting from elevated jugular venous pressure (JVP)]

Physical Examination

The sine qua non of constrictive physiology is elevated JVP. Classically, the JVP will exhibit a prominent y descent, reflecting rapid initial atrial emptying after the opening of the tricuspid valve (Figure 2-1e). This occurs as a result of elevated atrial pressure and unimpeded early ventricular diastolic filling. Often, the x descent is also prominent. This is to be distinguished from cardiac tamponade, in which the x descent is prominent but the y descent is blunted or absent, owing to the compressive effects of the pericardial fluid throughout the cardiac cycle. It may be difficult to detect these signs, especially during tachycardia.

As a result of pericardial constriction, the normal inspiratory decrease in intrathoracic pressure is not transmitted to the cardiac chambers, and RV volume therefore does not increase. The increased venous return instead results in a paradoxical increase in the JVP with inspiration (**Kussmaul sign**). This pattern is not seen with tamponade. **Pulsus paradoxus**, an exaggerated drop in the systemic BP with inspiration, is usually absent in constriction, whereas it is characteristically present during cardiac tamponade (see Table 33-2 and Chapter 32).

Cardiac auscultation may demonstrate an early, relatively high-pitched third heart sound, known as a **pericardial knock**. This sound occurs early in diastole as a result of the rapid cessation of ventricular filling as the pericardium is stretched to its limit. Other signs of right HF may be present, such as hepatic congestion, peripheral edema, and ascites. Left HF is less common but may be present.

Diagnostic Evaluation

The clinician should suspect this syndrome in any patient who presents with new-onset HF and a recent history of pericarditis. Although there is no diagnostic "gold standard," there are several diagnostic modalities that may aid in diagnosing this condition (Table 33-3). A CXR may reveal pericardial calcification in tuberculous pericarditis or other forms of long-standing pericardial constriction; however, CT scanning is a more accurate method of assessing pericardial thickness. An echocardiogram will reveal an abnormal diastolic filling pattern with diminished late diastolic ventricular filling. Cardiac catheterization will reveal:

- Elevated diastolic pressure in all cardiac chambers
- Rapid x and y descents on the right atrial and pulmonary capillary wedge pressures

TABLE 33-3

Some Typical Findings of Constrictive Pericarditis Using Various Diagnostic Modalities

Modality	Typical Findings
CXR	Normal cardiac size, calcification of the pericardium
CT scan	Thickened pericardium, dilated superior and inferior venae cavae
ECG	Low voltage of QRS complexes; commonly AF
Echocardiogram	Dilated IVC, augmented early diastolic transmitral flow, diastolic posterior-wall flattening, thickened pericardium
Cardiac catheterization	Elevated right and left heart diastolic pressures, elevated RA mean pressure, rapid y descent, equal LV and RV end-diastolic pressures, "dip-and-plateau" or "square-root" sign, normal CO

- Rapid early diastolic fall in ventricular pressure followed by a sustained elevation in pressure ("dip-and-plateau pattern"; see Figure 33-1)

The "dip" in the ventricular pressure tracing is the result of rapid, unimpeded, early diastolic ventricular relaxation, whereas the "plateau" reflects constant ventricular pressure once the ventricle expands to the limits of the constrictive pericardium. Occasionally, pericardial biopsy is required to confirm the diagnosis.

Treatment

Patients with limited symptoms of HF can usually be treated effectively with sodium restriction and diuretics. However, despite maximal medical therapy, many patients develop progressive symptomatic right and left HF and subsequently require surgical resection of the pericardium (pericardiectomy, or **pericardial stripping**). The operative mortality of pericardiectomy may be as high as 20%; however, over 90% of patients who survive surgery will improve significantly. The proper timing of surgery is controversial, but it should be performed before severe right HF develops.

KEY POINTS

1. Constrictive pericarditis is usually a sequela of acute pericarditis.
2. Classic physical findings of pericardial constriction include rapid x and y descents in the jugular venous waveform and a pericardial knock.
3. The thickened pericardium is best visualized by CT scanning.
4. The diagnosis of constrictive pericarditis can be suggested by echocardiography and confirmed with invasive measurement of intracardiac pressures (cardiac catheterization).
5. Medical treatment of pericardial constriction consists of diuretics and salt restriction; surgical pericardiectomy may be required to alleviate the hemodynamic disturbance.

Part Eight

Vascular Diseases

34 Hypertension

Elevation in BP above normal (120/80 mm Hg) has been linked in clinical studies to an increased risk of cardiovascular events. HTN is defined as an SBP >140 mm Hg or a DBP >90 mm Hg based on the average of two or more measurements on two or more occasions. The severity can be further classified according to the degree of systolic or diastolic pressure elevation (see Table 34-1).

Epidemiology

The estimated prevalence of HTN in the United States is 20 to 30%. It is more common in men than in women (up to the age of 55 years) and in African Americans than Caucasians; it increases in incidence with advancing age. Among patients with HTN, approximately 30% are unaware that they have elevated BP and only 25 to 30% of patients with HTN are optimally controlled with their present medical regimen.

Etiology

In the vast majority of patients, no cause for HTN can be determined (primary or essential HTN). Nonetheless, several risk factors for the development of essential HTN have been identified, including:

- Genetic predisposition (family history)
- Male gender
- Excessive alcohol consumption
- Obesity
- Inactivity
- Increased sodium intake
- African-American race

Secondary HTN is defined as HTN due to an identifiable cause and accounts for only 5 to 10% of cases. Etiologies include:

- Renovascular disease (renal artery stenosis, fibromuscular dysplasia)
- Renal parenchymal disease (glomerulonephritis, polycystic kidney disease)
- Endocrine disorders (primary hyperaldosteronism, Cushing syndrome, hyper- or hypothyroidism, hyperparathyriodism, pheochromocytoma)
- Alcohol and illicit drug use
- Coarctation of the aorta
- Obstructive sleep apnea
- Medications including oral contraceptives, NSAIDs, COX-2 inhibitors, sympathomimetics, adrenal steroids, tacrolimus, cyclosporine, and erythropoietin
- Over-the-counter preparations such as ephedra

Clinical Manifestations

The goals of the clinical evaluation of a person with HTN are to determine the presence and extent of

■ TABLE 34-1

Classification of Blood Pressure

Classification*	Systolic (mm Hg)		Diastolic (mm Hg)
Normal	<120	AND	<80
Pre-HTN	120–139	OR	80–89
Stage 1 HTN	140–159	OR	90–99
Stage 2 HTN	≥160	OR	≥100

*For adults who are not taking antihypertensive medications and are not acutely ill. If classification of SBP and DBP is discrepant, the higher classification is used.

TABLE 34-2

Target Organ Damage

Target Organ	Disease Manifestations
Heart	LVH, CHF, CMP, CAD
Brain	Hemorrhagic stroke, encephalopathy
Kidney	Proteinuria, renal failure, acute glomerulonephritis
Eye	Retinopathy, papilledema
Peripheral arteries	Aortic dissection, TIAs, claudication

target-organ damage (see Table 34-2), to identify secondary causes of HTN and precipitating or exacerbating factors, and to identify concomitant cardiovascular disease risk factors.

History

In general, HTN is a silent disease until complications develop, at which time the patient may report symptoms of cardiovascular, cerebrovascular, or peripherovascular disease. Nonetheless, the elevated pressure itself may cause headaches, chest pain, shortness of breath, or palpitations. Other important historic points that should be addressed include the following:

- Duration and degree of HTN
- Family history of HTN, CAD, stroke, DM, renal disease, or dyslipidemia
- History of tobacco, alcohol, or illicit drug use (including androgenic steroids) and use of herbal preparations (including sympathomimetics such as ephedrine)
- Level of physical activity
- Dietary intake of sodium, caffeine, and saturated fat
- Symptoms of target-organ damage
- Presence of other CAD risk factors (see Chapter 9)

A secondary cause of HTN should be suspected in patients with the following historical features:

- New-onset HTN in a patient <20 years old or >50 years old

Severe or refractory HTN despite maximal treatment with three or more antihypertensive agents

- An acute rise in BP over a previously stable baseline
- Moderate-to-severe HTN precipitating flash pulmonary edema
- Negative family history of HTN

Physical Examination

BP should be measured with a manual cuff with the patient in a seated position. Values should be confirmed in both arms. The physical examination should also be directed toward identifying signs of end-organ damage, including:

- Retinopathy (arteriolar narrowing, arteriovenous nicking, hemorrhages, exudates, papilledema)
- Vascular disease (arterial bruits, diminished peripheral pulses)
- Cardiac disease (displaced LV apex, S_3, S_4, pulmonary rales, elevated JVP)
- Neurologic disease (motor or sensory deficits)

Several physical findings suggest specific secondary causes of HTN, including thyromegaly, cutaneous striae (Cushing syndrome), abdominal bruits (renovascular disease), and arm-leg pressure discrepancy (aortic coarctation).

Diagnostic Evaluation

Routine testing in the initial evaluation of HTN should include a CBC, electrolytes, urinalysis, fasting glucose, lipid profile, and ECG. Additional testing should be directed at establishing a secondary cause or identifying specific target-organ damage, as directed by the history and physical examination.

Treatment

General Approach

General guidelines with regard to risk classification and treatment options for HTN are summarized in Table 34-3. The need for and intensity of antihypertensive therapy can be determined by considering the absolute level of BP elevation as well as a patient's cardiovascular risk factors and target-organ damage. Patients who have clinical evidence of cardiovascular or renal disease or who have DM are considered to be in the same high-risk group as patients who have target-organ damage. The presence of these conditions directs the choice of drug therapy; these patients are treated with medications specific to their disease, which offer proven mortality benefit based on clinical trials (see Table 34-4).

The goal of HTN therapy is to reduce BP to a level at which target-organ damage will be prevented or limited. The recommended goal BP levels are as follows:

- For uncomplicated HTN: BP <140/90 mm Hg
- For patients with DM or chronic renal disease: BP <130/80 mm Hg

■ TABLE 34-3

Treatment Recommendations in Hypertension

Risk	Prehypertensive (120–139/80–89)	Stage 1 (140–159/90–99)	Stage 2 (≥160/≥100)
Uncomplicated Hypertension	Lifestyle modifications	Drug therapy (usually thiazide)	Two agents for most patients (thiazide plus ACE-I, ARB, beta blocker, CCB)
DM, CHD, HF, chronic kidney disease, stroke, target-organ damage	Lifestyle modifications Agents for coexisting risks	Agents for coexisting risks plus other anti-HTN as needed	Agents for coexisting risk with additional anti-HTN as needed (ACE-I, ARB, beta blocker, CCB diuretics)

SOURCE: Modified from The Seventh Report of the Joint National Committee on the Prevention, Detection, Evaluation, and Treatment of High Blood Pressure (JNC VII), 2004.

Nonpharmacologic Therapy

Antihypertensive treatment generally begins with nonpharmacologic therapy and lifestyle modifications, including weight loss in obese patients, reduction of dietary sodium intake to <2 to 3 g/day, regular exercise, and avoidance of excess alcohol intake. All patients, regardless of their BP, should be counseled with regard to smoking cessation. Optimally, lifestyle changes can decrease SBP by 20 mm Hg, but actual BP reductions are usually more modest (2 to 4 mm Hg).

Pharmacologic Therapy

There are several classes of antihypertensive agents, including:

- Diuretics (e.g., hydrochlorothiazide, furosemide, spironolactone)
- Beta blockers (e.g., metoprolol, atenolol, propranolol)

■ TABLE 34-4

Indications for Specific Drug Therapy

Disease State	Agents of Choice
DM	ACE-I, ARB, beta blocker, diuretic, CCB
HF/CMP	ACE-I, ARB, beta blocker, diuretic, aldosterone antagonist
CHD	Beta blocker, ACE-I
Chronic kidney disease	ACE-I, ARB
Stroke	ACE-I, diuretic

SOURCE: Modified from The Seventh Report of the Joint National Committee on the Prevention, Detection, Evaluation, and Treatment of High Blood Pressure (JNC VII), 2004.

- CCBs (e.g., verapamil, diltiazem, nifedipine, amlodipine)
- ACE inhibitors (e.g., captopril, enalapril, lisinopril)
- Angiotensin-receptor blockers (e.g., losartan, valsartan)
- Alpha blockers (e.g., clonidine, prazosin)
- Mixed alpha and beta blockers (e.g., carvedilol, labetolol)
- Direct vasodilators (e.g., hydralazine, minoxidil)

Most antihypertensive agents will result in an adequate BP response in 40 to 60% of patients; however, much variability exists in individual responses to different agents. Patients who do not respond to one antihypertensive drug have a 50% chance of responding to a different agent.

The general recommendations for the initial treatment of uncomplicated HTN consist of monotherapy with a thiazide diuretic. However, in certain situations there are compelling indications for use of a specific agent (see Table 34-4). Several points regarding antihypertensive therapy are worth noting:

1. Medications should be started at lower doses and uptitrated every 1 to 2 weeks until the optimal effect is achieved.
2. If a person has no response to a particular agent after 2 to 3 weeks of therapy, a different agent should be substituted.
3. If a person responds to one agent but the BP is still not optimally controlled, a second agent of a different class should be added.
4. If combination therapy is required, the dose of the first agent should be maximized before initiating a second drug.

Aggressive pharmacologic therapy results in optimal BP control in 75 to 80% of patients; however, on

■ TABLE 34-5

Medications Used in the Treatment of Hypertensive Crises

Drug	Onset of Action	Duration of Action	Special Indications
Sodium nitroprusside	Immediate	1–2 min	Most hypertensive emergencies; use with caution in elevated ICP
Nitroglycerin	2–5 min	3–5 min	Myocardial ischemia
Labetalol	5–10 min	3–6 h	Most hypertensive emergencies except for acute HF
Nicardipine	5–10 min	1–4 h	Most hypertensive emergencies except for acute HF; use with caution in ischemia
Phentolamine	1–2 min	3–10 min	Catecholamine excess (pheochromocytoma, MAO interaction)
Hydralazine	0–20 min	3–8 h	Eclampsia
Esmolol	1–2 min	10–20 min	Aortic dissection, perioperative
Enalaprilat	15–30 min	6 h	Acute heart failure

average, at least three agents are required to achieve this result.

■ HYPERTENSIVE CRISIS

The term *hypertensive crisis* encompasses a variety of syndromes associated with marked elevation of BP (SBP >230 mm Hg, DBP >130 mm Hg), including:

- Hypertensive urgency: markedly elevated BP without acute target-organ damage
- Hypertensive emergency: markedly elevated BP with acute target-organ damage
- Accelerated HTN: markedly elevated BP with associated retinal hemorrhages or exudates
- Malignant HTN: markedly elevated BP with associated papilledema

Such profound HTN requires aggressive BP reduction. In the absence of symptoms or acute target-organ damage, BP should be decreased within hours to days. In the presence of symptoms or target-organ damage, immediate BP reduction is indicated. Hypertensive crises should be managed with IV agents to achieve an initial goal of not more than a 25% reduction in the mean arterial pressure in the first 2 hours (Table 34-5). BP should be further reduced toward 160/100 mm Hg over the next several hours. More rapid reductions in BP may precipitate cerebral hypoperfusion as a result of altered autoregulation of cerebral blood flow.

KEY POINTS

1. HTN is defined as an SBP >140 mm Hg or a DBP >90 mm Hg based on the average of two or more measurements on two or more occasions.
2. HTN is categorized as essential or secondary.
3. Treatment generally begins with lifestyle modifications unless the patient has multiple cardiovascular risk factors or stage 1 or greater HTN.
4. Goal BP is <140/90 in patients with uncomplicated HTN; the goal is <130/80 in patients with DM or chronic renal disease.
5. Drug therapy should be aimed at maximal BP reduction while minimizing side effects, treating concomitant conditions, and ensuring compliance.
6. Hypertensive crises are potentially life-threatening conditions that require immediate reduction in BP.

Peripheral Arterial Disorders

The peripheral arteries can be affected by a variety of disorders, including atherosclerosis, thromboembolic disease, and vasoconstrictive disorders. These conditions result in impaired blood flow to the brain or extremities and account for significant morbidity and mortality.

■ PERIPHERAL ARTERIAL DISEASE

Pathogenesis

PAD is most often a manifestation of atherosclerosis (see Chapter 9). In the peripheral vasculature, atheromatous lesions tend to develop at arterial branch points. The increased turbulence and shear stress in these areas result in intimal injury and stimulate plaque formation. The disease tends to be diffuse, affecting multiple arteries, which most often include:

- Femoral and popliteal arteries (80 to 90% of affected patients)
- Tibial, peroneal, and more distal arteries (40 to 50% of affected patients)
- Abdominal aorta and iliac arteries (30% of affected patients)

Risk Factors

The risk factors for PAD are the same as those for CAD and include:

- Advanced age
- HTN
- DM
- Dyslipidemia
- Male gender
- Cigarette smoking

Atherosclerotic PAD is frequently associated with coronary and carotid atherosclerotic disease. Therefore one should always look for evidence of CAD in patients presenting with PAD, and vice versa.

Clinical Manifestations

History

The principal symptom of PAD is intermittent claudication, a manifestation of skeletal muscle ischemia resulting from inadequate peripheral blood flow. The symptoms occur distal to the obstructing lesion and are usually described as a dull ache, cramp, or limb fatigue that occurs with exertion and resolves after a few minutes of rest. Discomfort may be limited to the calf in the case of femoropopliteal disease, or it may extend to the buttock, hip, and thigh in the presence of aortoiliac disease. This latter manifestation may be associated with impotence (**Leriche syndrome**). In severe occlusive PAD, the arterial blood supply may become inadequate to support resting metabolic demands, and patients may develop claudication at rest.

A thorough history includes a search for cardiac risk factors and symptoms of CAD, as these two disorders frequently coexist.

Physical Examination

Physical findings of PAD include:

- Diminished peripheral pulses with cool, pale extremities
- Vascular bruits
- Shiny, smooth, hairless skin (atrophic changes)
- **Dependent rubor** (reactive hyperemia of legs in dependent position)

Differential Diagnosis

True claudication must be distinguished from **pseudoclaudication** ("neurogenic claudication"). True claudication results from vascular compromise, is precipitated by walking, and resolves after standing still. Pseudoclaudication, a symptom of lumbar spinal stenosis, may mimic true claudication by causing exertional leg pain; however, pseudoclaudication resolves only after sitting down or changing position.

Diagnostic Evaluation

The diagnosis of PAD can usually be established by a thorough history and physical examination. Diagnostic testing is reserved for assessing the severity of the disease. The most commonly used test to assess PAD is the ankle-brachial index (ABI). Normally, the systolic blood pressure in the legs is higher than that in the arms and the ABI is greater than 1.0. Values less than 0.9 predict PAD with 95% sensitivity; values less than 0.5 are consistent with severe ischemia. Duplex ultrasonography can be useful in localizing the level of the disease and assessing its severity. MRA and contrast angiography are essential tests to define vascular anatomy in patients being considered for surgical revascularization.

Treatment

The treatment of PAD consists of nonpharmacologic, pharmacologic, and surgical therapies. Nonpharmacologic therapies should always be employed and include:

- Exercise therapy
- Risk-factor modification (smoking cessation, lipid-lowering therapy, aggressive blood sugar control, antihypertensive therapy)
- Meticulous foot care to avoid injury and infection

Exercise rehabilitation programs dramatically reduce symptoms and improve walking distance, likely through improved endothelial function and the formation of collateral vessels.

Antiplatelet agents (i.e., aspirin, dipyridamole, clopidogrel) have been the mainstay of medical therapy for PAD and may improve symptoms as well as decrease the need for surgical revascularization. Pentoxifylline (400 mg three times daily), a xanthine derivative, is thought to work by reducing the viscosity of blood and increasing flexibility of red blood cells. This agent appears to offer no advantage over exercise rehabilitation alone. Cilostazol (100 mg twice daily), a phosphodiesterase inhibitor that inhibits platelet aggregation and causes direct vasodilation, reduces claudication time by 30 to 60% compared with placebo and appears to be more effective

than pentoxifylline. Cilostazol should not be used in patients with HF, as other phosphosdiesterase inhibitors have been linked to increased mortality in HF patients. Several novel pharmacotherapies are under investigation, including serotonin, L-arginine, carnitine derivatives, and parenteral angiogenic growth factors (vascular endothelial growth factor, basic fibroblast growth factor).

Revascularization of peripheral arteries is indicated for patients with:

- Incapacitating claudication
- Rest pain
- Evidence of tissue necrosis

Revascularization may be performed percutaneously or through an open surgical procedure. The success and patency rates associated with percutaneous transluminal angioplasty (PTA) with stent implantation vary with the location of the vascular lesion. PTA and stent of the iliac arteries is associated with a >90% acute success rate and good long-term patency (80% remain patent after 1 year; 60% after 5 years). Less favorable outcomes are associated with femoral and popliteal interventions (65% patency at 1 year and 40% patency at 5 years).

Surgical revascularization procedures can be classified as aortoiliac or infrainguinal. Aortoiliac reconstruction is typically performed with placement of an aortobifemoral prosthetic bypass graft. Infrainguinal bypass procedures utilize saphenous vein grafts for the reconstruction. Long-term patency varies with location and type of graft utilized and ranges from 70 to 85% at 5 years.

■ ACUTE ARTERIAL OCCLUSION

Acute arterial occlusion is a medical emergency. It results in limb ischemia and requires emergent therapy to prevent limb loss.

Pathogenesis

Acute arterial occlusion can occur as a result of embolic disease, thrombotic disease, dissection, or trauma. Most arterial emboli originate in the heart, usually as a result of AF or mural thrombi in the LV. Less commonly, peripheral emboli may originate from thrombi associated with prosthetic heart valves, from valvular vegetations (endocarditis), or from atrial myxomas. In situ thrombosis of a peripheral artery may occur in patients with PAD, infrainguinal bypass grafts, and peripheral aneurysms, especially in patients with concomitant hypercoagulable states.

Clinical Manifestations

History and Physical Examination

The history and physical examination of the patient with acute arterial occlusion are characterized by the "six Ps" in the affected extremity:

- Pulselessness
- Pallor
- Pain
- Paresthesias
- Paralysis
- Poikilothermia (inability of the limb to self-regulate temperature)

A thorough history may disclose prior symptoms of a preexisting condition (e.g., AF, PAD, etc.). Additional physical findings may include muscle stiffness, absent deep tendon reflexes, cyanosis, and cutaneous mottling.

Diagnostic Evaluation

The clinical presentation should strongly suggest this diagnosis. Contrast angiography is typically used to confirm the diagnosis. Following definitive therapy for the acute occlusion, TEE should be performed in patients with a presumed cardiac source of the embolism.

Treatment

The initial management of acute arterial occlusion consists of analgesia and anticoagulation with unfractionated heparin. Intraarterial thrombolytic therapy has been used successfully to treat acute thrombotic occlusion and decreases the need for surgical thrombectomy by approximately 50%. In cases in which limb viability is threatened, expedient surgical thromboembolectomy or arterial bypass surgery is indicated. Following a thromboembolic vascular event, long-term anticoagulation with warfarin is usually warranted.

■ RAYNAUD PHENOMENON

Clinical Manifestations

The Raynaud phenomenon is a symptom or physical finding characterized by the sequential development of clearly demarcated digital blanching, cyanosis, and rubor (white-blue-red) on cold exposure. This episodic digital ischemia is attributed to arterial vasospasm. Raynaud disease, i.e., idiopathic or primary Raynaud phenomenon, most commonly occurs in young women (20 to 40 years old); it is bilateral, may involve the feet, and follows a benign course. Secondary Raynaud phenomenon occurs in association with a variety of systemic disorders, including collagen vascular diseases (e.g., SLE, progressive systemic sclerosis), vasculitis, pulmonary HTN, neurologic disorders, and blood dyscrasias. This form of Raynaud syndrome is more common in older men, is frequently unilateral, is usually limited to the hands, and may be associated with digital necrosis.

Treatment

Most patients with Raynaud phenomenon can be managed with reassurance and avoidance of unnecessary cold exposure. Pharmacotherapy should be instituted in severe cases. CCBs (e.g., nifedipine 10–30 mg three times daily, diltiazem 30–90 mg three times daily) have been shown to decrease the frequency and severity of attacks.

■ THROMBOANGIITIS OBLITERANS

Thromboangiitis obliterans (TAO), also known as Buerger disease, is a vasculitis of the small and medium-sized arteries and veins of the upper and lower extremities. Cerebral, visceral, and coronary vessels may also be involved. Young men (<45 years of age) are most commonly affected. The etiology of TAO is unknown, but there appears to be a definite relationship to cigarette smoking (in virtually all patients) and an increased incidence of HLA-B5 and HLA-A9 antigens in affected individuals.

Clinical Manifestations

Patients with TAO frequently present with the triad of claudication, Raynaud phenomenon, and migratory superficial thrombophlebitis. Physical examination typically reveals reduced or absent distal pulses (radial, ulnar, dorsalis pedis, posterior tibial). Trophic nail changes, digital ulcerations, and gangrene may develop in severe cases.

Diagnostic Evaluation

The diagnosis is suggested by the disorder's characteristic appearance on arteriography. Smooth, tapering segmental lesions of the distal vessels with surrounding collateral vessels at the site of occlusion are the hallmark of TAO. Definitive confirmation is obtained by excisional biopsy.

Treatment

No specific therapy exists for TAO. Smoking cessation appears moderately effective at halting disease progression. Surgical reconstruction is of limited applicability owing to the distal nature of the disease. In severe cases, amputation may be required.

KEY POINTS

1. PAD is frequently associated with coronary and cerebral vascular disease.
2. True claudication is a symptom of PAD and must be distinguished from pseudoclaudication, a symptom of lumbosacral spine disease.
3. Acute arterial occlusion is heralded by the "six Ps": pain, pulselessness, pallor, paresthesias, paralysis, and poikilothermia.
4. The Raynaud phenomenon is the result of vasospasm and produces sequential white, blue, and then red discoloration of the digits on exposure to the cold.
5. Thromboangiitis obliterans is almost universally a disease of young male smokers.

36 Diseases of the Aorta

The aorta, like other vascular structures, is subject to a variety of disorders, including atherosclerosis, aneurysm formation, dissection, inflammation, and collagen vascular diseases. Disease of this vessel may impair blood flow to one or more vital organs; the resulting symptoms depend on the particular vascular territory affected.

▇ AORTIC ANEURYSMS

An aneurysm is a focal (saccular) or diffuse (fusiform) area of vascular dilation. A true aneurysm is at least 50% greater in diameter than the normal vessel and involves all three layers of the vessel wall. This is in contrast to a false aneurysm (pseudoaneurysm), which is essentially a contained vascular rupture. The walls of a pseudoaneurysm do not include any of the normal vascular layers; rather, the pseudoaneurysm is contained by perivascular tissue. Aneurysms may arise at any point in the aorta; involvement of the abdominal aorta is the most common.

Epidemiology

The prevalence of abdominal aortic aneurysms in the United States is approximately 50 per 100,000 men and 10 per 100,000 women. The incidence increases significantly with age; more than 3% of people over the age of 50 years have abdominal aortic aneurysms. Thoracic aortic aneurysms are less common. In the United States alone, aortic aneurysms account for nearly 70,000 hospitalizations, 40,000 operations, and 20,000 deaths annually.

Risk Factors

Factors associated with a higher incidence of aortic aneurysms include:

- Smoking
- Male gender
- Advanced age
- HTN

Other cardiac risk factors (e.g., DM, hyperlipidemia) may contribute by accelerating the development of atherosclerosis. Genetic factors also play a role; over one-third of affected patients have a family history of aneurysmal disease.

Etiology

Several diseases are associated with the development of aortic aneurysms (Table 36-1). Atherosclerosis is the most common predisposing factor for the devel-

▇ TABLE 36-1

Diseases Associated With Aortic Aneurysms

Disease Category	Examples
Atherosclerosis	—
Cystic medial necrosis	Hypertension, Marfan syndrome, Ehlers-Danlos disease, Turner syndrome, osteogenesis imperfecta
Congenital abnormalities	Bicuspid or unicuspid AV, aortic coarctation
Infection	Syphilis, TB
Spondyloarthropathy	Reiter syndrome, ankylosing spondylitis, rheumatoid arthritis
Vasculitis	Takayasu arteritis, giant cell arteritis
Trauma	Blunt chest trauma, iatrogenic

opment of abdominal and descending thoracic aortic aneurysms. Cystic medial necrosis, as occurs with HTN and connective tissue disorders, is the most common cause of ascending aortic aneurysms.

Pathogenesis

Atherosclerosis clearly plays a large part in the formation of aortic aneurysms. These aneurysms have a predilection for the infrarenal abdominal aorta, owing in part to the absence of vasa vasorum in the media of this region of the aorta. Altered synthesis and expression of types I and III procollagen, destruction of elastin and collagen in the vascular media by cytokine-induced metalloproteinases, and medial neovascularization also contribute to the pathogenesis. These changes weaken the aortic wall, allowing it to expand. As the aorta enlarges, wall tension increases (LaPlace law), and progressive dilation ensues.

Clinical Manifestations

History

The majority of abdominal aortic aneurysms and almost half of thoracic aortic aneurysms are asymptomatic at the time of diagnosis. When symptoms are present, they relate to the size and location of the aneurysm.

Thoracic aneurysms may cause:

- Chest or back pain (compression of adjacent thoracic structures)
- Dyspnea (compression of phrenic nerve or tracheo-bronchial tree; aortic insufficiency)
- Dysphagia (esophageal compression)
- Hoarseness (compression of the left recurrent laryngeal nerve)
- Cough, wheezing, hemoptysis (compression of the tracheobronchial tree)
- Superior vena cava syndrome
- Symptoms of coronary, cerebral, renal, mesenteric, lower extremity, or spinal ischemia (rarely)

Abdominal aneurysms may cause:

- Abdominal, back, leg, groin, or flank pain
- Anorexia, nausea, vomiting (compression of the GI tract)
- Unilateral leg swelling (compression of the left iliac vein)

The pain of an aortic aneurysm is usually a steady, gnawing pain that is unaffected by exertion. An acute increase in the pain usually heralds aneurysmal expansion or rupture. Thrombus may form within an aneurysm and subsequently embolize, resulting in acute vascular occlusion (see Chapter 35).

Physical Examination

Physical findings of aortic aneurysms vary with the location of the aneurysm. Ascending aortic aneurysms may be associated with:

- A diastolic murmur of aortic regurgitation due to distortion of the aortic valve annulus
- A pulsatile mass in the sternal notch

Abdominal aortic aneurysms may be associated with:

- A pulsatile abdominal mass
- An abdominal bruit

Carotid and femoral bruits as well as diminished peripheral pulses are frequently present in patients with aortic aneurysms and are caused by coexistent peripheral vascular disease (see Chapters 35 and 37).

Diagnostic Evaluation

Asymptomatic thoracic aneurysms may be detected by routine CXR because they result in widening of the mediastinum, enlargement of the aortic knob, or displacement of the trachea. Abdominal aneurysms may also be an incidental finding noted by calcification of a dilated aorta on abdominal radiographs. In patients with suspected thoracic aortic aneurysms, CT with IV contrast and MRA are both accurate methods of assessing aneurysmal size and determining its location with regard to branch vessels. Ultrasound is the usual initial imaging modality for the diagnosis of abdominal aortic aneurysms (sensitivity approaches 100%), and it can be used as a screening tool in high-risk patients. If an aneurysm is detected by ultrasound, another imaging modality such as CT can be used to further delineate its extent. Angiography remains the preferred modality for imaging aortic aneurysms before corrective surgery.

Approximately 25% of patients with thoracic aortic aneurysms have coexistent abdominal aneurysms, and more than 10% of patients with aortic aneurysms have peripheral vascular aneurysms. Therefore a full vascular evaluation is warranted when an aortic aneurysm is identified.

Natural History

The major risks associated with aortic aneurysms are dissection (see below) and vascular rupture. The risk of rupture is directly related to:

- The size of the aneurysm [risk is very low for aneurysms <4 cm in diameter and high for abdominal aneurysms >5 cm in diameter (2-year risk >20%) or thoracic aneurysms >6 cm in diameter (risk of rupture ~30%)]
- The rate of expansion of the aneurysm (risk increased if expansion >0.5 cm/6 months)
- The presence of symptoms

Treatment

Surgical correction is the definitive therapy for aortic aneurysms. Indications for surgery include:

- The presence of symptoms attributable to the aneurysm
- Abdominal aortic aneurysms >5 cm
- Thoracic aortic aneurysms >6 cm (>5.5 cm in Marfan syndrome)
- Rapidly expanding aneurysms (>0.5 cm/year)
- Thrombotic or embolic complications

Endovascular stent grafting is a novel, less invasive alternative for the repair of aortic aneurysms. Successful repair is achieved in approximately 80 to 90% of cases, with a mortality rate of 9 to 10%; this represents a lower short-term mortality compared with open surgical repair. The long-term outcome of the endovascular approach compared with that of surgery remains uncertain. This technique is currently applied to a subset of abdominal aneurysms with favorable anatomy and remains investigational in thoracic aneurysm repair.

Smaller, asymptomatic aneurysms may be managed medically with aggressive BP control and beta-blocker therapy. Beta blockers decrease shear stress in the aorta and may decrease the rate of aneurysmal expansion and risk of rupture. Reduction of other cardiovascular risk factors is also essential (see Chapter 9). In patients managed medically, serial imaging every 6 months (usually with CT scanning for thoracic aneurysms or ultrasound for abdominal aneurysms) is required to assess for aneurysmal expansion.

Prognosis

Some 60% of patients who suffer a ruptured aortic aneurysm die before reaching the hospital and 50% of the remainder die perioperatively. Elective thoracic aneurysm repair is associated with a 30-day mortality that approaches 10% and a significant risk of morbidity, namely stroke and renal failure. The mortality of abdominal aortic aneurysm repair is somewhat less (2 to 5%).

■ AORTIC DISSECTION

An aortic dissection is a tear of the intimal lining of the aorta that allows intraluminal blood to enter the vascular wall and then propagate down a dissection plane between the intima and media of the vessel. More than 2,000 cases occur in the United States each year.

Classification

Aortic dissections are classified according to their anatomic location (see Figure 36-1) and their duration. About 65% of aortic dissections begin in the ascending aorta, 20% in the descending thoracic aorta (distal to the left subclavian artery at the ligamentum arteriosum), and 10% in the aortic arch. Only 5% originate in the abdominal aorta. Dissections that have been present for less than 2 weeks are classified as acute, while dissections of greater than 2 weeks' duration are considered chronic. Both prognosis and management vary with the different types of aortic dissections (see below).

Pathogenesis

The intimal tear may occur following rupture of an atherosclerotic plaque or as a result of stretching of an aortic aneurysm. It may also follow rupture of the vasa vasorum within the aortic media (see Figure 36-2). This latter mechanism results in hemorrhage within the vascular media (an intramural hematoma) which may then rupture into the vascular lumen, creating an intimal tear. Once the dissection plane is established, it may propagate proximally or distally, thereby creating a false channel. This channel may subsequently thrombose

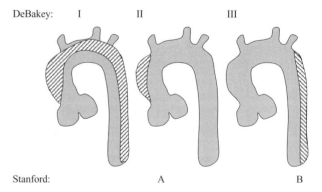

Figure 36-1 • Anatomic classifications of aortic dissections. DeBakey classes I and II and Stanford class A involve the ascending aorta. DeBakey class III and Stanford class B involve only the descending aorta. Hatched areas represent the false lumen.

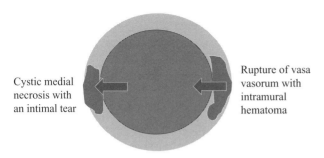

Cystic medial
necrosis with
an intimal tear

Rupture of vasa
vasorum with
intramural
hematoma

Figure 36-2 • Pathogenesis of aortic dissection.

or may rupture back into the vascular space, allowing continued flow in both the true and false lumens.

Several conditions predispose to aortic dissection, including:

- Aortic aneurysms (mainly atherosclerotic)
- Connective tissue diseases (Marfan syndrome, Ehlers-Danlos syndrome)
- Trauma

Clinical Manifestations

History

More than 90% of patients with acute aortic dissection present with the abrupt onset of severe pain localized to the chest or back and described as sharp, "ripping," or "tearing." The pain often radiates to the neck, jaw, flanks, or legs. Less common symptoms include:

- Syncope
- CHF (acute aortic valve insufficiency)
- Stroke (carotid artery dissection or impaired cerebral blood flow)
- Paraplegia (spinal artery occlusion)
- MI (coronary artery occlusion)
- SCD (pericardial tamponade, aortic rupture)

Physical Examination

HTN is the most common finding in patients with distal dissections, whereas those with proximal dissections frequently present with hypotension as a result of acute aortic insufficiency or pericardial tamponade. Other physical findings may include:

- Pulse deficits, asymmetric extremity blood pressures (>30 mm Hg difference), or acute limb ischemia (occlusion of limb vessel by dissection flap)
- Diastolic murmur of aortic insufficiency
- Left pleural effusion (hemothorax from rupture of aneurysm into the pleural space)

- Paraparesis, paraplegia, focal neurologic deficits
- Cardiac tamponade (rupture into the pericardial space)

Rarely, patients with dissection of the aorta may present with hoarseness, hemoptysis, a pulsating neck mass, Horner syndrome, hematemesis, or upper airway obstruction.

Diagnostic Evaluation

CXR often provides the first clues to the diagnosis of aortic dissections by revealing:

- Widening of the mediastinum (Figure 36-3)
- "Calcium sign" (separation of intimal calcification from outer aortic soft tissue border)
- Pleural effusion
- Tracheal deviation

Routine blood tests are typically nondiagnostic, although a novel immunoassay for smooth muscle myosin heavy chain has recently been introduced and appears to be a promising diagnostic technique in acute dissections.

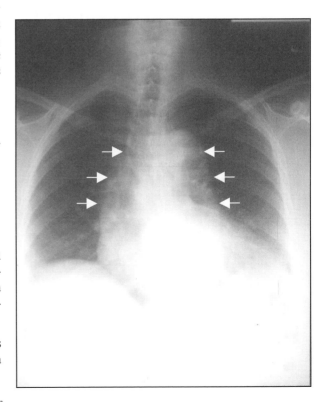

Figure 36-3 • CXR of a patient with an acute aortic dissection. Note the marked widening of the mediastinal shadow (arrows).

TABLE 36-2

Diagnostic Tests in the Evaluation of Aortic Dissection

Test	Advantages	Limitations	Sensitivity/Specificity
TEE	Performed at bedside; rapid; readily available; can assess LV function, valvular function, and pericardial disease; no contrast required; reasonable cost	Distal dissections may be missed; specificity dependent on strictness of diagnostic criteria; requires conscious sedation	Sensitivity 98% Specificity 77–97%
Contrast-enhanced CT (I$^+$ CT)	Rapid; readily available; can assess entire aorta; noninvasive; reasonable cost	Intimal flap often not identified; site of entry rarely seen; requires IV contrast; no information about aortic regurgitation	Sensitivity 85–95% Specificity 87–100%
MRA	Fairly rapid; noninvasive; no contrast required; can assess entire aorta and its branches; can assess LV function and aortic regurgitation	Not ideal for very unstable patients as patients are inaccessible during study; metal objects cannot be in vicinity of scanner; moderate cost	Sensitivity 98% Specificity 98%
Aortography	Fairly rapid; can assess entire aorta and its branches; can assess LV function and AR	False-negative results occur with simultaneous opacification of true and false lumens; invasive; requires IV contrast; high cost	Sensitivity 85–90% Specificity 94%

Several imaging modalities, including CT, MRI, and echocardiography, have been employed to aid in the rapid diagnosis of this disorder (see Table 36-2). Selection of a diagnostic test requires knowledge of the testing and expertise available at the institution as well as consideration of the patient's clinical status. In critically ill, hemodynamically unstable patients, TEE is the test of choice because it is rapid, portable, and highly sensitive for identifying thoracic aortic dissections (Figure 36-4). In more stable patients and those with suspected abdominal aortic dissections, CT or MRI is invaluable and can define the presence and extent of the dissection.

Treatment

Prompt, aggressive medical therapy aimed at lowering BP in hypertensive patients and decreasing LV contractility is crucial to the management of aortic dissections. All patients should be treated with intravenous beta blockers (e.g., labetalol, metoprolol, esmolol) to decrease the rate of pressure development (dP/dT) within the aorta, even if they are normotensive. Intravenous vasodilators (e.g., nitroprusside, enalaprilat) can rapidly lower BP. However, It is recommended that therapy with vasodilators be preceded by the administration of beta blockers, because marked vasodilation can result in reflex activation of

the sympathetic nervous system with enhanced contractility and increased shear stress (thereby propagating the dissection).

The overall mortality of an untreated aortic dissection is ~1%/hour for the first 48 hours and 65 to 75% in the first 2 weeks. Mortality of ascending aortic dissections is significantly improved with emergent surgical repair (~25% with surgery vs. ~60% with medical therapy). Conversely, descending aortic

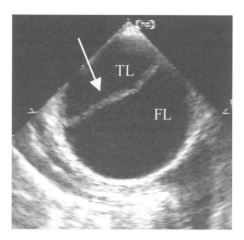

Figure 36-4 • TEE in a patient with a dissection of the descending thoracic aorta. An intimal flap (arrow) separates the true lumen (TL) from the false lumen (FL).

dissections are better managed without surgery unless vascular compromise is present (mortality ~10% with medical management vs. ~30% with surgery).

Surgical therapy includes resection of the damaged aortic segment, decompression of the false channel, and often resuspension of the aortic valve. Indications for surgery include:

- Acute ascending aortic dissection
- Any aortic dissection in a patient with Marfan syndrome
- Acute distal dissections complicated by vascular compromise, aneurysm formation, rupture or impending rupture, or retrograde propagation to the ascending aorta

As in the elective repair of aortic aneurysms, the use of endovascular stents in the treatment of acute aortic dissection is under investigation.

AORTITIS

Takayasu arteritis and giant-cell arteritis are the principal inflammatory diseases of the aorta. Aortitis can also occur in diseases such as SLE, syphilis, Wegener granulomatosis, Behçet disease, and Cogan syndrome and as a complication of Kawasaki disease. Systemic manifestations including fevers, malaise, fatigue, and weight loss are common. The aortic inflammation may narrow the aorta or its major branches and result in limb or organ ischemia; this may manifest as MI, limb claudication, HTN, or stroke. Treatment usually includes glucocorticoid therapy; however, there may be recurrences.

KEY POINTS

1. Leaking/ruptured aortic aneurysms and acute ascending aortic dissections require emergent surgical treatment.
2. Ascending aortic aneurysms are usually the result of cystic medial necrosis, whereas descending aortic aneurysms are usually atherosclerotic.
3. Asymptomatic thoracic aortic aneurysms should undergo surgical repair if they are >6 cm, whereas asymptomatic abdominal aortic aneurysms should undergo surgical repair if they are >5 cm.
4. Ascending aortic dissections require surgical repair, whereas descending aortic dissections are usually managed medically.
5. Takayasu arteritis and giant-cell arteritis are the principal inflammatory diseases of the aorta.

37 Carotid Arterial Disease

Cerebrovascular disease (CVD) is the third leading cause of death in the United States. A stroke carries an acute mortality of 20%, has a 5-year mortality of 50%, and produces substantial morbidity in survivors. Carotid artery disease represents a major cause of CVD. This chapter discusses the evaluation and management of carotid arterial disease but does not discuss the management of the neurologic syndromes that result.

Pathophysiology

The pathophysiology of carotid disease is that of atherosclerosis (see Chapter 9). The most common site of atheromatous lesion formation in the cerebral circulation is within 2 cm of the origin of the internal carotid arteries. Lesions that impair cerebral blood flow and result in cerebral ischemia can produce neurologic symptoms. The ischemia may result from either a severe flow-limiting carotid stenosis with inadequate collateral circulation or from an embolism originating from the site of the stenosis.

A carotid stenosis causes local acceleration of blood flow that can be heard as a bruit over the involved vessel. Among patients with carotid bruits, only 35 to 40% have hemodynamically significant carotid artery disease. Moreover, the absence of a carotid bruit does not exclude the presence of significant carotid artery disease. Patients with carotid bruits have an increased risk of TIA or stroke; however, these events are not always in the vascular territory supplied by the affected artery.

Clinical Manifestations

History

The vast majority of patients with carotid artery disease are asymptomatic. Symptoms, when present, occur as a result of cerebral ischemia and reflect the specific cerebral territory involved. Common presenting symptoms include:

- Arm and/or leg weakness
- Change in vision
- Difficulty speaking
- Difficulty walking
- Unilateral facial droop

Less common symptoms include headache, confusion, and seizure. Loss of consciousness is a distinctly uncommon presentation of carotid disease owing to the fact that it requires either bilateral cortical ischemia or brainstem ischemia, neither of which should occur in the setting of unilateral carotid disease. Many patients do not recognize their own neurologic deficits and are instead brought to medical attention at the insistence of others.

The clinical syndromes resulting from carotid arterial disease may be classified on the basis of the duration of the associated neurologic deficit.

- A **transient ischemic attack** is an ischemic neurologic symptom lasting less than 24 hours.
- A **reversible ischemic neurologic deficit (RIND)** is an ischemic event of 24 to 72 hours in duration.
- A permanent neurologic deficit is termed a **cerebrovascular accident (CVA)** or **stroke**.

Physical Examination

In the absence of a cerebral ischemic event, the physical examination may be completely normal, although a carotid bruit may be noted. The specific neurologic abnormalities present during a TIA or following a CVA vary depending on the location and extent of cerebral ischemia/infarction present. Common findings include:

- Contralateral homonymous hemianopsia
- Hemiparesis
- Hemisensory loss
- Aphasia (dominant-hemisphere ischemia)
- Hemineglect (nondominant-hemisphere ischemia)
- Transient monocular blindness (amaurosis fugax)
- Constructional apraxia (nondominant-hemisphere ischemia)

Careful physical examination may also disclose evidence of coronary or peripheral vascular disease, as these conditions often coexist.

Diagnostic Evaluation

Imaging of the carotid arteries is warranted both in patients with asymptomatic carotid bruits and in those who have suffered a transient or permanent cerebral ischemic event. Carotid duplex ultrasound is the usual initial test following a TIA/CVA and can be used as a screening test in patients with suspected carotid disease. Although reasonably accurate (sensitivity 91 to 94%; specificity 95 to 99%), it can only visualize the cervical portion of the carotid artery. MRA and CT are more sensitive studies and can image the intracranial as well as the carotid vessels. However, these studies are more expensive and less readily available. Additionally, MRA cannot be performed in patients with pacemakers or other metal implants, and CT angiography is invasive and requires the use of IV contrast. Cerebral angiography remains the "gold standard" for imaging the carotid arteries; however, it is usually reserved for patients who are undergoing carotid endarterectomy (see below).

Treatment

The treatment of carotid artery disease depends on the presence or absence of symptoms and the severity of the stenosis. Nonpharmacologic therapy is applied to all patient groups with carotid artery disease and consists of aggressive risk-factor modification (BP control, blood sugar control, smoking cessation, and lipid-lowering therapy).

Antiplatelet therapy is the mainstay of medical management for carotid artery disease. Aspirin has been shown clearly to decrease the risk of subsequent stroke in patients who have suffered a TIA or CVA. The appropriate dose is between 75 and 325 mg/day. The efficacy of stroke prevention with clopidogrel (75 mg/day) is at least equal to that of aspirin and may exceed it; a combination of aspirin and dipyridamole is an alternative antiplatelet regimen. The utility of these agents in patients with asymptomatic carotid disease is not clear. Warfarin is not routinely indicated in the therapy of carotid artery disease (in the absence of stroke), but it is often used in patients with very severe stenoses awaiting surgery and in those who have recurrent ischemic events despite antiplatelet therapy.

Surgical therapy for carotid artery stenosis consists of resection of the carotid plaque, i.e., carotid endarterectomy (CEA). Long-term antiplatelet therapy is an obligatory adjunct to this surgery. CEA clearly reduces the long-term risk of CVA in patients with symptomatic carotid disease. The data are less clear for patients with asymptomatic carotid stenoses, although patients with moderate to severe carotid artery stenoses (>60%) likely benefit. Table 37-1 summarizes the currently accepted criteria for CEA in symptomatic and asymptomatic carotid disease. PTCA and carotid stent placement hold promise for the treatment of carotid disease, although these procedures may be associated with a higher procedure-related stroke rate than is CEA. In general, these percutaneous procedures are reserved for patients who are not felt to be candidates for CEA owing to comorbid illness.

■ TABLE 37-1

Recommendations Regarding Carotid Endarterectomy in Patients with Carotid Artery Disease Based on Stenosis Severity and the Presence or Absence of Symptoms

	CEA Not Indicated	CEA Acceptable but of No Proven Benefit	CEA Beneficial
Symptomatic	<30% stenosis (**NNT* 67**)	30–69% stenosis (**NNT 20**)	70–99% stenosis[†] (**NNT 8**)
Asymptomatic	<60% stenosis (**NNT 83**)		60–99% stenosis[‡] (**NNT 48**)

*NNT signifies the number needed to treat to prevent one ischemic stroke.
†Provided surgical risk <6%.
‡Provided surgical risk <3%.

KEY POINTS

1. Carotid artery disease is predominantly the result of atherosclerosis.
2. Significant stenosis of the carotid artery may occur in the absence of symptoms.
3. Neurologic symptoms resulting from carotid artery disease may be transient (TIA, RIND) or permanent (CVA).
4. All patients with symptomatic carotid disease should receive antiplatelet therapy.
5. Carotid endarterectomy is indicated in patients with symptomatic moderate to severe carotid artery stenoses (>70%) and should be considered in asymptomatic patients with >60% carotid artery stenosis.

Chapter 38

Deep Venous Thrombosis and Pulmonary Embolic Disease

■ VENOUS THROMBOEMBOLIC DISEASE

Venous thromboembolism (VTE) accounts for significant morbidity and mortality. Over 500,000 cases of pulmonary embolism (PE) occur in the United States annually, accounting for about 200,000 deaths each year. The mortality rate of untreated PE is approximately 30%; this is due, in large part, to recurrent emboli. Despite advances in diagnostic modalities and therapeutic strategies, it is estimated that the majority of patients with PE remain undiagnosed.

Pathogenesis

Venous thrombosis most commonly involves the deep veins of the lower extremities, although the superficial veins, veins of the upper extremity, and pelvic and renal veins may also be involved. Predisposing factors involve stasis, vascular injury, and hypercoagulability (the Virchow triad). Both hereditary and acquired factors contribute (see Box 38-1). Venous thrombosis is usually associated with inflammation of the vessel wall (thrombophlebitis). The thrombi may detach, embolize through the venous system, and lodge in the pulmonary arteries. Large thrombi may lodge in the main pulmonary artery bifurcation, causing hemodynamic instability (saddle embolus), whereas smaller emboli lodge in distal pulmonary arterial branches and may be clinically silent.

Occlusion of small pulmonary arteries results in increased pulmonary vascular resistance (both directly, and indirectly via release of vasoactive substances from the thrombus), pulmonary HTN, RV hypertrophy, and eventually RV failure. The PE also impairs gas exchange in the affected lung regions, resulting in hypoxemia and an increased alveolar-arterial oxygen gradient (A-a gradient). Pulmonary infarction occurs infrequently (<10% of pulmonary emboli).

Clinical Manifestations

History

The most common presenting complaint associated with a DVT is calf pain. Additionally, patients may note unilateral leg swelling, erythema or warmth, and low-grade fevers. In obtaining a history from a patient with DVT, it is important to note the following:

- History of trauma or other injury
- History of recent prolonged immobility
- Use of prescription medications (including oral contraceptive pills), recreational drugs, or tobacco
- Prior history of thrombosis or abnormal bleeding
- History of malignancy
- Family history of thrombosis

Patients with recurrent DVT frequently have a hypercoagulable state. Patients with underlying carcinoma (especially adenocarcinomas) may have a migratory superficial thrombophlebitis (Trousseau syndrome).

The most common presenting symptom of PE is sudden dyspnea, which occurs in approximately 80% of patients. Additional symptoms include:

- Pleuritic chest pain (66%; associated with pulmonary infarction)
- Cough (20%)
- Hemoptysis (10%)
- Syncope (10%)

Physical Examination

Physical findings associated with DVT may include the following:

BOX 38-1 CAUSES OF VENOUS THROMBOEMBOLIC DISEASE

Hereditary hypercoagulable states
Factor V Leiden mutation
Activated protein-C resistance
Protein-C deficiency
Protein-S deficiency
Antithrombin III deficiency
Prothrombin G20210A mutation
Hyperhomocyst(e)inemia
Antiphospholipid antibody syndrome
Plasminogen deficiency
Dysfibrinogenemia
Factor XII deficiency
Inherited thrombophilia
Elevated factor VIII coagulant activity

Acquired conditions
Stasis:
    Immobilization (stroke, spinal cord injury, prolonged travel)
    Obesity
    Pregnancy
    Advanced age
    Heart failure
Vascular injury:
    Trauma
    Surgery
    Indwelling venous catheters
    Prior DVT
Hypercoagulability:
    Surgery
    Malignancy
    Oral contraceptives
    Smoking
    Pregnancy
    Nephrotic syndrome

- Calf asymmetry, erythema, warmth, and/or tenderness
- Pedal edema
- Homans sign (calf pain with resisted dorsiflexion of the foot)
- Venous engorgement
- Palpable thrombosed vein (a cord) in the posterior calf
- Phlegmasia cerulea dolens (cyanotic hue due to deoxygenated hemoglobin in stagnant veins)
- Phlegmasia alba dolens (pallor associated with massive edema)

The physical examination of patients with PE may be normal but often demonstrates signs of pulmonary HTN or right HF, including:

- Tachypnea (60%)
- Tachycardia (40%)
- Elevated JVP with prominent V waves
- Right-sided S_3 or S_4
- Murmur of tricuspid regurgitation
- Accentuated pulmonic component of S_2 (P_2)
- RV heave

The lung fields are usually clear, although a pulmonary rub may be heard over the involved area of lung when pulmonary infarction has occurred.

Differential Diagnosis

The differential diagnosis of DVT includes cellulitis, venous insufficiency, ruptured Baker cyst, lymphedema, and muscular injury. The differential diagnosis of PE includes pneumonia, pleurisy, pneumothorax, MI, pericarditis, CHF, and anxiety.

Diagnostic Evaluation (See Figure 38-1)

Duplex venous ultrasonography is the most common test used to confirm the diagnosis of DVT and has a

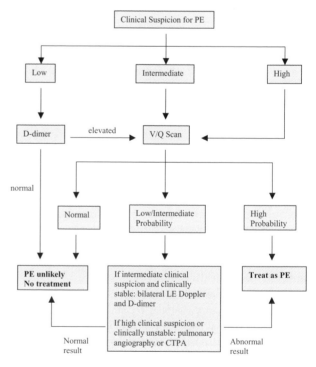

Figure 38-1 • Diagnostic algorithm for patients with suspected PE. CTPA: CT of the chest with IV injection of contrast.

sensitivity and specificity of >95%. Other noninvasive tests (e.g., impedance plethysmography) are used less frequently. Contrast venography remains the "gold standard" for the diagnosis of DVT (sensitivity and specificity 100%) but is typically reserved for cases in which noninvasive testing is equivocal.

In patients with PE, arterial blood gas analysis typically demonstrates a respiratory alkalosis, hypocapnea, and hypoxemia. Additionally, the A-a gradient is increased (>10 mm Hg). The A-a gradient can be calculated by the following formula:

$$A\text{-a gradient} = [(P_{atm} - P_{H_2O})\,(F_{IO_2}) \\ -(P_{CO_2}/0.8)] - P_{aO_2}$$

Where P_{atm} is atmospheric pressure (760 mm Hg at sea level), P_{H_2O} is the partial pressure of water in the atmosphere (47 mm Hg), F_{IO_2} is the percent oxygen in the inspired air (21% in room air), P_{CO_2} is the partial pressure of carbon dioxide in the blood, and P_{aO_2} is the partial pressure of oxygen in the blood.

The ECG is abnormal in the majority of patients with an acute PE and may show a deep S wave in lead I and a deep Q-wave and T-wave inversion in lead III (S_1-Q_3-T_3). Other frequent patterns include sinus tachycardia, an incomplete or complete RBBB, or T-wave inversions in the inferior leads (II, III, aVF) or anterior leads (V_1 to V_4).

Chest radiography is frequently normal in patients with PE but may reveal decreased vascular markings in the affected lung regions (Westermark sign), a wedge-shaped peripheral infiltrate (Hampton hump), or an enlarged right descending PA (Palla sign). V/Q lung scan is the usual initial diagnostic test for PE. Using two different radioactive tracers (one injected intravenously and one inhaled), blood flow and ventilation in each area of the lung are compared. Lack of perfusion in an area that is ventilated normally (V/Q mismatch) is consistent with PE. Normal and near-normal tests virtually exclude the diagnosis, while a high-probability result is confirmatory. However, in patients for whom there is high clinical suspicion of PE, a low- or intermediate-probability scan is unhelpful, as at least 40% of these patients have a PE.

CT of the pulmonary arteries with IV contrast (CTPA; also called spiral CT or PE protocol CT) and MRA with gadolinium enhancement can confirm or exclude the diagnosis if the V/Q scan is equivocal, but may miss small peripheral emboli. A CTPA is generally the test of choice in patients with intrinsic lung disease and an abnormal chest radiograph. Pulmonary angiography (catheterization of the pulmonary arteries and injection of contrast) remains the "gold standard" for diagnosis of PE.

Other tests that may be helpful in the evaluation of PE include:

- Echocardiography—demonstrates signs of pulmonary hypertension and/or right ventricular dysfunction
- Lower extremity duplex ultrasonography—a negative result does not exclude the diagnosis of PE as up to 50% of patients with PE have no evidence of DVT
- D-dimer (a fibrin degradation product)—a normal value, if obtained by the enzyme-linked immunosorbent assay (ELISA) technique, essentially excludes PE with a negative predictive value of ~90%. The negative predictive value is even higher when combined with a normal lower extremity duplex. D-dimer is elevated in patients with recent surgery, MI, malignancy, or infection. Positive results in these settings are not diagnostic of PE.

Treatment

In patients with suspected DVT or PE, anticoagulant therapy should be started immediately and supplemental oxygen and pain management instituted as needed. It is imperative that therapeutic anticoagulation (1.5 to 2.0 times the control PTT value if unfractionated heparin is used) be achieved in the first 24 hours to decrease the risk of recurrent DVT/PE and postphlebitic syndrome. Unfractionated heparin may be used initially (using a weight-based protocol), although LMWH may be more effective. Advantages of LMWH include its greater bioavailability, ease of administration (subcutaneous injection), reliable anticoagulant effect, lack of need for laboratory monitoring, and lower incidence of heparin-induced thrombocytopenia.

Oral anticoagulation with warfarin may be begun concurrently with heparin but should overlap with heparin therapy for 5 to 7 days to avoid the transient hypercoagulability that may occur after warfarin initiation. Heparin may be discontinued once the INR is therapeutic (2.0 to 3.0). Anticoagulation should be continued for 3 to 6 months in patients presenting with their first DVT and for 6 months in patients with PE. Prolonged therapy may be required in patients with recurrent DVT/PE, underlying malignancy, or primary hypercoagulable states. Patients

BOX 38-2	INDICATIONS FOR PLACEMENT OF AN INFERIOR VENA CAVA FILTER

Recurrent PE on therapeutic anticoagulation
Contraindications to anticoagulation
Active bleeding that is life-threatening
Postsurgical (relative)
Thrombocytopenia (spontaneous or heparin-induced)
Prophylaxis in high-risk patients
Extensive venous thrombosis
Severe pulmonary HTN, cor pulmonale

with recurrent DVT despite therapeutic anticoagulation and those with contraindications to anticoagulation may benefit from placement of an IVC filter (see Box 38-2).

Patients presenting with massive PE associated with hemodynamic instability should be treated with thrombolytic therapy. If this is contraindicated or unsuccessful, percutaneous or open surgical thrombectomy should be considered.

The treatment of DVT limited to the calf is controversial. These thrombi pose a much lower risk of embolism, although 10 to 15% will progress to the thigh. Conservative therapy with NSAIDs is the usual course, coupled with serial noninvasive studies (weekly for 2 to 3 weeks) to identify thrombi that propagate proximally and therefore warrant anticoagulation.

Prophylaxis of Deep Venous Thrombosis

Prophylaxis against DVT is critical for reducing the morbidity and mortality of this disease and should be considered in high-risk clinical situations (hospitalization, postoperative states, prolonged immobility, etc.). Prophylactic therapy may consist of external pneumatic compression or low-dose subcutaneous administration of unfractionated heparin (5,000 units twice daily) or LMWH (e.g., enoxaparin 30 mg twice daily or 40 mg once daily).

KEY POINTS

1. Predisposing factors for DVT include stasis, vascular injury, and hypercoagulability.
2. Approximately 80% of patients with PE present with dyspnea.
3. The initial diagnostic test of choice for DVT is duplex ultrasonography, whereas V/Q scan is the test of choice for PE.
4. Once DVT or PE is suspected, anticoagulation with unfractionated heparin or LMWH should be started immediately; therapeutic levels should be established within 24 hours. Warfarin should be initiated soon after heparin therapy.
5. Patients with recurrent DVT or underlying hypercoagulable state require long-term anticoagulation.
6. Thrombolytic therapy or surgical thrombectomy should be considered for patients with hemodynamically significant PE.
7. DVT prophylaxis is important in high-risk patients.

Pulmonary Hypertension

Pulmonary HTN is a disorder defined by a mean PA pressure >25 mm Hg at rest or >30 mm Hg with exercise (PA mean = 1/3 PA systolic pressure +2/3 PA diastolic pressure). A variety of disorders can result in pulmonary HTN (**secondary pulmonary HTN**, or SPH) by producing alterations in pulmonary blood flow, pulmonary vascular tone, pulmonary venous pressure, or the size of the pulmonary vascular bed. When pulmonary HTN occurs in the absence of an identifiable cause, it is referred to as **primary pulmonary HTN** (PPH).

Epidemiology and Pathogenesis

The incidence of PPH is estimated at two cases per million people per year. PPH classically afflicts young and middle-aged women. Its etiology is unknown, but a familial component has been described, suggesting a genetic susceptibility. Current theories implicate the interaction between endothelial and smooth muscle cells, in addition to an imbalance of vasoactive amines, in the pathogenesis of PPH. The classic histopathologic finding in PPH consists of intimal proliferation, in situ thrombosis, and plexogenic arteriopathy.

Secondary pulmonary HTN may result from:

1. **Increased pulmonary blood flow** associated with:

- Intracardiac shunts (ASD, VSD)
- PDA

2. **Hypoxic vasoconstriction** associated with:

- Emphysema
- Obstructive sleep apnea and other hypoventilation syndromes
- High altitude

3. **Pulmonary venous HTN** associated with:

- MV disease (stenosis or regurgitation)
- LV failure
- Pulmonary venous thrombosis
- Constrictive pericarditis
- Congenital anomalies (e.g., cor triatriatum)

4. **A decrease in the size of the pulmonary vascular bed** associated with:

- COPD
- Connective tissue disorders
- Vasculitis (e.g., SLE, systemic sclerosis)
- HIV infection
- PE disease
- Toxic injury (e.g., crack cocaine, L-tryptophan, fenfluramine, rapeseed oil)
- Liver dysfunction (hepatopulmonary syndrome)

Clinical Manifestations

History

Patients with pulmonary HTN commonly present with advanced disease because of the insidious progression of their symptoms. Symptoms generally include:

- Dyspnea at rest and/or with exertion (occurs in >95% of patients)
- Fatigue, lethargy
- Exertional syncope (due to an inability to augment cardiac output)
- Chest pain (due to PA "stretch" or RV ischemia)
- Cough, hemoptysis
- Hoarseness (due to compression of the left recurrent laryngeal nerve by the dilated PA)
- Anorexia, right-upper-quadrant pain (from liver congestion)
- Peripheral edema (due to right HF)

In evaluating a patient with suspected pulmonary HTN, a detailed history must be obtained and should include questions about the following: use of appetite suppressants or IV drugs, smoking, HIV risk factors, symptoms of liver disease, connective tissue disorders, venous thrombotic disease, and lung disease.

Physical Examination

The physical findings in pulmonary HTN occur as a result of either RV strain or RV failure (cor pulmonale) secondary to chronically elevated PA pressure. Hypoxia (either ambulatory or nocturnal) is a uniform finding. Other physical findings include:

- Tachypnea
- Elevated JVP
- Loud pulmonic component of the P_2
- Palpable P_2
- Tricuspid regurgitation
- RV S_3 and/or S_4
- Left parasternal (RV) lift
- Hepatomegaly, ascites
- Pulsatile liver (with severe tricuspid regurgitation)
- Peripheral edema

Differential Diagnosis

The differential diagnosis of pulmonary HTN is similar to the differential diagnosis of dyspnea (see Chapter 1) and includes cardiac (myocardial and valvular diseases), pulmonary (pulmonary parenchymal and vascular diseases), and systemic (anemia, physical deconditioning) disorders.

Diagnostic Evaluation

Several diagnostic studies provide indirect evidence of pulmonary HTN. The ECG may reveal right-axis deviation, RV hypertrophy or strain, RA enlargement, or RBBB (see Figure 39-1). Chest radiography may demonstrate enlargement of the central pulmonary arteries or RV and pruning of the peripheral pulmonary vessels. Signs of chronic RV pressure overload apparent by echocardiography include RV hypertrophy and dilation, RA enlargement, abnormal interventricular septal flattening, and tricuspid regurgitation. The PA pressure can be estimated during Doppler echocardiography by measuring the velocity of the tricuspid regurgitation jet and converting this velocity into a pressure using the equation $P = 4V^2$ (97% correlation with measurement by PA catheter). Direct transduction of the PA pressure can be obtained using a PA catheter (Swan-Ganz catheter); this is the "gold standard" for the diagnosis of pulmonary HTN.

In the case of SPH, additional laboratory studies should be obtained in an attempt to identify the underlying process. These studies may include arterial blood gases, LFTs, HIV antibody assays, connective

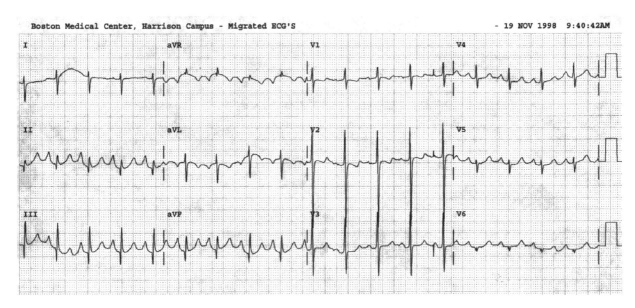

Figure 39-1 • ECG of a patient with pulmonary HTN. Characteristic features include right axis deviation (QRS axis is +130 degrees), RA enlargement (P wave in lead II >0.25 mV), and RVH (R > S in V_1, S > R in V_6).

tissue serology, pulmonary function tests, sleep studies, V/Q lung scanning, or pulmonary angiography. There is no specific test available to diagnose PPH; this is a diagnosis of exclusion.

Treatment

Primary pulmonary HTN is an incurable disease with a poor prognosis (median survival of 2 to 3 years from the time of diagnosis). It is only in the last 15 years that advances in medical and surgical therapies have been able to alter the natural history of this disease.

Vasoconstriction is thought to play an important role in the pathogenesis of PPH. Accordingly, treatment with vasodilators has received a great deal of attention, although not all patients exhibit a uniform response to vasodilator therapy. The oral vasodilators of choice are CCBs such as nifedipine or diltiazem. These agents result in sustained clinical improvement in approximately 25 to 30% of patients.

Epoprostenol (prostacyclin), a potent vasodilator that acts by increasing intracellular levels of cAMP, has been found to produce both acute and sustained hemodynamic improvement in patients with PPH. It is administered as a continuous infusion (inhaled forms are available in Europe) and has been shown to improve exercise tolerance and prolong survival. Continuous epoprostenol therapy is currently used either as primary treatment or as a bridge to lung transplantation in patients with PPH, depending on the degree of observed hemodynamic improvement. Bosentan is an oral antagonist of endothelin-1, which is a potent pulmonary vasoconstrictor. Studies show a favorable effect on exercise tolerance and clinical outcomes, although experience with this agent is limited.

Retrospective analysis of small, nonrandomized studies suggests that chronic anticoagulation in patients with PPH improves survival. Therefore the general consensus is to treat these patients with warfarin to achieve an INR of 1.5 to 2.5. Single-lung and combined heart-lung transplantation remain the only definitive therapies for PPH. One-year survival following lung transplantation approaches 65 to 70%.

The mainstay of treatment of SPH is treatment of the underlying disease. Accepted general treatment modalities include supplemental oxygen for patients with hypoxemia, diuretics for symptomatic relief of ascites and hepatic congestion, and anticoagulation for patients at high risk for thromboembolic events. Specific therapies aimed at treating or correcting the underlying disorder (e.g., valve replacement for mitral disease, surgical correction of intracardiac shunts,

maximization of medical therapy for left HF) may lead to normalization of pulmonary pressures and marked improvement in symptoms. Other treatment options of less clear benefit in SPH include CCBs and other vasodilators. Patients with certain forms of SPH that have histopathologic findings in common with PPH (connective tissue disorders, HIV, hepatopulmonary syndrome) have shown improvement in hemodynamics, exercise tolerance, and survival on epoprostenol therapy.

KEY POINTS

1. Pulmonary HTN is defined as a mean pulmonary pressure greater than 25 mm Hg at rest or greater than 30 mm Hg with exercise.
2. Primary pulmonary HTN is a diagnosis of exclusion and is most commonly seen in young and middle-aged women.
3. Secondary pulmonary HTN may result from a variety of cardiovascular, pulmonary, and systemic disorders.
4. PA catheterization is the "gold standard" for the diagnosis of PH, but elevated pulmonary pressures can often be identified by echocardiography.
5. Primary pulmonary HTN is an incurable disease. Vasodilators (CCBs or epoprostenol) are the mainstay of therapy; transplantation is the definitive treatment.
6. The treatment of SPH relies primarily on treatment of the underlying condition.

Part Nine

Other Important Cardiac Conditions

Chapter 40

Preoperative Cardiac Evaluation

Internists and cardiologists are frequently consulted regarding the preoperative evaluation of patients undergoing noncardiac surgery. This process involves assessing the risk of a given patient for developing an adverse cardiac event (MI, heart HF, or death) during the perioperative period and formulating recommendations aimed at minimizing this risk. In general, a physician cannot "clear" a patient for a surgical procedure (there is never a zero risk of cardiac or other adverse events during surgery), and the patient or his or her family must understand and be willing to accept the level of risk as determined by the preoperative assessment.

Presurgical patients should be evaluated within the broader context of their medical problems, and diagnostic tests or therapeutic interventions should not be performed unless the treating physician would consider pursuing the workup in the absence of the planned procedure. In general, the treatment and evaluation of cardiac diseases are the same perioperatively as they are in the nonoperative setting. Furthermore, preoperative testing should be performed only if the results of the test will affect patient management.

■ PREDICTORS OF RISK

Several factors are taken into account in determining the overall risk of a surgical procedure: patient-specific factors (known as clinical predictors), the specific type of surgery planned, and the patient's exercise capacity.

Patient-Specific Risks

The initial evaluation of the preoperative patient should include a complete history and physical examination, with careful attention to identifying the presence of cardiovascular disease and medical comorbidities known to be associated with increased perioperative risk (see Table 40-1). A 12-lead ECG is essential to document prior infarction, active ischemia, or arrhythmia (including conduction system disease).

The presence of major clinical predictors of risk should prompt delay or cancellation of surgery until the cardiac condition is fully evaluated and stabilized.

■ TABLE 40-1

Clinical Predictors of Increased Perioperative Cardiovascular Risk

Major predictors	Unstable coronary syndromes (acute or recent MI, UA) Decompensated HF Arrhythmia with potential hemodynamic compromise (high-grade AV block, symptomatic ventricular arrhythmias, atrial arrhythmias with uncontrolled ventricular rate) Severe valvular disease
Intermediate predictors	Mild angina (class I–II) Prior MI History of HF, currently compensated DM Renal insufficiency (creatinine >2)
Minor predictors	Older age Abnormal ECG Rhythm other than sinus Poor exercise tolerance Stroke Uncontrolled hypertension

Patients with decompensated HF should have an assessment of their cardiac function (i.e., echocardiogram) if it is not already known, and medical management of their heart failure should be maximized before proceeding to surgery. Patients with active ischemic heart disease should be considered for cardiac catheterization and revascularization provided that the surgery is not urgent/emergent.

Surgery-Specific Risk

Not all surgical procedures carry the same potential for adverse cardiovascular events. For example, emergent operations and procedures involving prolonged anesthesia or major volume shifts carry a risk that can be above 5%, whereas biopsies and endoscopy are associated with a low risk (less than 1%; see Table 40-2).

Functional Status

After patient- and surgery-specific risks have been assessed, the overall perioperative risk can be further defined by considering the patient's exercise capacity. Patients who routinely engage in moderate exertion during their daily lives have a much lower perioperative risk than do their counterparts who can only exert themselves to a minor degree. In general, if an individual has no major or intermediate clinical risk predictors and can achieve a workload of at least 4 METs without untoward cardiac or pulmonary symptoms,

noncardiac surgery is considered safe. Examples of 4 METs of activity include climbing one flight of stairs or walking at 4 mph. Eating equals 1 MET, and strenuous sports are usually above 10 METS.

■ AN ALGORITHMIC APPROACH

Once the patient's clinical risk predictors, the nature of the planned procedure, and the patient's functional status have been clarified, recommendations regarding the need for further cardiac testing and the timing of surgery can be made. The algorithm in Figure 40-1 is a well-established and widely used tool to help synthesize overall cardiac risk and summarize appropriate courses of action in several specific situations. It should be noted that patients who have undergone coronary revascularization within the preceding 5 years or have had a cardiac catheterization or stress test with good results within the preceding 2 years do not need further coronary risk stratification preoperatively unless their symptoms or exercise capacity have changed significantly.

■ DIAGNOSTIC EVALUATION (SEE ALSO CHAPTER 4: STRESS TESTING)

Further diagnostic evaluation is sometimes warranted to clarify the presence and severity of CAD and determine the appropriate treatment approach prior to elective surgery. Patients with major clinical predictors do not require further testing; they require aggressive treatment of their heart disease. Patient with only minor clinical predictors of risk rarely if ever require further cardiac testing preoperatively. In general, noninvasive testing for ischemia should be considered if two of the following three factors are present:

- Intermediate clinical predictors
- Planned high-risk surgery
- Low functional capacity

However, noninvasive tests should be performed only when their results will affect the patient's perioperative management. Based on the results of this testing, coronary angiography and revascularization (i.e., invasive evaluation) may be considered.

■ OTHER CARDIAC CONDITIONS

In addition to possible stress testing to evaluate myocardial ischemia, other cardiovascular conditions should be addressed and managed preoperatively. HTN should

■ TABLE 40-2	
Risk of Adverse Cardiac Event Associated with Specific Surgeries	
High risk (>5%)	Emergent, major surgery (especially in the elderly)
	Major vascular surgery, including aortic
	Peripheral vascular procedures
	Prolonged procedures with large fluid shifts or high-volume blood loss
Intermediate risk (1–5%)	Carotid endarterectomy
	Head and neck operations
	Intrathoracic and intraperitoneal operations
	Orthopedic surgery
	Prostate surgery
Low risk (<1%)	Endoscopy
	Cataract surgery
	Breast surgery
	Biopsies, other superficial procedures

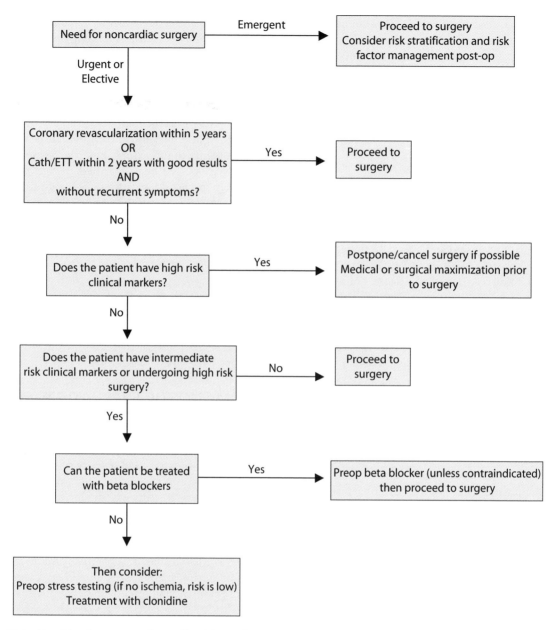

Figure 40-1 • Algorithm for preoperative cardiac risk stratification.

be controlled (ideally with a regimen including beta blockers) and valvular lesions fully assessed. In general, stenotic valvular lesions are tolerated less well perioperatively than are regurgitant lesions; valvular stenosis may need to be corrected (i.e., with balloon valvuloplasty or valve replacement) prior to elective noncardiac surgery. Hemodynamic monitoring in patients with symptomatic regurgitant lesions, recent MI, or CMP can be achieved during and after surgery with a PA catheter (see Chapter 6), although this type of invasive monitoring has not to been shown to reduce perioperative events and its use is controversial. Patients with tachyarrhythmias (e.g., AF) must be stabilized with medications (such as beta blockers) preoperatively, and patients with high-degree HB should be considered for temporary or permanent pacemaker implantation preoperatively.

PERIOPERATIVE MEDICAL THERAPY

Patients who need medications for the control of chronic cardiac conditions preoperatively will definitely require these medications to maintain a stable cardiac status perioperatively. It is essential that all chronic cardiac medications be continued throughout the perioperative period unless there are compelling reasons to withhold them. If the patient is unable to take medications orally, IV or transcutaneous formulations should be substituted.

Beta blockers have been shown to decrease the incidence of perioperative cardiovascular events in a wide range of patients who have ischemic heart disease or are at risk for it. In high-risk patients (i.e, those with ischemia, uncontrolled HTN, or major risk factors for coronary disease) beta blockade should be initiated several days to weeks before elective procedures and continued perioperatively. In these patients, the goal resting heart rate is between 50 and 60 bpm in the perioperative period. Clonidine is an alternative therapy in patients who are intolerant of beta blockers.

THE ROLE OF REVASCULARIZATION

Patients who have undergone coronary revascularization have a lower risk of perioperative complications when they undergo subsequent noncardiac surgery. However, when PCI is performed with intracoronary stent placement 4 to 6 weeks prior to the noncardiac surgery, the risk of perioperative complications is increased. Specifically, there is an increased risk of MI (resulting from stent thrombosis) and major bleeding (resulting from the obligatory use of combined antiplatelet therapy after coronary stenting). Therefore preoperative PCI/stenting is appropriate only if the noncardiac surgery can be delayed for at least 4 to 6 weeks to allow the patient to benefit from the revascularization procedure. Use of the new drug-eluting stents may require even longer periods of delay.

For example, a patient with CAD who is scheduled for colectomy for colon cancer should not undergo cardiac catheterization and PCI in the absence of an unstable coronary syndrome. The invasive approach would require combined antiplatelet therapy for an extended period (minimum 4 weeks), thereby postponing a potentially curative operation. In general, coronary revascularization should be performed preoperatively only in patients with very unstable coronary disease or a very high ischemic burden on noninvasive testing.

SURVEILLENCE

It is essential that patients who are seen for a preoperative evaluation be followed closely in the postoperative period. This ensures that recommendations are followed and complications identified as early as possible. In patients with ischemic disease, an ECG should be checked routinely immediately after surgery and on the following day to assess for an occult ischemic event. New recommendations should be made depending on the patient's clinical course, and the patient's usual medications should be restarted as soon as possible after surgery.

KEY POINTS

1. Assessment of perioperative cardiovascular risk involves consideration of the patient's clinical predictors and the risk of the surgery.
2. Diagnostic tests or therapeutic interventions should not be performed simply to "get the patient through" the surgery.
3. Noninvasive (stress testing) or invasive (cardiac catheterization) evaluation is sometimes warranted to clarify and/or treat cardiac ischemia prior to elective procedures.
4. Perioperative beta blockade should be considered in all patients with ischemic heart disease or at risk for it.
5. PCI should be avoided preoperatively unless the patient is extremely unstable or the surgery can be delayed for 4 to 6 weeks.
6. Postoperative surveillance is essential for the early recognition of adverse cardiac events.

Chapter 41

Congenital Heart Disease

CONGENITAL CARDIAC SHUNTS

Intracardiac shunts are the second most common congenital heart defects; only bicuspid aortic valves are more common. VSDs account for 30% of all CHD and are common findings in infants and children. Some 50 to 70% of VSDs close spontaneously during childhood; thus they are rarely first diagnosed in adults. ASDs and PDAs each account for 10% of CHD. ASDs are the most common CHDs diagnosed in adulthood but are infrequently diagnosed in infancy.

Pathogenesis

Prior to birth, the pulmonary and systemic circulation communicate. Blood entering the RA is directed across the foramen ovale into the LA, and blood entering the PA flows through the ductus arteriosus into the aorta. These communications help to limit blood flow to the pulmonary system, since the lungs are nonfunctional prior to birth. Shortly after birth, these anatomic connections usually seal off.

Occasionally the formation of the interatrial septum is incomplete, resulting in a defect (ASD) that allows for interatrial shunting of blood (Figure 41-1). The defect may be of three general types, based on location:

- Sinus venosus defect (at the superior aspect of the septum near the vena cava)
- Ostium secundum defect (at the site of the fossa ovalis)
- Ostium primum defect (at the inferior aspect of the interatrial septum near the AV plane)

Identification of the particular type of ASD is important because each is associated with specific concomitant congenital abnormalities (see Table 41-1).

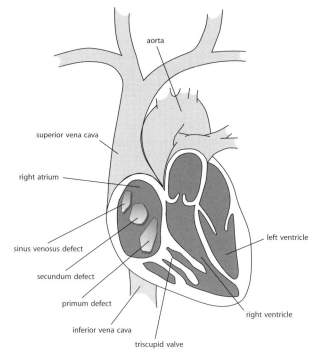

Figure 41-1 • Diagram of the various types of atrial septal defects.

In approximately 25% of patients, the interatrial septum forms completely but the foramen ovale fails to seal off following birth. This does not lead to shunting of blood in the resting state but can lead to shunt flow if the RA pressure exceeds the LA pressure (patent foramen ovale).

The interventricular septum may also fail to form correctly, resulting in a VSD. VSDs are of two main types:

- Membranous VSD (located high in the septum)
- Muscular VSD (located in the mid- to distal septum)

■ TABLE 41-1

Types of Atrial Septal Defects and Associated Abnormalities

Type of ASD	Relative Prevalence	Associated Abnormalities	Classic ECG Findings
Ostium primum	20%	Cleft mitral valve, Down syndrome	Incomplete RBBB, left axis deviation, first-degree AV block
Ostium secundum	70%	Mitral valve prolapse	rSr' in V_1
Sinus venosus	10%	Anomalous pulmonary venous return	None

Last, in some infants, the ductus arteriosus fails to constrict after birth and remains patent (PDA).

ASDs, VSDs, and PDAs allow for the abnormal flow of blood between the right and left circulation. Because the pressure in the left side of the heart is higher than that in the right, the shunt flow is usually from left to right and results in increased flow in the pulmonary circulation (Qp) compared with that in the systemic circulation (Qs). The ratio of these flows (Qp:Qs) is a method of quantifying shunt severity. Over time, the increased pulmonary flow results in pulmonary HTN and right HF. Rarely, the right heart pressure may then exceed the left heart pressure, resulting in right-to-left shunting of blood (Eisenmenger syndrome; see below).

Clinical Manifestations

Infants and children with ASDs are usually asymptomatic but may occasionally present with signs of CHF. Large VSDs tend to produce HF at a young age.

Adults with an ASD, PDA, or small VSD usually present with either arrhythmias (e.g., AF) or symptoms of progressive right HF and pulmonary HTN, including:

- Dyspnea with exertion
- Peripheral edema
- Fatigue
- Chest pain

Patients with intracardiac shunts may occasionally present with a stroke caused by a thromboembolism that enters the systemic circulation through the defect (paradoxical embolus). Physical examination of patients with cardiac shunts may reveal signs of right HF. The characteristic findings on cardiac examination are outlined in Table 41-2.

Diagnostic Evaluation

Patients with suspected cardiac shunts should undergo echocardiography to locate the defect (TEE may be

■ TABLE 41-2

Some Physical Characteristics of Atrial Septal Defect, Ventricular Septal Defect, and Patent Ductus Arteriosus

Defect	Physical Examination Findings	Useful Diagnostic Modalities
ASD	Fixed split S_2 Midsystolic pulmonary ejection murmur Prominent RV impulse Cyanosis (if element of R-to-L shunt) Tricuspid diastolic flow murmur	Echocardiography ECG (rSr' in V_1, RV strain pattern) Cardiac catheterization CXR
VSD	Loud holosystolic murmur at LSB Thrill over precordium Prominent RV impulse	Echocardiography Cardiac catheterization CXR
PDA	Wide pulse pressure Continuous (systolic and diastolic) murmur at second left ICS	Echocardiography Cardiac catheterization MRA

required to visualize small defects). The extent of shunt flow should be quantified by measurement of Qp:Qs. If echocardiography yields borderline or equivocal findings, cardiac catheterization and measurement of intracardiac oxygen saturations can be performed.

Treatment

Patients with small shunts may tolerate them well, have no long-term ill effects, and require no specific therapy aside from endocarditis prophylaxis (not necessary for patients with ASDs). Patients with larger shunts may develop progressive pulmonary HTN and subsequent right HF. In these patients, closure of the defect should be considered before irreversible right HF occurs.

In patients with ASDs, the defect should be closed if the pulmonary blood flow exceeds the systemic blood flow by at least 50% (i.e., the Qp:Qs is >1.5:1.0), if echocardiography reveals right heart dilation or dysfunction, or if the patient has suffered a paradoxical embolism. Available closure techniques include:

- Percutaneous closure with catheter-based devices (usually for ASDs <2 cm in diameter)
- Primary surgical closure without a patch (small defects)
- Surgical closure with a patch (larger defects)

Management of a VSD is similar, with closure recommended when the Qp:Qs exceeds 1.5 to 2.0:1. Surgical closure of a VSD is the standard therapy.

In the absence of severe pulmonary HTN and right HF, a PDA in a full-term infant is an indication for closure. Surgical ligation is the usual technique; percutaneous methods are still investigational. In some infants, constriction of the PDA may be stimulated by the use of prostaglandin inhibitors (e.g., indomethacin). Patients with large, uncorrected PDAs rarely survive into adulthood.

CYANOTIC HEART DISEASE

Although many forms of congenital cyanotic heart disease are fatal in childhood, several disorders (including Eisenmenger syndrome, tetralogy of Fallot, and corrected transposition) are compatible with survival to adulthood.

■ EISENMENGER SYNDROME

Patients who are born with a large VSD, PDA, or (rarely) a large secundum ASD initially have a substantial left-to-right shunt. The resultant marked increase in pulmonary flow produces irreversible pulmonary HTN. As right heart pressure rises, it may exceed left heart pressure, resulting in reversal of the shunt (i.e., right-to-left). This directional change shunts deoxygenated blood to the systemic circulation, leading to cyanosis.

Physical Examination

Prominent cyanosis and digital clubbing are usually present. An RV heave and loud P_2 (pulmonary HTN) are typical.

Diagnostic Evaluation

The ECG demonstrates RVH. Chest radiography reveals prominent central pulmonary arteries with peripheral arterial pruning and RV enlargement. Echocardiography confirms the diagnosis and demonstrates right-to-left shunt flow, pulmonary HTN, and RVH.

Treatment

Surgical repair of the shunt is not possible after irreversible pulmonary HTN develops. Vasodilator therapy should be avoided, as this will exacerbate the shunting. The only effective therapy is heart-lung or single-lung transplantation and closure of the defect.

Prognosis

Patients may survive into the sixth decade but usually develop RV failure in their forties. Hypoxia and ventricular arrhythmias are the common causes of death.

■ TETRALOGY OF FALLOT (TOF)

TOF is characterized by:

- VSD
- Overriding aorta
- Obstruction to RV outflow
- RVH

Incidence

TOF accounts for 10% of all congenital cardiac abnormalities but is the most common congenital abnormality causing cyanosis after 1 year of age. Most patients with uncorrected TOF do not survive to adulthood; only 6% survive to age 30.

Physiology

TOF results from anterior displacement of the ventricular septum with an associated membranous VSD. The aorta thus straddles the septum (overriding aorta), allowing flow from both ventricles to enter the systemic circulation. In addition, there is a varying degree of RV outflow tract obstruction, resulting in RVH. These abnormalities impair blood flow through the pulmonary system and allow flow of deoxygenated blood from the RV to the aorta, resulting in systemic hypoxemia and cyanosis.

The degree of cyanosis depends directly on two factors:

• Severity of RV outflow obstruction
• SVR

More severe RV outflow obstruction and low SVR favor flow of deoxygenated blood from the RV to the aorta, increasing cyanosis. However, if SVR is increased, RV blood flows preferentially to the PA, and oxygenation improves.

Clinical Manifestations

Most children with TOF are cyanotic at birth. They usually develop dyspnea with exertion and often learn to squat after exercise, thereby increasing their SVR, increasing pulmonary blood flow, and reducing fatigue and cyanosis. Episodic, sudden increases in the shunt may occur, resulting in worsened cyanosis and tachypnea ("Tet fits"). These episodes may progress to syncope, seizure, or death. Physical examination reveals a systolic ejection murmur caused by stenosis of the RV outflow tract. A precordial thrill may be present. The second heart sound is single, as P_2 is absent. A prominent RV heave may be present, as may digital clubbing, the latter resulting from chronic hypoxemia.

Diagnostic Evaluation

ECG may reveal evidence of RA enlargement and RVH. CXR usually demonstrates right heart enlarge-

ment, resulting in a characteristic "boot-shaped" cardiac silhouette. Echocardiography will demonstrate the classic anatomic abnormalities, which can be confirmed by cardiac catheterization.

Treatment

Surgical correction early in infancy is the treatment of choice. The feasibility of surgery depends on the size of the RV outflow tract and the PAs. A severely hypoplastic RV outflow tract or PA atresia may not allow for complete surgical repair. In these patients, palliative surgical therapy can be performed to create a systemic-to-PA anastomosis (Blalock-Taussig shunt, Watterson shunt, or Pott shunt), allowing increased pulmonary blood flow and improved oxygenation.

■ CORRECTED TRANSPOSITIONS

Complete transposition of the great arteries (the aorta arises from the RV; the PA arises from the LV) is a universally fatal syndrome if not surgically corrected at birth. In congenitally corrected transposition, there is AV and VA discordance (essentially the ventricles have switched position). Blood flows through the circulation in the appropriate direction; however, the morphologic RV (in the anatomic LV position) pumps blood to the systemic circulation and the morphologic LV pumps blood to the pulmonary circulation. There is frequently an associated VSD, pulmonary stenosis, and complete HB.

Clinical Manifestations

Patients with congenitally corrected transposition without associated anomalies may survive into the sixth decade but often develop left-sided HF, as the morphologic RV is unable to maintain systemic pressures. Patients with associated VSDs have varying degrees of cyanosis.

Treatment

Surgical repair of the VSD and pulmonary stenosis, when present, is the treatment of choice. The left AV valve frequently becomes regurgitant and requires replacement.

KEY POINTS

1. ASD, VSD, and PDA allow for left-to-right shunting of blood and may present as pulmonary HTN, right HF, or an asymptomatic murmur.

2. The three types of ASDs ostium primum, ostium secundum, and sinus venosus. The most common type is ostium secundum.

3. VSDs may occur in the membranous or the muscular regions of the interventricular septum.

4. ASDs should be closed if the Qp:Qs is >1.5:1 or RV failure develops.

5. Large VSDs require surgery during infancy, whereas small VSDs may require no specific therapy and may close spontaneously before adulthood.

6. PDAs produce a continuous "machinery-like" murmur and should be surgically closed unless severe pulmonary HTN and right HF are present.

7. Eisenmenger syndrome consists of pulmonary hypertension and right-to-left shunting through an ASD, VSD, or PDA.

8. Tetralogy of Fallot is the most common cause of cyanotic CHD after 1 year of age and consists of RVH, VSD, overriding aorta, and pulmonic outflow obstruction.

9. The degree of cyanosis in TOF is dependent on the severity of the pulmonic outflow obstruction and the systemic vascular resistance.

10. Surgical correction early in infancy and childhood is the cornerstone of therapy for TOF.

Pregnancy and Cardiovascular Disease

Significant circulatory changes occur during pregnancy and the peripartum period and can precipitate clinical deterioration in the presence of preexisting CVD. In addition, pregnancy itself may be an etiologic factor in the development of certain cardiovascular disorders, including HTN and dilated CMP. An understanding of this altered cardiovascular physiology is essential to the management of the pregnant cardiac patient.

■ CARDIOVASCULAR PHYSIOLOGY DURING PREGNANCY

Blood volume, HR, SV, and CO increase substantially during pregnancy. On average, blood volume increases by 40%, accounting in part for an increase in CO of 30 to 50%. BP tends to decline during the first trimester, reaching a nadir during the second trimester and returning to normal toward the end of the pregnancy. These hemodynamic changes are summarized in Table 42-1.

Despite the increase in blood volume, venous return is reduced during late pregnancy as a result of compression of the inferior vena cava by the gravid uterus. This compression is relieved after delivery, and, when combined with the shifting of blood from the contracting uterus into the systemic circulation, results in an acute rise in preload, SV, and CO. These volume shifts may result in HF in the immediate postpartum period, especially in patients with depressed LV function.

■ CLINICAL MANIFESTATIONS

The normal hemodynamic changes of pregnancy may result in signs and symptoms that mimic or obscure cardiac disease, including:

■ TABLE 42-1

Hemodynamic Changes During Normal Pregnancy

	Trimester		
	First	Second	Third
Blood volume	↑	↑↑	↑↑↑
Stroke volume	↑	↑↑↑	↑, ↔, or ↓
HR	↑	↑↑	↑↑ to ↑↑↑
CO	↑	↑↑ to ↑↑	↑↑ to ↑↑↑
SBP	↔	↓	↔
DBP	↓	↓↓	↓
Pulse pressure	↑	↑↑	↔
SVR	↓	↓↓↓	↓↓

- Fatigue, decreased exercise capacity
- Dyspnea (due to hormonal changes and diaphragmatic elevation)
- Orthopnea (due to diaphragmatic elevation)
- Light-headedness, presyncope (due to compression of the vena cava with decreased venous return)
- Palpitations (due to sinus tachycardia)
- Elevated JVP and edema (due to fluid retention)
- Displaced PMI
- Third and/or fourth heart sounds
- Systolic flow murmurs (due to increased SV)

Physical findings seen almost exclusively in pregnancy include:

- Cervical venous hum (continuous murmur in the right supraclavicular fossa)
- Mammary souffle (continuous murmur over the breast)

Diastolic and systolic murmurs that are greater than II/VI in intensity are rarely related solely to pregnancy and warrant further evaluation.

DIAGNOSTIC CARDIAC TESTING IN PREGNANCY

ECG changes in normal pregnancy include sinus tachycardia, QRS-axis shift, and premature atrial and ventricular complexes. ST-T changes are not routinely seen as part of normal pregnancy and warrant further evaluation. Echocardiography is safe in pregnancy and frequently reveals dilation of the atrial and/or ventricular chamber; a small pericardial effusion; and mild MV, TV, and PV regurgitation. Chest radiography is generally avoided during pregnancy; when performed, it may reveal cardiomegaly, increased pulmonary markings, and small pleural effusions.

PREEXISTING CARDIAC DISEASE AND PREGNANCY

Congenital Heart Disease

Maternal prognosis is influenced by the type of CHD, previous surgical repair, severity of cyanosis, pulmonary vascular resistance, and functional capacity. In general, a good maternal outcome can be expected in most patients with:

- Noncyanotic CHD
- Surgically corrected CHD
- Small uncorrected ASDs *or* VSDs
- PDA
- PS
- Uncomplicated coarctation of the aorta

Patients with uncorrected or partially corrected TOF do not tolerate pregnancy well. The increase in blood volume and venous return to the RA, combined with a drop in SVR, can produce or exacerbate right-to-left shunting and cyanosis in these patients. Eisenmenger syndrome continues to be associated with high maternal morbidity and mortality; pregnancy should be avoided by patients with this condition and elective termination should be considered for those who are already pregnant.

Valvular Heart Disease

Mitral and aortic regurgitation is usually well tolerated during pregnancy owing to the reduction in SVR. Symptomatic patients can be treated with diuretics, digoxin, and/or hydralazine. Mild AS (valve area >1.0 cm^2) and mild MS (valve area >1.5 cm^2) is generally well tolerated during pregnancy; more severe valvular stenosis is often problematic. Patients with stenotic valvular disease who develop severe symptoms despite medical therapy may require surgical valve repair or percutaneous balloon valvuloplasty. Those managed medically often require invasive hemodynamic monitoring with a PA catheter in the peripartum period. Termination of the pregnancy is occasionally required.

Hypertension

Women with chronic HTN have a higher risk of peripartum complications, including fetal growth retardation, placental abruption, premature delivery, acute renal failure, and hypertensive crisis. Drug therapy for HTN during pregnancy is recommended for a DBP >100 mm Hg, or >90 mm Hg in patients with renal disease or evidence of end-organ involvement (see Table 42-2).

PREGNANCY-RELATED CARDIOVASCULAR DISORDERS

Preeclampsia is characterized by HTN associated with proteinuria, edema, or both. HTN in preeclampsia is defined as either (1) an increase in SBP of >30 mm Hg or (2) an increase in DBP of >15 mm Hg over baseline values obtained prior to 20 weeks' gestation. If BPs prior to the 20th week of gestation are not known, a blood pressure of $>140/90$ mm Hg is diagnostic. Drug therapy and hospitalization are recommended for preeclamptic patients. Eclampsia is defined as preeclampsia complicated by seizure.

Peripartum Cardiomyopathy

Peripartum CMP is a form of dilated CMP that usually becomes apparent by the third trimester. The reported incidence in the United States is 1 in 10,000 pregnancies. Its etiology is unknown. Treatment of resultant HF includes use of diuretics, digoxin, and vasodilators (such as hydralazine). Patients should also receive anticoagulant therapy postpartum because of an increased incidence of thromboembolic events. Varying degrees of recovery of LV function may occur after delivery. Subsequent pregnancies are associated with a high risk of relapse, in addition to maternal

■ TABLE 42-2

Cardiovascular Agents in Pregnancy

Medication	Safety	Comment
Alpha blocker (methyldopa)	Yes	Safety and efficacy supported in randomized trials
Beta blockers (metoprolol and atenolol)	Yes in late pregnancy	Fetal growth retardation noted when used in early or mid gestation
Alpha-beta blocker (labetalol)	Unknown	Lack of data; concern for maternal hepatotoxicity
Vasodilator (hydralazine)	Yes	Rare cases of neonatal thrombocytopenia
ACE-I	No	Fetal death or renal failure in newborns
Diuretics	Yes and no	May continue if prescribed before gestation; thiazides may result in low birth weight, hypoglycemia, and bone marrow suppression in fetus
CCBs	Probably, in late pregnancy	No human studies; no clear adverse effects in second and third trimesters
Digoxin	Unknown	No data supporting use in pregnancy; should be avoided unless absolutely necessary; may cause low birth weight
Amiodarone	No	Contraindicated due to growth retardation, prematurity, and fetal hypothyroidism
Heparin	Yes	May cause prematurity, fetal thrombocytopenia, or osteopenia
Warfarin	No	Hemorrhage, skeletal problems

morbidity and mortality. Further pregnancies should be discouraged in patients with persistent LV dysfunction, while patients with recovered LV function should be counseled regarding their increased risk of relapse.

KEY POINTS

1. Substantial hemodynamic changes occur during pregnancy, including increased HR, increased SV, increased CO, and decreased SVR.
2. Symptoms and signs of normal pregnancy may mimic or obscure cardiac disease.
3. Preexisting cardiac conditions, especially HF, may be exacerbated by the altered physiology of pregnancy. Regurgitant valvular disease is usually tolerated well, while stenotic valvular disease may be problematic and result in HF during the pregnancy.
4. HTN, preeclampsia, and peripartum CMP may complicate gestation.

Traumatic Heart Disease

Cardiac trauma is a leading causes of death among individuals sustaining violent injuries, such as motor vehicle accidents and gunshot or stab wounds. Iatrogenic cardiac trauma can also occur, caused by the use of intravascular and intracardiac catheters or from the performance of closed chest compressions during cardiopulmonary resuscitation (CPR). Cardiac injuries can be separated into two major types: **nonpenetrating** and **penetrating**.

Nonpenetrating Cardiac Injury

Nonpenetrating injuries most commonly result from:

- Impact during a motor vehicle accident with resultant compression of the chest from the steering wheel
- Blows to the chest by any kind of blunt object or missile (e.g., a clenched fist or sporting equipment)
- External chest compression during CPR

Blunt trauma can result in injuries to the myocardium, pericardium, endocardial structures, coronary arteries, and aorta (see Box 43-1).

Clinical Manifestations

Cardiac injury should be suspected in patients with an appropriate mechanism of injury, even in the absence of other overt chest trauma. Traumatic **cardiac rupture** usually results in exsanguination or cardiac tamponade and is almost always fatal. Cardiac rupture can either occur immediately on injury (acute laceration) or be delayed (e.g., contusion leading to hemorrhage, necrosis, and subsequent rupture) and can affect any cardiac chamber. Rupture of the papillary muscles, chordae tendineae, or any of the valve leaflets results

in acute valvular insufficiency with HF, hemodynamic instability, and a new murmur. Rupture of the interventricular septum may present similarly but may be relatively well tolerated. Rupture of the pericardium can present as circulatory collapse owing to cardiac herniation through the pericardial sac.

Less severe blunt injuries may lead to **myocardial contusion**, the presentation of which varies depending

BOX 43-1	TYPES OF CARDIAC INJURIES RESULTING FROM BLUNT TRAUMA

Myocardium
1. Contusion
2. Rupture
3. Septal perforation (VSD)
4. Ventricular aneurysm or pseudoaneurysm

Pericardium
1. Pericarditis
2. Postpericardiotomy syndrome
3. Constrictive pericarditis
4. Pericardial laceration
5. Cardiac herniation
6. Hemopericardium or tamponade

Endocardial structures
1. Papillary muscle rupture
2. Rupture of chordae tendineae
3. Valvular leaflet rupture

Coronary artery
1. Thrombosis and MI
2. Laceration
3. Fistula

on the location and extent of injury. The RV is most frequently involved owing to its anterior location; the interventricular septum and LV apex are less frequently affected. The most common symptom of cardiac contusion is precordial pain similar to that of MI. Patients with extensive contusion may present with shock resulting from RV and/or LV failure.

Diagnostic Evaluation

The ECG may be helpful in suspected cases of cardiac contusion. Initially, it may demonstrate nonspecific ST-T-wave abnormalities or findings of pericarditis. Subsequently, ECG findings similar to those of MI may evolve. A variety of supraventricular or ventricular arrhythmias may occur, and transient or persistent RBBB may develop. Markers of myocardial injury (CK-MB fraction and cardiac troponins) will be elevated in myocardial contusion.

2D echocardiography is very helpful in evaluating cardiac injuries. This study can identify pericardial effusions and determine their hemodynamic significance, identify structural injuries (myocardial or valvular rupture, intracardiac shunts), and demonstrate poorly functioning myocardium in the region of a cardiac contusion.

Treatment

Patients with ventricular free-wall rupture or valvular rupture require emergent surgery, whereas those with rupture of the interventricular septum can often initially be managed conservatively; small VSDs often close spontaneously. The treatment of patients with myocardial contusion is similar to that of patients with MI except that anticoagulation is contraindicated in the setting of contusion. These patients should receive supportive care and observation, including close monitoring for arrhythmias and potential late complications.

■ PENETRATING CARDIAC INJURY

Most penetrating cardiac injuries are caused by sharp objects (such as knives or ice picks) and missiles (mostly bullets). As in myocardial contusion, the chamber most commonly involved is the RV, owing to its anterior location. In contrast to blunt trauma, penetrating cardiac wounds generally involve concomitant laceration of both the pericardium and myocardium. Gunshot wounds tend to cause extensive tissue destruction and bleeding along the path of the projectile, whereas stab wounds may seal quickly before disastrous complications occur.

Clinical Manifestations

The clinical presentation depends on the type, location, and extent of injury. Pericardial laceration is common, and the nature of this wound (open or closed) determines whether intrapericardial blood drains freely into the chest, resulting in extensive hemorrhage and hemothorax, or collects in the pericardial space, resulting in cardiac tamponade. Although severe penetrating injuries to the heart generally result in immediate shock or death, one must maintain a high index of suspicion in hemodynamically stable patients with penetrating injuries to the chest that involve the lungs and other organs. Delayed clinical manifestations of cardiac injury include infection, retained foreign bodies, and arrhythmias.

Diagnostic Evaluation

2D echocardiography is the diagnostic test of choice for the evaluation of penetrating cardiac trauma and can be invaluable in recognizing pericardial effusion, intracardiac shunts (ASD or VSD), foreign bodies, and valvular disruption. If echocardiography is not immediately available, emergent thoracotomy should be performed to allow for the direct visualization of cardiac injury.

Treatment

The definitive therapy for severe hemorrhage accompanying cardiac injuries is immediate thoracotomy and cardiorrhaphy. The heart and its surrounding structures are inspected carefully and repaired according to the particular injury present. Treatment for retained foreign bodies is more controversial; the risk of the operation should be weighed against the risk of future embolization or infection. ASD, VSD, and valvular regurgitation, when diagnosed as late complications, are corrected only if symptoms warrant operative repair.

KEY POINTS

1. Nonpenetrating cardiac injuries are most commonly due to motor vehicle accidents.
2. Blunt chest trauma can lead to cardiac rupture, valvular disruption, pericardial effusion, and myocardial contusion.
3. Myocardial contusion may mimic MI in both symptoms and associated complications. The treatment of contusion is similar to the medical treatment of infarction except that anticoagulation is contraindicated in the setting of contusion.
4. Penetrating cardiac injuries usually result from knife and gunshot wounds and if severe lead to immediate shock or death. Survivors usually require emergent thoracotomy and cardiorrhaphy.

44 Cardiac Tumors

Primary tumors of the heart are rare, with an incidence of less than 0.3% by autopsy, and may be benign or malignant (see Box 44-1). Of the primary cardiac tumors, myxomas are the most common. Other benign tumors include papillary fibroelastomas, lipomas, and rhabdomyomas. Angiosarcomas, rhabdomyosarcomas, mesotheliomas, and fibrosarcomas account for the majority of malignant primary cardiac tumors in adults. Metastatic tumors to the heart are far more common and may involve the myocardium, pericardium, or endocardial surface. The most common primary source of metastatic cardiac tumors is the lung, followed by the breast and kidney. Cardiac involvement may also occur with melanomas and lymphomas. Carcinoid tumors are rare neuroendocrine tissues that usually originate in part of the GI tract or the bronchi. Secretion of serotonin and other vasoactive metabolites by these tumors causes carcinoid syndrome (see below) and induces fibrotic scarring of the TV and PV, resulting in tricuspid regurgitation and PS.

Clinical Manifestations

History

The specific signs and symptoms of cardiac tumors are more dependent on their anatomic location than on their histologic type. One notable exception is cardiac myxomas, which are frequently associated with nonspecific systemic symptoms such as fever, malaise, weight loss, arthralgias, and rash.

Tumors arising on the endocardial surface of the heart commonly present with symptoms of PE (right-sided tumors), or systemic or cerebral emboli (left-sided tumors). These result from embolization of tumor fragments or of thrombi from the surface of the tumor.

LA tumors (predominantly myxomas) often mimic MV disease. These tumors may prolapse into the MV

BOX 44-1	PRIMARY CARDIAC TUMORS

Benign
1. Myxoma
2. Lipoma
3. Papillary fibroelastoma
4. Rhabdomyoma
5. Fibroma
6. Hemangioma
7. Teratoma (in childhood)
8. Mesothelioma of the AV node
9. Granular cell tumor

Malignant
1. Angiosarcoma
2. Rhabdomyosarcoma
3. Mesothelioma
4. Fibrosarcoma
5. Malignant lymphoma
6. Osteosarcoma
7. Thymoma
8. Neurogenic sarcoma
9. Malignant teratoma (in childhood)

orifice during diastole, thereby impairing LV filling, mimicking MS, and resulting in symptoms of CHF. Patients who have such tumors may report symptoms that occur in relation to body position. RA tumors are frequently asymptomatic but may produce symptoms of right HF if they are large. Myxomas occur more frequently in the LA, and sarcomas are more commonly found in the RA.

LV tumors are often asymptomatic unless significant obstruction of the LVOT or impairment of myocardial function causing left HF is present. Systemic embolization may also occur. RV tumors often present with right HF; however, they may present with syncope or SCD when RV outflow tract obstruction is present.

Intramyocardial tumors most commonly result in rhythm or conduction disturbances and may produce palpitations or syncope. They can occasionally present as SCD due to cardiac rupture. Pericardial tumors result in the accumulation of blood or exudative fluid in the pericardial space and may produce symptoms of pericarditis or pericardial tamponade (see Chapters 31 and 32).

Carcinoid heart disease is usually associated with signs and symptoms of carcinoid syndrome: flushing, diarrhea, bronchospasm, and hypotension. If severe tricuspid regurgitation develops, right sided HF (elevated neck veins, pedal edema) may ensue.

Physical Examination

The physical examination of patients with cardiac tumors is often unremarkable. However, several findings may be noted, including:

- A tumor plop, an early diastolic sound frequently confused with an OS or an S_3, may be heard in patients with large atrial tumors.
- Systolic or diastolic murmurs mimicking MR or stenosis may be present with LA tumors.
- Signs of HF may be present with large tumors of any cardiac chamber.

With metastatic cardiac tumors, signs of the primary tumor may be identifiable on examination.

Diagnostic Evaluation

Routine laboratory testing is not usually helpful in the diagnosis of cardiac tumors. Nonetheless, cardiac myxomas are often associated with anemia and an elevated ESR. These findings likely result from production of interleukin-6 by the myxoma.

The diagnosis of cardiac tumor is usually made by 2D echocardiography. A TTE can provide information about tumor size, site of attachment, and mobility. When the transthoracic study is not definitive, TEE can provide improved resolution of the tumor and its attachment (see Figure 44-1) and can detect smaller tumor masses not readily seen by TTE. Cardiac CT and MRI are useful in determining the degree of myocardial tumor invasion and identifying involvement of pericardial and extracardiac structures. In addition, cardiac MRI provides better definition of tumor prolapse and secondary valve obstruction and can differentiate thrombi from tumors. Cardiac catheterization and angiography are not necessary in the evaluation of

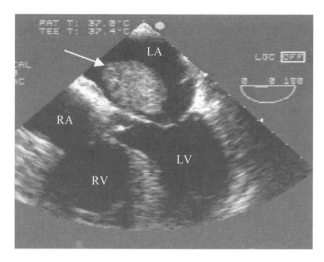

Figure 44-1 • TEE demonstrating a large (4.5 × 3.5 cm) atrial myxoma arising from the interatrial septum.

most cases of cardiac tumors except to exclude coexisting CAD that may warrant revascularization at the time of tumor resection.

Treatment

For benign cardiac tumors, operative excision is the treatment of choice and is curative in most cases. Peripheral embolization or dispersion of micrometastases remains the major surgical risk. Long-term prognosis is good, although myxomas may recur after initial resection.

Owing to extensive tissue involvement or distal metastases, operative resection is not an effective treatment for the majority of malignant primary or metastatic cardiac tumors. Prognosis is poor in general, with overall survival of 1 to 3 years following partial resection, chemotherapy, radiation, or combinations of these treatment modalities. Malignant pericardial effusions frequently recur after initial drainage and may require surgical pericardiotomy (the creation of a "pericardial window").

KEY POINTS

1. Primary cardiac tumors are rare.
2. The most common primary cardiac tumor is an atrial myxoma.
3. The most common tumors to metastasize to the heart are lung, breast, and renal carcinomas, melanomas, and lymphomas.
4. Symptoms of cardiac tumors usually relate to their anatomic position rather than their histologic type.

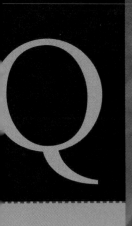

Questions

1. A 67-year-old man with a history of calf claudication and an abdominal aortic aneurysm repair presents to your office for a routine visit. He has no known CAD, DM, or family history of premature CAD. He stopped smoking 3 years ago. His BP is 128/70 mm Hg on an ACE inhibitor. His other medications include aspirin and multivitamins. His physical examination is notable for diminished bilateral dorsalis pedis and posterior tibial pulses. His wife mentions that his diet is "terrible," and she is concerned that his cholesterol level might be high. A fasting lipid profile is as follows:

Plasma total cholesterol	196 mg/dL
Plasma LDL cholesterol	140 mg/dL
Plasma HDL cholesterol	35 mg/dL
Serum TGs	105 mg/dL

   In addition to initiating therapeutic lifestyle changes, what is the most appropriate management?
   a. Repeat lipid profile in 3 months; target LDL <130 mg/dL
   b. Repeat lipid profile in 3 months; target LDL <100 mg/dL
   c. Initiate HMG-CoA reductase inhibitor; target LDL <100 mg/dL
   d. Repeat lipid profile in 3 to 5 years
   e. Initiate a fibric-acid derivative

2. A 25-year-old woman presents to your clinic after "passing out." She was standing in line at a bank when she developed nausea and had a "warm sensation all over." She subsequently became light-headed and lost consciousness for approximately 30 to 40 seconds, following which she awoke and was aware of her surroundings. Witnesses told her that she attempted to hold onto a counter prior to collapsing. She denies previous syncopal episodes. Examination reveals normal BP and HR. Her pulmonary, cardiac, and neurologic examinations are all normal. Hematocrit, BUN, creatinine, and electrolytes are all normal. An echocardiogram and ECG performed in your office are unremarkable.

   What is the most appropriate next test to perform in this patient's evaluation?
   a. Holter monitoring
   b. Electrophysiologic study
   c. CT scan of the head
   d. Tilt-table testing
   e. CSM

3. A 35-year-old nonsmoking man without significant past medical history presents with chest pain and exertional dyspnea. Review of symptoms is notable for a 1-week history of antecedent flu-like symptoms. Physical examination reveals a JVP of 14 cm H_2O and rales halfway up the lung fields bilaterally. An S_3 and a III/VI holosystolic murmur at the apex are noted, as is pitting edema of bilateral lower extremities. ECG reveals diffuse ST-T-wave abnormalities. The initial CPK is 586, with an index of 7%. The most likely diagnosis is:
   a. PE
   b. AMI
   c. Viral pericarditis
   d. Viral myocarditis
   e. HCM

4. You are are asked to evaluate a 56-year-old man who has recently developed intermittent chest pain. He has a history of HTN, smoking, and GERD. Over the past 3 weeks he has noted several episodes of right-sided chest pain that occur at rest, are associated with mild diaphoresis, last 5 to 10 minutes, and resolve spontaneously. He has not noted exertional symptoms. His BP is 140/80 mm Hg and his HR is 70 bpm. He has a prominent S4 but an otherwise normal examination. An ECG reveals normal sinus rhythm and LVH with a "strain" pattern (anterolateral ST-T abnormalities). You make the diagnosis of atypical chest pain and schedule him for a stress test. Which of the following is the most appropriate type of stress test for this patient?
   a. Exercise ECG
   b. Dobutamine echocardiogram

c. Adenosine stress with nuclear imaging
d. 24-hour ambulatory ECG monitoring
e. Exercise stress with nuclear imaging

5. A 63-year-old man, a smoker, presents to your clinic for a regularly scheduled appointment. On examination, his blood pressure is 140/90 mm Hg; his pulse is 70 bpm and regular. His respiratory rate is 20. There is no jugular venous distention. His carotid pulses are 1+ bilaterally without bruits. Examination of his chest reveals diffusely decreased breath sounds with scattered rhonchi. Precordial examination is unremarkable. Abdominal examination reveals a pulsatile mass with an associated bruit. Peripheral pulses are diminished but symmetric. You obtain an abdominal ultrasound that reveals an abdominal aortic aneurysm. Which of the following factors would prompt you to recommend elective surgical repair?
a. Absence of symptoms
b. Coexistent CAD
c. Family history of abdominal aneurysm
d. Aneurysm diameter of 6 cm
e. Concomitant peripheral vascular disease

Select one of the following for questions 6 to 8:
a. Acute MI
b. UA
c. Stable angina
d. PE
e. Spontaneous pneumothorax
f. Pericarditis
g. Costochondritis
h. Aortic dissection
i. Coronary artery spasm

6. A 60-year-old man with a history of hypercholesterolemia and smoking reports a 2-year history of substernal chest discomfort precipitated by exertion and relieved by rest. In the past several weeks, the pain has become more frequent and is precipitated by less exertion. What is the most likely diagnosis?

7. A 45-year-old man presents with sudden, severe, sharp chest pain that radiates to his back. On examination, his weight is 160 lb; his height is 72 in. His heart rate is 110 bpm. His BP is 124/70 in the left arm and barely palpable in the right arm. What is the most likely cause of his chest pain?

8. A 36-year-old man presents with intermittent, sharp, mid-sternal chest pain. The pain is somewhat worse with inspiration and associated with mild dyspnea. Several weeks prior, he and his children had "cold" symptoms. What is the most likely diagnosis?

9. A 41-year-old man, a smoker, is referred to your clinic for the evaluation of claudication. This began several months ago

and has steadily progressed since that time. Additional questioning reveals symptoms of cold-induced vasospasm. He has no history of diabetes or hypertension. On physical examination, the patient is found to be thin and in no acute distress. His BP is 140/80 mm Hg and his pulse is 68 bpm. His chest is clear and cardiac examination is unremarkable. His abdomen is soft and nontender without masses or bruits. His extremities are warm but with diminished radial, dorsalis pedis, and posterior tibial pulses. Which of the following is the most effective treatment of this condition?
a. Atenolol 50 mg qd
b. Diltiazem 30 mg qid
c. Assessment of ankle-brachial indices
d. Smoking cessation
e. Surgical revascularization

10. A 70-year-old woman is admitted for progressive dyspnea. Physical examination reveals moderate respiratory distress. Her heart rate is 110 bpm and her BP is 105/60 mm Hg, but the systolic pressure falls to 90 mm Hg with inspiration. Her radial pulse is regular but the pulse volume varies significantly with the respiratory cycle. Her JVP is elevated and there is moderate lower extremity edema. Chest examination reveals faint crackles at the base of the left lung. Heart sounds are poorly heard and there are no murmurs. The best method to confirm your presumed diagnosis is:
a. CXR
b. TTE
c. Pulmonary arterial catheterization
d. V/Q scan
e. CT scan of the chest

11. A 60-year-old man, a smoker, presents with intermittent fevers over a several week period. He has no significant past medical history but was told that he had a murmur at some point in the past. His temperature is 100°F, HR 85 bpm, and BP 135/70 mm Hg. Physical examination reveals digital clubbing and splenomegaly. Small, erythematous, nontender spots are noted over the palmar aspect of his hands. His lungs are clear to auscultation. Cardiac examination reveals a midsystolic click and a faint apical holosystolic murmur. What is the most likely diagnosis?
a. Pneumonia
b. Viral syndrome
c. Infectious endocarditis
d. Pericarditis
e. Congenital cardiac shunt

12. A 44-year-old woman presents to the ED with increased pedal edema. She has a history of smoking, HTN, and CHF resulting from a nonischemic cardiomyopathy. Her medications include a diuretic, a beta blocker, and a birth control pill. She lives in Mexico and recently traveled to the United States to visit family. Shortly after her arrival she

noted increased pedal edema. She denies chest pain or change in her baseline dyspnea and has been compliant with her medications.

On examination, she is in no respiratory distress. Her BP is 130/70 mm Hg. Her pulse is 88 bpm and regular. Her JVP is elevated at 8 cm H_2O without HJR. Chest examination reveals clear lung fields. Precordial examination is remarkably only for a soft S_3. The abdominal examination is benign. There is 1+ edema of the right lower extremity. The left lower extremity demonstrates 2 to 3+ edema with mild erythema. What is the most appropriate next step in this patient's management?
a. Administer IV diuretics
b. Obtain blood cultures and start IV antibiotics
c. Obtain bilateral lower extremity ultrasound studies
d. Check 24-hour urine protein excretion
e. Start an ACE inhibitor and arrange follow-up with a local physician

13. A 69-year-old man is referred to you after an episode of syncope. While walking on the beach in Florida, he had sudden loss of consciousness and awoke to find his family looking down at him. He does not recall the event, but his daughter states that he "fell over" without warning. He has never had syncope in the past but does admit to occasional chest pain and exertional dyspnea. Physical examination reveals a BP of 132/76 mm Hg and a HR of 72 bpm. His lungs are clear. His carotid pulses are diminished and there is a loud, late-peaking systolic ejection murmur over the sternal border near the second intercostal space. The second heart sound is faintly audible. Pulses are 1+ in all four extremities; there is no edema.

The most likely cause of this patient's syncope is:
a. AMI
b. AS
c. Orthostatic hypotension
d. Vasovagal syncope
e. MS

14. A 75-year-old woman with chronic AF presents to the ambulatory care clinic complaining of 1 week of fatigue and intermittent dizziness. She had previously been very active and usually walks around a small park every day. She denies any dyspnea or angina and reports no episodes of syncope. Her only other medical history is hypertension, for which she takes hydrochlorothiazide. She also takes warfarin for her AF. An ECG in the clinic reveals AF with an average HR of 38 bpm. The next appropriate step in the management of this patient would be:
a. Holter monitoring
b. Echocardiogram
c. Implantation of a pacemaker
d. Implantation of an ICD
e. No therapy other than reassurance

15. A 35-year-old woman with systemic lupus erythematosus complains of sharp left chest pain that is aggravated by breathing. She admits to having felt "under the weather" for the past week with a mild nonproductive cough and rhinorrhea. She has also noted mild dyspnea with exertion. She denies any recent injury or other focal pains. Her lupus has been relatively quiescent and has not required treatment for several years. Physical examination demonstrates a temperature of 38.0°C, BP of 140/82 mm Hg, and HR of 80 bpm. Her JVP is normal and her lungs are clear to auscultation. Cardiac examination reveals normal heart sounds and a faint, coarse murmur that is difficult to characterize. Her ECG is shown (see Figure Q-15). The most likely diagnosis is:
a. AMI
b. Acute pericarditis
c. MS
d. PE
e. Pneumonia

16. A 44-year-old man with alcoholic cardiomyopathy presents with dyspnea and increasing edema. Review of symptoms is notable for orthopnea and PND. On examination he is in moderate respiratory distress. BP is 110/83 mm Hg, pulse is 100 bpm and regular, respiratory rate is 24/min, and oxygen saturation is 93% on room air. JVP is markedly elevated and HJR is present. Examination of the chest reveals bibasilar rales. Precordial examination demonstrates tachycardia, a prominent S_3, and a II/VI holosystolic murmur at the apex. His extremities are cool and he has severe pedal edema. He is admitted to the coronary care unit, and right heart catheterization is performed. Initial pressures are as follows:

RA: 20 mm Hg
PA: 72/36 mm Hg
PCW: 33 mm Hg
CO: 2.2 L/min
SVR: 2,218 dynes/sec/cm^{-5}

In addition to oxygen and diuresis, the initial management of this patient should include:
a. Enalapril and metoprolol
b. Dopamine and dobutamine
c. Dobutamine and sodium nitroprusside
d. digoxin and IV NTG
e. Intraaortic balloon pump

17. A 72-year-old man is referred for the evaluation of exertional dyspnea. History is notable for PND, orthopnea, lower extremity edema, and increasing abdominal girth. On examination, the patient appears comfortable, with BP of 130/80 mm Hg, HR of 90 bpm, respiratory rate of 24/min, and an oxygen saturation of 94% on room air. His JVP is elevated and increases during inspiration. There are decreased breath sounds and dullness to percussion at the lung bases. Precordial examination is notable for a nondisplaced PMI

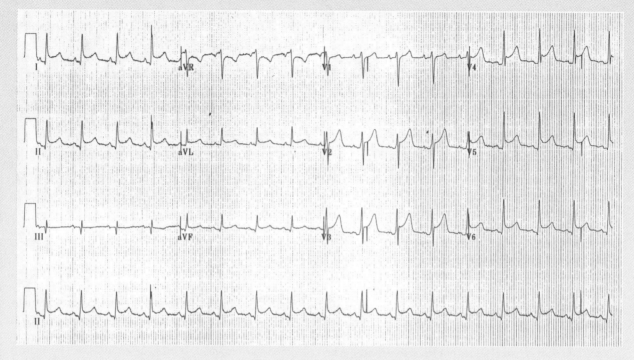

Figure Q-15 •

and normal S_1 and S_2 without additional heart sounds or murmurs. His abdomen is distended and liver enlarged. There is severe bilateral lower extremity edema.

CXR: Normal cardiac silhouette. Bilateral pleural effusions.

ECG: Sinus rhythm at 90 bpm. Low limb-lead voltage and poor R-wave progression.

Echocardiogram: Thickened LV and RV with mildly reduced systolic function. There is no significant valvular disease. A small pericardial effusion is noted. The most likely diagnosis is:

a. Idiopathic dilated CMP
b. Restrictive CMP
c. Constrictive pericarditis due to undiagnosed connective tissue disease
d. High output failure
e. Pericardial tamponade

18. A 34-year-old woman without significant past medical history is referred to your clinic for the evaluation of exertional dyspnea. She reports a 2-month history of progressive dyspnea and decline in exercise tolerance. She denies PND, orthopnea, or edema. She does not smoke and denies any history of recreational drug use.

Her BP is 130/90 mm Hg; pulse, 90 bpm; respiratory rate, 20/min; and oxygen saturation, 94% on room air. JVP is 10 cm H_2O without HJR. Her lungs are clear. Precordial examination is notable for a prominent parasternal impulse, a loud S_2, and a holosystolic murmur at the left lower sternal border that increases slightly with inspiration. Her extremities are without clubbing, cyanosis, or edema.

All laboratory tests are normal. CXR reveals loss of the retrosternal airspace and prominent central vasculature. Her ECG demonstrates normal sinus rhythm at 90 bpm, a QRS axis of +110 degrees, and RA enlargement.

The most likely cause of this patient's dyspnea is:

a. CAD
b. Asthma
c. Pulmonary HTN
d. Anemia
e. Acute PE

Select one of the following for questions 19 to 21:

a. AS
b. AR
c. MS
d. MR
e. ASD
f. PDA
g. HOCM

19. A 36-year-old woman from Trinidad presents with intermittent palpitations, which she has had for several months. She also notes dyspnea on exertion and occasional orthopnea. Examination demonstrates an HR of 100 bpm and BP of 110/60. Her lungs are clear but her JVP is elevated at 8 mm Hg. She has a loud S_2 and a low-pitched diastolic murmur

at the cardiac apex. An additional sound is heard shortly after the S_2. What is the cause of her murmur?

20. A 75-year-old man presents for evaluation of dyspnea. He reports several years of occasional exertional chest pain and the recent onset of dyspnea both on exertion and at rest. He admits to a single episode of light-headedness while climbing stairs several weeks prior. Examination reveals a soft S_2, a III/VI, and a crescendo-decrescendo systolic murmur at the upper sternal border that radiates to his carotids. What is the cause of his murmur?

21. A 40-year-old man presents for evaluation of a murmur. He has a history of HTN, for which he has been treated with diuretics. His brother died suddenly at 38 years of age. On examination, his BP is 148/90 mm Hg. There is a III/VI mid-peaking systolic murmur along his left sternal border that increases in intensity during the strain phase of Valsalva. What is the cause of his murmur?

22. A 65-year-old man presents with fevers, chills, weight loss, and malaise. His examination demonstrates splinter hemorrhages in his nail beds and conjunctival petechiae. A III/VI HSM is heard at the cardiac apex. Echocardiography demonstrates a vegetation on his mitral valve and moderate MR. Blood cultures are obtained and grow *Streptococcus bovis*. He is placed on appropriate antibiotics and remains hemodynamically stable. Further evaluation at this stage should include:
   a. TEE
   b. Thoracic CT scan
   c. CT scan of the head
   d. Cardiac catheterization
   e. Colonoscopy

23. A 62-year-old woman presents to the ED of a community hospital complaining of dyspnea and diaphoresis over the last 2 hours. When questioned, she also admits to mild chest heaviness and an uncomfortable feeling in her left shoulder. She has a history of HTN, type 2 DM, and former tobacco use.

   On physical examination, her pulse rate is 96 bpm and regular, respiratory rate is 20/min, and BP is 110/65 mm Hg. Lungs are clear to auscultation. There is an S_4, but no murmur is detected. Her ECG is shown (see Figure Q-23). What is the most likely diagnosis?
   a. Pericarditis
   b. AMI
   c. UA
   d. LBBB
   e. PE

24. A 65-year-old woman is admitted to the hospital for progressive dyspnea and fatigue. She has a history of smoking and lung cancer. Initial evaluation demonstrated a BP of 110/75 mm Hg, a HR of 88 bpm, and a room-air oxygen saturation of 95%. Her examination reveals decreased breath sounds at the left lower lung field and distant heart sounds. Initial laboratory evaluation is significant for a hematocrit of 27% (normal: 42 to 52%). Initial CXR demonstrates a left pleural effusion and a large cardiac silhouette.

   She is treated with transfusion therapy. During her hospitalization, she develops acute hypotension with a BP of 80/50 mm Hg and an HR of 115 bpm. Her room-air oxygen saturation is unchanged. She feels light-headed but denies chest pain. Cardiac examination reveals faint heart sounds and elevated JVP. Her lung examination is unchanged from the previous. The intervention likely to be of most benefit to this patient is:
   a. Cardiac catheterization
   b. IV antibiotics

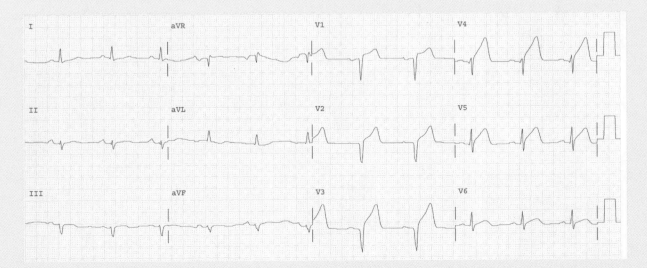

Figure Q-23 •

c. Pericardiocentesis
d. IV heparin
e. Thoracentesis

25. A 50-year-old man presents to the urgent care clinic for evaluation of substernal chest pain. Over the past 2 weeks, he has experienced similar chest discomfort that is brought on by light exertion, relieved with rest, and has increased in frequency and duration. He describes having had an episode of chest pain at rest, lasting for 40 minutes, which prompted him to seek medical care. He is currently pain-free. He smokes 1 pack of cigarettes a day and reports that his younger brother had suffered a "heart attack" at age 40.

   On examination, his pulse rate is 80/min and regular; respiratory rate, 20/min; BP, 150/95 mm Hg; and oxygen saturation 98% on room air. An S_4 gallop is present, but the rest of his physical examination is unremarkable. An ECG reveals normal sinus rhythm with LV hypertrophy but without significant ST-segment abnormalities.

   You send him to the ED immediately for further evaluation. CXR and all laboratory tests, including cardiac enzymes, are normal. What is the most likely diagnosis?
   a. AMI
   b. UA
   c. Stable angina
   d. Acute pericarditis
   e. PE

26. A 65-year-old man with type 2 DM presents with recurrent exertional chest discomfort that is felt to be consistent with angina pectoris. His medications include aspirin, atenolol, captopril, isosorbide mononitrate, glyburide, simvastatin, and an H_2 blocker. His pulse rate is 64/min and BP 130/75 mm Hg. A subsequent ETT induces 3 mm of ST-segment depression after 3 minutes of exercise. Cardiac catheterization is performed promptly and reveals high-grade obstruction (>75%) of the proximal LAD and RCA. LV function by echocardiography is mildly depressed, with an EF of 45%. Which of the following should you recommend?
   a. PTCA +/− stent implantation
   b. Continuation of current medical therapy
   c. Transmyocardial laser revascularization
   d. CABG
   e. Intensification of current medical therapy

27. A 73-year-old man with a history of HTN and peripheral vascular disease presents with an acute onset of chest pain. The pain was initially epigastric but then settled between his shoulder blades. On physical examination, he appears quite anxious. His BP is 190/90 mm Hg in both arms. Pulse is 98 bpm and regular. Respiratory rate is 20/min. His jugular veins are not distended and his lungs are clear. Precordial examination reveals an S_4. No murmur

is noted. Abdominal examination is notable for moderate tenderness with deep palpation and a periumbilical bruit. His right dorsalis pedis and posterior tibial pulses are 1+.

   Laboratory studies include the following:

   BUN: 40
   Creatinine: 1.5
   Hematocrit: 34%
   ECG: Sinus tachycardia, LVH, no acute ischemic changes.

   The most likely diagnosis is:
   a. Aortic dissection
   b. AMI
   c. Acute arterial embolus
   d. PE
   e. Pancreatitis

28. You are asked to consult on the case of a 70-year-old man who was admitted to the CCU following resuscitation from a cardiac arrest. He was initially unresponsive, but after 5 days regained all neurologic function. He has no known prior cardiac history but admits to occasional dyspnea on exertion and pedal edema. The initial ECG reveals sinus rhythm with an LBBB. Laboratory evaluation in the CCU failed to demonstrate evidence of AMI. An echocardiogram was performed and demonstrated severely impaired LV function (LVEF 25%). Coronary angiography revealed only mild atherosclerotic disease of his coronary arteries.

   In addition to optimizing medical therapy, you would recommend:
   a. Holter monitoring
   b. Exercise stress testing
   c. Implantation of an ICD
   d. Electrophysiologic study
   e. Implantation of a pacemaker

29. A 48-year-old obese man presents to the ED with dyspnea, which began suddenly while he was sitting and watching television. He notes associated left lateral chest pain that is worse when he breathes deep. He denies fevers, chills, or cough. He appears to be in moderate respiratory distress. BP is 110/70 mm Hg; pulse, regular at 104 bpm and respiratory rate 28/min. His oxygen saturation is 93% on room air. JVP is 9 cm H_2O without HJR. His chest is clear, and his precordial examination is normal aside from tachycardia. His extremities are symmetric without edema or calf tenderness. CXR is normal and ECG shows no ST- or T-wave abnormalities. The most likely diagnosis is:
   a. Pneumonia
   b. Pneumothorax
   c. Pleurisy
   d. PE
   e. Pericarditis

30. A 32-year-old woman with progressive dyspnea undergoes PA catheterization, which demonstrates a PA pressure

of 76/45 mm Hg. Echocardiography demonstrates normal LV function but moderate RV dysfunction and tricuspid regurgitation. An extensive evaluation does not reveal an obvious underlying cause and she is diagnosed with primary pulmonary HTN. The initial treatment of choice is:

a. An ACE inhibitor
b. A vasodilating calcium channel blocker (i.e., nifedipine)
c. A beta blocker
d. epoprostenol
e. Lung transplantation

31. A 64-year-old man with HTN and dyslipidemia presents to the ED with dyspnea. He has not had chest pain, abdominal pain, back pain, headache, visual changes, or paresthesias. His only medications are atenolol and simvastatin. He does not smoke and denies illicit drug use.

He appears in severe respiratory distress. His BP is 230/120 mm Hg in both arms; his pulse is 92 bpm and regular. Funduscopic examination reveals changes consistent with hypertensive retinopathy. JVP is 12 cm H_2O. Lung examination reveals rales nearly to the apices bilaterally. Precordial examination demonstrates a prominent S_4 and a hyperdynamic apex without appreciable murmurs. Neurologic examination is nonfocal.

Laboratory studies are pertinent for a creatinine of 1.5 and trace protein in the urinalysis. ECG reveals LV hypertrophy with repolarization abnormalities.

The most appropriate initial management of this patient should include:

a. Oxygen, IV furosemide
b. Oxygen, IV furosemide, SL NTG
c. Oxygen, IV furosemide, IV sodium nitroprusside
d. Oxygen, IV furosemide, morphine
e. Oxygen, IV furosemide, oral metoprolol

32. A 35-year-old construction worker reports having had fevers and chills for several days. Examination reveals a temperature of 102°F, HR of 110 bpm, and BP of 120/85 mm Hg. His teeth are in poor condition. His lungs are clear, and cardiac examination is unremarkable. Blood cultures are drawn and grow *Streptococcus viridans*. He is diagnosed with SBE. Despite antibiotics, the patient continues to have persistent fever and develops acute dyspnea on the fifth hospital day. Physical examination is likely to reveal:

a. An HSM at the apex
b. An early-peaking, crescendo-decrescendo murmur at the upper sternal border
c. Weak and delayed carotid upstrokes
d. An apical middiastolic murmur with presystolic accentuation and an OS
e. A three-component pericardial friction rub

33. A 70-year-old man called EMS after having had anterior chest pain for 2 hours. He was found to have a BP of 104/74 mm Hg and a HR of 110 bpm. He was given oxygen and chewable aspirin in the ambulance with minimal improvement in his symptoms and was brought to the ED, where an ECG revealed an acute STEMI. Initial therapy for this patient should include:

a. Beta blockers and heparin
b. Calcium channel blockers and heparin
c. NSAIDs
d. Nitrates and IV diuretics
e. Dopamine and IV nitrates

34. A 45-year-old woman with a history of DM and HTN presents reporting several days of progressive shortness of breath. Her initial BP is 80/50 mm Hg with an HR of 120 bpm. Her CXR reveals diffuse patchy infiltrates and a right-sided pleural effusion. ECG reveals sinus tachycardia without significant ST abnormalities. She develops progressive respiratory distress and is intubated and sent to the ICU. A PA catheter is placed to improve hemodynamic management. The initial pressures are as follows:

RA: 4 mm Hg
PA: 28/10 mm Hg
PCW: 8 mm Hg
CO: 7.2 L/min
SVR: 622 dynes/sec/cm^{-5}

These findings are most consistent with what underlying process?

a. Cardiogenic shock
b. Hypovolemic shock
c. Pericardial tamponade
d. Septic shock
e. PE

35. A 45-year-old woman from Haiti arrives at your clinic complaining of dyspnea and a dry cough, which she has had for 2 to 3 months. She has been unable to walk more than about 200 ft before developing severe shortness of breath. She denies any fevers but has episodic night sweats. She tells you that she has been in the United States for about 6 weeks. Physical examination demonstrates elevated JVP with prominent waveforms. Notably, there is an increase in the venous distention with inspiration. Her heart sounds are faint, with an early diastolic third sound present. No murmur is heard. The right upper quadrant is tender and the liver pulsatile. ECG reveals sinus tachycardia but is otherwise normal. CXR reveals mild scarring of the right upper lobe of the lungs and a normal-sized cardiac silhouette. The PPD is positive.

The most likely cause of her dyspnea is:

a. Pericardial tamponade
b. Pulmonary tuberculosis
c. Constrictive pericarditis
d. Acute pericarditis
e. Severe MS

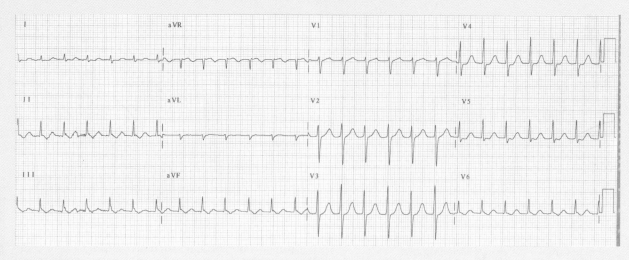

Figure Q-36 •

36. A 60-year-old woman is seen in the ED for the acute onset of palpitations without dyspnea or chest discomfort. She has no known cardiac history. She states the palpitations began an hour prior to her arrival at the ED and recalls no inciting factors. She admits to mild associated light-headedness. Her BP is 140/80 mm Hg. There is no increase in her JVP and her lungs are clear. Cardiac examination reveals no abnormal sounds. ECG in the ED is shown (see Figure Q-36).

CSM is attempted and has no effect. Which of the following is the next best treatment option:
a. Oral nifedipine
b. Electrical cardioversion
c. IV lidocaine
d. IV diltiazem
e. IV enalaprilat

37. A 37-year-old woman arrives at your clinic reporting a 6-month history of progressive dyspnea on exertion as well as fatigue. She also notes occasional irregular palpitations and the recent onset of pedal edema. Her past medical history is significant for asthma and a childhood murmur. She has not seen a physician in many years. On examination, her HR is 75 bpm and irregularly irregular. BP is 135/60 mm Hg. Her JVP is 10 cm H$_2$O. Palpation of her precordium reveals a prominent left parasternal impulse. She has a normal S$_1$ and a prominent S$_2$. The second heart sound is persistently split, without respiratory variation. There is a 2/6 systolic ejection murmur localized to the base of her heart. Her PMI is normal. The liver is enlarged to 3 cm below the costal margin and is pulsatile. ECG reveals AF and an incomplete RBBB.

The most likely cause of her right HF is:
a. PPH
b. ASD

c. VSD
d. AS
e. Aortic coarctation

38. A 15-year-old girl is evaluated for a fever and joint pains. Three weeks earlier, she had a sore throat that resolved without treatment. Four days ago, she developed pain and swelling of the right ankle and the right elbow. Today she complains of pain and swelling of the left knee. Physical examination reveals a temperature of 101°F and an HR of 110. A soft HSM and an S$_3$ are audible at the cardiac apex. The left knee is erythematous and tender; it has an effusion. Laboratory evaluation demonstrates an elevated antistreptococcal antibody. You make the clinical diagnosis of acute rheumatic fever.

In regard to this patient, which of the following statements is true?
a. Blood cultures are likely to be positive for group A streptococci.
b. Cardiac examination is also likely to disclose an OS and a low-pitched middiastolic murmur at the cardiac apex.
c. Acute antibiotic treatment is not required, as the patient's sore throat has resolved.
d. She should receive benzathine PCN every 3 weeks until she is 25 years old.
e. She may have residual deformity of her left knee.

39. A 56-year-old man, a smoker, presents to the ED with UA. He is treated with aspirin, LMWH, and beta blockers, with resolution of his symptoms. ECG is without acute ischemic changes. Which of the following is the most appropriate next step in his management?
a. Emergent cardiac catheterization
b. Administration of thrombolytic therapy

c. Observe on telemetry and obtain further serum cardiac markers

d. Immediate ETT with nuclear imaging for diagnosis

e. TTE

40. A 58-year-old postmenopausal woman comes to your office for a routine physical examination. She does not have a history of CAD or DM. She smokes one pack of cigarettes per day. Family history is negative for premature CAD. Her physical examination is unremarkable. BP is 130/85 mm Hg.

Laboratory data show:

Plasma glucose (fasting)	100 mg/dL
Plasma total cholesterol	238 mg/dL
Plasma HDLc	45 mg/dL
Plasma LDLc	166 mg/dL
Serum TGs	135 mg/dL
LFTs	normal

Which of the following is most appropriate?

a. No specific therapy

b. Smoking cessation and repeat lipid profile in 3 months

c. Smoking cessation and TLC with a goal LDL of 160 mg/dL

d. Smoking cessation, TLC, and repeat lipid profile in 3 months, with a goal LDL of <130 mg/dL

e. Initiation of pharmacologic therapy with a goal LDL of <100 mg/dL

41. A 55-year-old man is admitted to the CCU with an inferior wall MI. He receives IV TPA with successful reperfusion and resolution of STE. On his third hospital day, he develops sudden onset of shortness of breath without any chest discomfort. His current medications are aspirin, metoprolol, captopril, and simvastatin. His pulse rate is 110/min and regular; respiratory rate, 32/min; and BP, 100/70 mm Hg. Oxygen saturation is 90% on room air. Rales are present bilaterally. Cardiac examination reveals a III-IV/VI HSM heard best at the apex with radiation to the axilla and back. An S_3 gallop is present. ECG shows sinus tachycardia, with inferior Q waves and T-wave inversions but it is unchanged compared with an earlier ECG. What is the most likely diagnosis?

a. Ventricular septal rupture

b. LV free wall rupture

c. Papillary muscle rupture with acute MR

d. Recurrent MI

e. PE

42. A 55-year-old man with a history of DM presents to your office for a routine physical examination; you note his BP to be 145/90 mm Hg. His BMI is normal. He does not smoke, has normal cholesterol, and has no family history of CAD. His only medication is metformin. Two weeks later he returns and a repeat BP is 140/95 mm Hg bilaterally. The next step in management is:

a. Instruction in TLS, including low-salt diet and exercise; return for follow-up in 3 months

b. Initiation of HCTZ

c. Initiation of atenolol and HCTZ

d. Initiation of lisinopril

e. HCTZ and stress testing to evaluate for coronary ischemia

43. A 58-year-old postmenopausal woman with history of chronic stable angina, HTN, and type 2 DM presents to your office for a routine visit. Her anginal symptoms have remained stable since her last visit 3 months earlier. She walks briskly for 45 minutes three to five times per week. She does not smoke and is compliant with her medications, which include aspirin, atenolol, lisinopril, and insulin. On examination, her pulse rate is 60/min and BP 118/75 mm Hg. Fasting laboratory data are notable for a Hb_{A1C} of 7.2%, blood glucose of 150 mg/dL, total cholesterol of 200 mg/dL, HDL of 35 mg/dL, and LDL of 140 mg/dL. Which of the following would be most appropriate?

a. Addition of clopidogrel

b. Initiation of HMG-CoA reductase inhibitor ("statin")

c. Increase atenolol

d. Increase lisinopril

e. Increase insulin

44. A 26-year-old woman who is in the second trimester of her first pregnancy is referred to you because of a cardiac murmur. She is asymptomatic aside from exertional fatigue. On physical examination, her pulse rate is 85 bpm and BP is 116/64 mm Hg. Jugular venous pressure is 6 to 7 cm H_2O. Lungs are clear. Cardiac examination reveals a hyperdynamic apex and a grade II/VI early-peaking systolic ejection murmur heard best at the upper left sternal border. S_1 and S_2 are normal. Additional heart sounds are not heard. Mild bilateral lower extremity edema is present. ECG is essentially normal. Which of the following is most appropriate?

a. Obtain a CXR to evaluate the cardiac silhouette.

b. Start diuretic therapy.

c. Obtain an echocardiogram to evaluate for structural cardiac abnormalities.

d. Antibiotic prophylaxis for endocarditis.

e. No specific cardiac therapy.

f. Obtain lower extremity vascular ultrasound to rule out DVT.

45. A 70-year-old man presents with complaints of dyspnea and a pounding sensation in his neck, which he has noted over the past several months. He has not seen a physician in over 20 years. He notes that when was under the care of a physician, he was on two antihypertensive agents but stopped taking them when they ran out because he "felt fine."

On physical examination, his BP is 190/55 mm Hg and his pulse rate is 88/min. He has a bounding carotid pulse. The cardiac apical impulse is hyperdynamic and laterally displaced. On auscultation, S_1 is soft and a high-pitched descrescendo diastolic murmur is heard in the third left intercostal space. Lungs are clear to auscultation. His extremities are without edema; however, visible pulsations in his nail beds are noted.

What is the most likely etiology of his symptoms?

a. AS
b. AI
c. MS
d. Mitral insufficiency
e. Tricuspid insufficiency

46. A 46-year-old man presents to the ED with intermittent episodes of chest pain, initially on exertion and now occurring at rest. His initial examination and ECG are normal. He is treated with oxygen, aspirin, beta blockers, and heparin. While waiting to be admitted, he develops recurrent chest pressure radiating to his neck and associated with diaphoresis. A repeat ECG is obtained (see Figure Q-46). His chest pain is relieved by two tablets of SL NTG; however, a subsequent ECG is unchanged. Which of the following would you recommend?

a. Administration of thrombolytic therapy
b. Administration of a GP IIB-IIIA inhibitor, then urgent cardiac catheterization
c. Administration of NSAIDs
d. Administration of IV NTG
e. Observation for 24 hours, followed by an ETT

47. A 27-year-old IV drug user presents complaining of fevers, hemoptysis, and pleuritic chest pain over the preceding 2 weeks. On physical examination, his temperature is 38.2°C, pulse rate is 100/min, and BP is 110/68. His LV impulse is normal and no murmurs are appreciated on cardiac auscultation. His lungs are clear to auscultation. Three sets of blood cultures are positive for *Staphylococcus aureus* and echocardiography shows a tricuspid valve vegetation with trace tricuspid regurgitation. He is started on IV antibiotic therapy with nafcillin. Despite 2 weeks of appropriate antibiotic therapy, he continues to have intermittent fevers and has developed a grade 2/6 pansystolic murmur along his left sternal border as well as a first-degree AV block on his ECG. His repeat blood cultures remain positive for *S. aureus*.

Which diagnostic test is most appropriate at this time?

a. TEE
b. TTE
c. Electrophysiologic study
d. Bronchoscopy
e. Cardiac catheterization

48. A 62-year-old woman is hospitalized with increasing dyspnea, increasing abdominal girth, and bilateral lower extremity edema. She also complains that she has gained 17 lb over the past week, despite being compliant with her medications, and notes that she has to sleep sitting in a chair because she cannot breathe when she lies flat. She denies any chest pain. She is on diabetic medications as well as a beta blocker and ACE inhibitor for HTN.

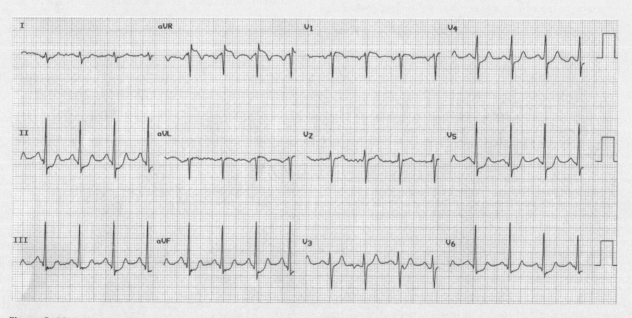

Figure Q-46 •

On physical examination, her BP is 108/50 mm Hg and her pulse 52 bpm. Her oxygen saturation is 88% on room air and 96% on 2-L nasal cannula. Her JVP is estimated at 14 cm H_2O. Cardiac auscultation demonstrates an S_3. She has crackles throughout both lung fields. Her lower extremities are cool, with 3+ bilateral pitting edema. Laboratory values are significant for a BUN/creatinine of 20/1.3. An echocardiogram demonstrates an estimated LVEF of 10%.

She is admitted with decompensated HF and started on IV diuretics in addition to continuation of her home medical regimen. Despite 3 days of aggressive IV diuretics, she continues to gain weight. Her BUN/creatinine is now 36/3.1, her BP is 100/54 mm Hg, and her oxygen saturation is 96% on 2-L nasal cannula.

What is the next step in this patient's management?
a. Hemodialysis
b. PA catheter placement
c. Coronary angiography
d. Dobutamine echocardiogram
e. Exercise echocardiogram

49. A 28-year-old woman with a history of rheumatic MS presents to your office for a yearly examination. Which of the following abnormalities would you expect to find on her physical examination?
a. High-pitched descrescendo diastolic murmur at the third left intercostal space
b. Pulsus parvus et tardus
c. Crisp additional heart sound after S_2 heard best with the diaphragm of the stethoscope at the apex
d. Midsystolic click at the apex
e. Increased pulsus paradoxus

50. A 21-year-old woman is diagnosed with a PDA. This patient is at greatest risk for
a. MI
b. Endocarditis
c. Aortic dissection
d. Pericardial tamponade
e. PE

51. An 82-year-old woman presents to the ED with light-headedness, which she has felt for the past several weeks. Symptoms are worse with exertion. She denies chest pain, dyspnea, or syncope. She has mild HTN, which is treated with HCTZ. She has had no recent travel or illness. BP is 130/90, HR 38 and regular. Her neck veins are not elevated, but intermittent prominent waves are visible. The first heart sound is variable in intensity. Her lungs are clear. Laboratory data, including electrolytes and cardiac enzymes, are normal. Her ECG is shown (Figure Q-51). The most appropriate management includes:
a. Atropine
b. Emergent transvenous temporary pacing wire
c. Observation on telemetry and serial cardiac enzymes
d. Urgent permanent pacemaker implantation
e. Discharge home with Holter monitor

QUESTIONS

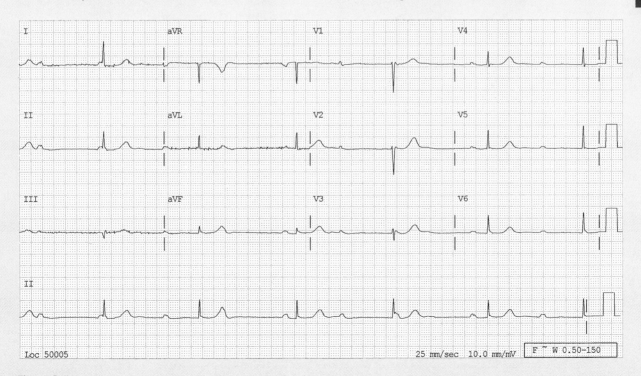

Figure Q-51 •

52. A 75-year-old man is brought to the ED by his family after having had several episodes of slurred speech at home. His history is notable for HTN, tobacco abuse, and DM, which has been marginally controlled with diet. He is currently asymptomatic, with a BP of 150/80 mm Hg and a normal neurologic examination. Cardiac examination reveals an S_4 gallop but no murmurs. Carotid bruits are heard bilaterally. ECG demonstrates normal sinus rhythm without ST- or T-wave changes. CT of the head is pending. Appropriate initial evaluation and treatment include:
a. IV heparin if CT is negative for intracranial hemorrhage
b. Antiplatelet therapy, BP control, and carotid ultrasound
c. Lumbar puncture
d. Antiplatelet therapy and echocardiogram
e. BP control and MRI of the brain

53. A 24-year-old woman who was the unbelted driver in a motor vehicle collision is brought to the ED by ambulance. She is awake and alert despite hitting the steering wheel and windshield on impact. Her HR and BP are stable, and her JVP is not elevated. There is mild bruising over her shoulders and midchest and a laceration on her forehead. CXR reveals a fractured rib and ECG reveals a right bundle branch pattern. In addition to the remainder of the trauma workup, the following tests should be performed:
a. Echocardiogram
b. Electrophysiologic study
c. Cardiac catheterization
d. Holter monitoring after discharge
e. Cardiac MRI

54. A 37-year-old woman comes to your office with the chief complaint of palpitations. Symptoms occur once or twice a week for about 30 minutes at a time; they are associated with light-headedness and a sense of anxiety. She notes occasional brief episodes of sharp chest pain but denies dyspnea or syncope. On physical examination, her HR is 60 bpm and regular, BP 125/80 mm Hg. Cardiac examination is notable for a normal S_1 and S_2 and an extra sound in midsystole. There is no murmur. Routine laboratory studies are normal, including CBC and TSH. The next step in management would be:
a. Reassurance
b. Holter monitor
c. Event monitor
d. Echocardiogram and event monitor
e. Tilt-table testing

55. A 78-year-old man is sent to you for consultation prior to elective total knee replacement. He has been fairly healthy but does have DM and a long smoking history. Up until 6 months ago he was active, but he has recently been limited by knee pain, so that he can walk only a block or two at a time. He denies a history of chest pain, CHF, valvular disease,

or syncope. He is taking glyburide and lisinopril. On physical examination, his BP is 140/85 mm Hg; HR is 75 bpm. No murmurs or gallops are appreciated on cardiac examination. His JVP is not elevated, his lungs are clear, and there is no lower extremity edema. ECG shows normal sinus rhythm without Q waves or ST-T-wave changes. The orthopedic surgeon is awaiting your clearance to set a date for the surgery. The most appropriate recommendations are:
a. Proceed to surgery without further recommendations
b. Start beta blockers and have the patient return for follow-up BP measurements
c. Cardiac catheterization prior to surgery
d. Pharmacologic nuclear stress testing prior to surgery
e. Echocardiogram

56. A 61-year-old woman is admitted to the CCU after an anterior STEMI and LAD stenting. She has been free of chest pain with a stable HR and BP. You are on call the first night of her hospital stay and the nurse asks you to look at an "abnormal rhythm" (Figure Q-56). The next step should be:
a. IV lidocaine
b. DC cardioversion
c. Continued close observation
d. Repeat cardiac catheterization
e. Restart IV heparin

57. A 45-year-old man presents for an initial office visit. He has no medical problems, but his family history is notable for the early death of his father. On physical examination, he is 6'2" tall and weighs 165 lb. His BP is 112/45 mm Hg. Cardiac examination is regular with a normal S_1 and S_2, a midsystolic click, a late systolic murmur at the apex, and an early diastolic murmur heard at the left midsternal border. His lungs are clear and there is no peripheral edema. ECG is unremarkable. In addition to routine health maintenance, which of the following tests should be performed first:
a. TEE
b. TTE
c. Cardiac catheterization
d. CT of the chest
e. MRA of the chest

58. A 55-year-old woman is admitted with dyspnea and abdominal pain. She reports several months of palpitations, diarrhea, and facial flushing, with a recent onset of abdominal distention and lower extremity edema. Physical examination reveals ruddy complexion, HR 90, BP 125/70. JVP is 15 cm H_2O with positive HJR. There is an HSM at the left lower sternal border and a right-sided S_3. The liver is enlarged, mildly tender, and pulsatile; there is ascites and marked lower extremity edema bilaterally. The most appropriate diagnostic tests include:
a. Abdominal CT scan and measurement of urinary metanephrines
b. Abdominal ultrasound and LFTs

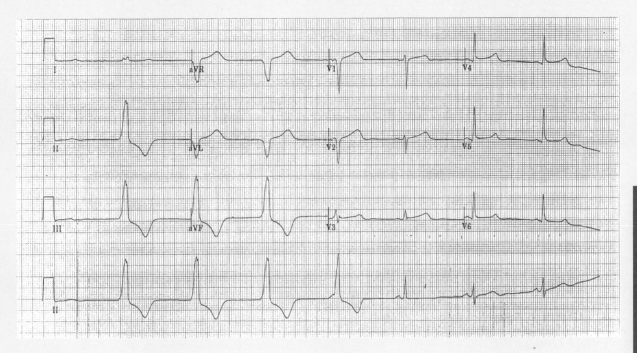

Figure Q-56 •

c. RHC
d. Echocardiogram and 24-hour urine for 5-HIAA
e. Lower extremity ultrasound

59. A 36-year-old woman presents to the urgent care clinic for further evaluation of HTN. She has had yearly physicals and has never been noted to have HTN in the past. She has been taking her BP at a local grocery store and over the past several months has noted a gradual rise, with recent values as high as 180/100 mm Hg. She has no history of DM, smoking, high cholesterol, or family history of HTN and denies chest pain, dyspnea, claudication, or neurologic symptoms. She is taking no medications or over-the-counter preparations. Today, her BP is 170/90 mm Hg in both arms. She is in no distress and is not obese. Cardiac examination is unremarkable; radial and femoral pulses are equal. What is the most likely diagnosis?
a. Cushing syndrome
b. Essential hypertension
c. Coarctation of the aorta
d. Fibromuscular dysplasia of the renal arteries
e. Pheochromocytoma

60. A 31-year-old woman from India presents with several months of increasing lower extremity edema and dyspnea on exertion. She also notes that her voice has become hoarse. Her hemodynamic tracing is shown (see Figure Q-60).
    What is the diagnosis?
a. AS
b. AI

c. MS
d. Mitral insufficiency
e. Tricuspid insufficiency

61. A 77-year-old man with a history of an ischemic cardiomyopathy and prior CABG comes to clinic with complaints of dyspnea on exertion and fatigue. He notes dyspnea after walking less than a block or climbing one flight of stairs.

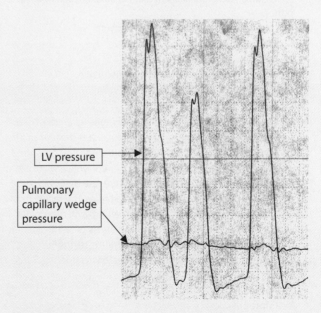

LV pressure

Pulmonary capillary wedge pressure

Figure Q-60 •

His symptoms have persisted despite treatment with metoprolol XL 100 mg daily, lisinopril 40 mg daily, amlodipine 5 mg daily, digoxin 0.125 mg daily, aspirin 81 mg daily, furosemide 40 mg twice daily, spironolactone 25 mg daily, and isosorbide mononitrate 120 mg daily. He had undergone cardiac catheterization 2 weeks earlier, which demonstrated severe native three-vessel CAD with patent bypass grafts. An echocardiogram at that time revealed a dilated LV cavity with an LVEF of 20% and mild MR. There was no significant change from an echocardiogram 1 year prior.

On physical examination, his BP is 112/70 mm Hg and his HR is 56 bpm. His oxygen saturation is 99% on room air. His JVP is at 8 cm H_2O. Carotid pulses are normal. His LV impulse is laterally displaced and a soft S_3 is audible. There are crackles just at the right base of his lung field. His extremities are warm and dry, with trace bipedal edema. ECG demonstrates an LBBB with a QRS interval of 140 ms.

What is the next step in this patient's management?

a. Admit to the hospital for IV diuresis
b. Exercise nuclear test
c. Refer for biventricular pacer evaluation
d. Repeat echocardiogram
e. Admit to the hospital for a trial of nesiritide

62. A 34-year-old woman with a bicuspid AV is referred for AV replacement. By TTE, she has normal LV systolic function with an AV area of 0.6 cm^2. She is otherwise in good health and denies any history of bleeding problems. She is newly married and hopes to have at least two children. All laboratory work is normal.

What is the preferred type of prosthetic valve for this patient?

a. Carpenter-Edwards porcine xenograft
b. Bjork-Shiley single tilting-disc valve
c. Starr-Edwards ball-in-cage valve
d. St-Jude Medical bileaflet tilting-disc valve
e. Medtronic-Hall single tilting-disc valve

63. You are seeing a 38-year-old woman who is in the third trimester of her third pregnancy. She has a history of mild HTN which was treated with HCZT, although this was discontinued by her obstetrician. She is currently asymptomatic. On physical examination, her pulse rate is 84/min, and her BP is 140/96 mm Hg on multiple readings. The rest of her examination is unremarkable other than a gravid uterus. Her serum creatinine is normal. No proteinuria is present.

In addition to recommending sodium restriction and rest, which of the following antihypertensive medications would you prescribe at this time?

a. Atenolol
b. Captopril
c. HCZT

d. Methyldopa
e. Labetalol

64. A 65-year-old man with a history of hypertension presents with tearing chest pain that radiates to his back. He undergoes a CT scan that demonstrates a descending aortic dissection originating just distal to the aortic arch and extending to the aortic bifurcation. No significant vascular obstruction is seen. The most appropriate initial therapy for this patient should include:

a. Thrombolytic therapy
b. Heparin
c. Emergent surgical intervention
d. Labetalol and nitroprusside
e. IV fluids and narcotic analgesics

65. You are called to evaluate a 67-year-old woman who developed sudden dyspnea and pleuritic chest pain 48 hours after undergoing hip replacement surgery. Her BP is 132/88 mm Hg; HR, 104 bpm; and O_2 saturation, 95%. You suspect that she has had a PE. The most appropriate initial diagnostic study to confirm the diagnosis is:

a. Sputum culture
b. Arterial blood gas
c. Echocardiogram
d. Lower extremity ultrasound
e. V/Q scan

66. A 65-year-old man with a history of HTN and DM presents with an acute STEMI. He is treated with oxygen, aspirin, sublingual nitroglycerin, morphine, and IV beta blockers. Despite this, he continues to complain of severe chest discomfort and has persistent ECG changes. Further history reveals that he suffered a mild stroke 6 months earlier. What is the most appropriate next step in management?

a. Increase analgesics (morphine sulfate) until discomfort resolves.
b. Obtain a chest CT to rule out aortic dissection.
c. Administer IV thrombolytic therapy.
d. Arrange transfer to a tertiary care hospital for primary angioplasty.
e. Obtain V/Q scan to rule out PE.

67. A 62-year-old woman presents with several months of progressive edema, fatigue, and a 20-lb weight gain. Her past history is significant for TB, for which she received treatment for 20 years prior. Her examination reveals resting tachycardia, clear lungs, prominent jugular venous waveforms that increase with inspiration, hepatic engorgement, and 3+ pedal edema. You suspect that she has pericardial constriction. Which of the following would be the best method to confirm the diagnosis?

a. CT scan of the chest
b. ECG

c. CXR

d. Bronchoscopy

e. Cardiac catheterization

68. A 26-year-old woman presents for a routine physical examination. She has no significant prior history and her vital signs are normal. Her cardiac examination reveals a split S_2 that does not normalize with maneuvers, and there is a II/VII SEM at the left upper sternal border. You suspect that she has an ASD. The most appropriate initial method to confirm your suspected diagnosis is:

a. Echocardiogram

b. Exercise stress test

c. Cardiac catheterization

d. CXR

e. Cardiac MRI

69. A 34-year-old man with a history of a bicuspid AV is diagnosed with endocarditis. Despite 2 weeks of appropriate antibiotic therapy, he has persistent fevers and bacteremia. A diagnostic study is performed and a paravalvular abscess discovered. What is the next step in this patient's management?

a. Continue current antibiotic therapy

b. Add gentamicin

c. Change nafcillin to vancomycin

d. Change nafcillin to ceftriaxone

e. Refer for surgery

70. A 19-year-old woman presents with increasing dyspnea on exertion and chest pain. She has been told since childhood that she has a "heart murmur." On physical examination, her arterial pulse is brisk, with a wide pulse pressure. She has a prominent RV heave and a prominent P_2. A loud, machinery-like, continuous (systolic and diastolic) murmur is heard at the second left intercostal space. Interestingly, she has clubbing and cyanosis of her toes but not her fingers (differential cyanosis).

What is the most likely diagnosis?

a. PDA

b. ASD

c. VSD

d. Tetralogy of Fallot

e. Pulmonary stenosis

71. A 72-year-old man with a history of HTN and cigarette smoking presents with transient right arm weakness and slurred speech. Examination reveals a BP of 122/72 mm Hg. A neurologic examination reveals no focal abnormality. A carotid ultrasound is obtained and reveals 30% stenosis of the right internal carotid artery and 75% stenosis of the left internal carotid artery. The best long-term management strategy is:

a. Aggressive risk-factor modification to prevent further cerebral events

b. Warfarin therapy

c. Serial MRA of the carotid arteries

d. Referral for carotid endarterectomy

e. Combination antiplatelet therapy with aspirin and clopidogrel

72. A 69-year-old woman presents to the ED reporting substernal chest tightness associated with nausea and diaphoresis for the preceding 3 hours. Her history is significant for HTN. Her medications include diltiazem. On physical examination, her pulse rate is 100/min and BP is 120/75 mm Hg. Jugular venous pressure is 10 cm H_2O. Lungs are clear to auscultation. Cardiac examination reveals a regular rhythm without murmurs or gallops. ECG shows 2-mm STE in II, III, and aVF with ST-segment depression in V_2. CXR is normal. SL NTG is administered. She becomes pale, clammy, and light-headed. Repeat BP is 80/60 mm Hg. She is placed in the Trendelenburg position and an IV fluid bolus is given. Her BP increases to 90/62 mm Hg. What is the most likely diagnosis?

a. Acute inferior MI with RV infarct

b. Aortic dissection

c. PE

d. Cardiac tamponade

e. Papillary muscle rupture with MR

73. An 85-year-old man is brought to the ED by his family because of severe abdominal pain. His medical history is notable for HTN, DM, and CAD, with a CABG 10 years earlier. His wife reports that he has been complaining of intermittent chest pressure with exertion for 2 weeks. On examination, he is very uncomfortable. HR 110, BP 90/50. Cardiac examination is unremarkable. Abdomen is diffusely tender, with a 6-cm pulsatile mass in the epigastric area. The ED physician confirms her suspicion of a leaking abdominal aortic aneurysm with a CT scan and calls you to stratify the patient in terms of risk prior to potential vascular surgery. Your recommendations include the following:

a. Proceed to surgery without further cardiac workup and with intraoperative invasive hemodynamic monitoring

b. Intensive beta blockade for a goal HR <60 bpm prior to surgery

c. Bedside echocardiogram

d. Adenosine nuclear scan prior to surgery

e. Urgent cardiac catheterization

74. A 21-year-old man presents with exertional dyspnea and presyncope. He is quite athletic; however, he notes that over the past several months he has become light-headed and short of breath when playing competitive sports. His BP is 116/78 mm Hg. There is no increase in his JVP. His lungs are clear. His LV impulse is prominent. There is a normal S_1 and S_2 with a soft S_4. There is a II/VI systolic murmur at the left sternal border that does not radiate but worsens during the strain phase of Valsalva. An ECG reveals LV hypertrophy. An echocardiogram is performed and reveals moderate LVH and RVH with a dynamic gradient in the LVOT. The best medical management of this condition is:

a. Diuretics
b. Calcium channel blockers
c. ACE inhibitors
d. Nitroglycerin
e. Antiplatelet agents

75. A 68-year-old man from Trinidad presents for his first medical evaluation after moving to the United States. He has a history of HTN and was told several years ago that he had an irregular heartbeat. He denies any history of chest pain, dyspnea, palpitations, or syncope. His only medication is metoprolol. His examination is significant only for a BP of 124/78 mm Hg and an irregularly irregular rhythm. An ECG reveals AF with a ventricular rate of 76 bpm. The most appropriate course of treatment for this patient is:

a. Admit to the hospital for electrical cardioversion.
b. Start aspirin and continue metoprolol.
c. Add digoxin to the metoprolol.
d. Start amiodarone and warfarin and plan electrical cardioversion in 3 to 4 weeks.
e. Start warfarin and continue metoprolol.

A Answers

1. c (Chapter 10)

Recognize CHD risk equivalents according to current guidelines. PAD, abdominal aortic aneurysm, symptomatic carotid artery disease, and DM are considered CHD risk equivalents. The goal LDL level should be less than 100 mg/dL in these patients. In patients at very high risk (including those who have had a recent MI, have CAD combined with DM, or have poorly controlled risk factors), a lower LDL goal should be considered (<70 mg/dL). In addition to TLC, drug therapy should also be considered in such patients. In order to achieve the LDL goal, a 30% reduction in LDL level is necessary; TLC alone is unlikely to achieve this level. HMG-CoA reductase inhibitors lower LDL levels effectively (18 to 55%). Fibric-acid derivatives lower TGs effectively but their LDL reduction is relatively small (5 to 20%).

2. d (Chapter 23)

Recognize the presentation of vasovagal syncope and know the appropriate diagnostic test. This type of syncope is common in younger patients and is frequently associated with a stressful event or prolonged standing. It is often preceded by light-headedness, dizziness, and vasodilation ("warm feeling"). Other causes to be considered in this patient include HCM, congenital long-QT syndrome, and seizure, although the normal ECG and echocardiogram exclude the first two options, and the history does not suggest seizure activity. The best test to confirm the diagnosis of vasovagal syncope is a tilt-table test. In this setting it is 70 to 75% sensitive. EPS is not indicated in syncope patients without structural heart disease as the test is neither sensitive nor specific. CT of the head is usually unhelpful in the evaluation of syncope unless the patient has neurologic signs or symptoms. Holter monitoring is useful if bradyarrhythmias and tachyarrhythmias are suspected. This patient's history is not suggestive of carotid sinus hypersensitivity syndrome; thus CSM is not indicated.

3. d (Chapter 18)

Recognize the presentation of viral myocarditis. The typical patient with acute myocarditis is an otherwise healthy young adult. Although the clinical presentation varies widely, symptomatic patients usually present with HF of recent onset. Other presenting symptoms include palpitations, chest pain, syncope, and SCD. Patients may recall a preceding viral syndrome. Echocardiography typically demonstrates ventricular systolic dysfunction, which may be either global or regional. Acute myocarditis can mimic AMI (chest pain, ST-T-wave changes, myocardial enzyme elevation, and regional wall-motion abnormalities on echocardiogram). A careful history must be obtained to distinguish between the two entities. Pericarditis usually presents with chest pain and diffuse STE but does not cause HF. Neither pericarditis nor HCM is associated with an elevation in CK-MB. PE rarely results in left HF or significant CK-MB elevation.

4. e (Chapter 4)

Determine the appropriate stress-test modality and recognize the indications for adding an imaging modality to a stress test. In general, if a patient can exercise, an exercise test should be performed. If the patient cannot exercise, pharmacologic stress testing is required (adenosine, dipyridamole, or dobutamine). If an exercise test is performed and there are no significant ST abnormalities on the resting ECG, then ECG monitoring alone is usually adequate for the detection of ischemia. However, if there are abnormal ST segments on the resting ECG (e.g., LBBB, LVH with a "strain" pattern, digoxin effect, persistent ST depression, paced rhythm), the ECG is not adequate to identify ischemia and an imaging modality is necessary. The use of echocardiographic or nuclear imaging improves the sensitivity and specificity of the test in this setting. If pharmacologic stress testing is performed, an imaging modality is always required.

5. d (Chapter 36)

Recognize indications for surgical repair of abdominal aneurysms. These include diameter >5.5 cm, rate of growth >0.5 cm in 6 months, symptoms, and thrombotic or embolic complications. Randomized trials have compared surgery with watchful waiting in patients with asymptomatic aneurysms of < 5.5 cm and have not found a survival benefit with early surgery. Small, asymptomatic aneurysms may be managed medically with aggressive BP control and beta-blocker therapy. Beta blockers decrease shear stress in the aorta and may decrease the rate of aneurysm expansion and risk of rupture. In patients managed medically, serial imaging is required to assess for aneurysm expansion. Patients with coexisting CAD may need to undergo coronary revascularization prior to aneurysm repair.

6. b (Chapter 12)

7. h (Chapter 36)

8. f (Chapter 31)

Anginal chest pain is usually a midsternal or left-sided discomfort that comes on with exertion and is relieved with rest. Stable angina occurs at a reproducible level of exertion. US is that which occurs at rest, with increased frequency, or with less exertion. The pain of MI is similar to that of angina but is more severe and prolonged. An aortic dissection usually causes severe, sharp, sometimes tearing pain that radiates to the back. It may be associated with pulse discrepancies owing to impairment of blood flow in branch vessels. Pericardial pain is usually pleuritic and positional; it may be associated with a friction rub. Pericarditis is often preceded by a viral illness. Pain from a PE or pneumothorax may mimic angina but is usually pleuritic and associated with dyspnea. Chest pain from coronary spasm tends to occur at rest, with variable relationship to exertion.

9. d (Chapter 35)

Diagnose and manage TAO. TAO, also known as *Buerger disease,* is a vasculitis of the small and medium-sized arteries and veins of the upper and lower extremities. Cerebral, visceral, and coronary vessels may also be involved. Young male smokers (< 45 years of age) are most commonly affected. Patients with TAO frequently present with the triad of claudication, Raynaud phenomenon, and migratory superficial thrombophlebitis. Physical examination typically reveals reduced or absent distal pulses, trophic nail changes, digital ulcerations, and digital gangrene. The etiology of TAO is unknown, but there appears to be a definite relationship to cigarette smoking and an increased incidence of HLA-B5 and HLA-A9 antigens in patients with the disease. There is no specific therapy for TAO. Smoking cessation appears to be moderately effective at halting disease progression. Surgical reconstruction is of limited applicability due to the distal nature of the disease. In severe cases, amputation may be required.

10. b (Chapter 32)

Recognize the presentation of pericardial tamponade and know the appropriate test to confirm the diagnosis. This patient

has the classic features of tamponade, with mild hypotension, quiet heart sounds, and elevated JVP (the Beck triad). Additionally, there is marked respiratory variation in her pulse volume and systolic BP (pulsus paradoxus) and findings consistent with right HF. The systolic pressure normally may fall by as much as 10 mm Hg during inspiration (pulsus paradoxus) but frequently falls by >15 mm Hg during tamponade. An exaggerated pulsus paradoxus may also be seen in constrictive pericarditis, or severe airway obstruction. Tamponade is a diagnosis made on clinical grounds but is best confirmed with a TTE. This study will reveal the size of the pericardial effusion as well as demonstrate evidence of increased intrapericardial pressure (e.g., dilated IVC; RA or RV inversion; marked variability of mitral valve inflow). A CXR or CT scan can reveal evidence of a pericardial effusion but cannot distinguish between an effusion and tamponade physiology. A PA catheter will demonstrate equilibration of diastolic pressures in the setting of tamponade; however, it is an invasive study and requires much more time than an echocardiogram and is rarely necessary to confirm the diagnosis. A V/Q scan is not indicated in the evaluation of tamponade; it is useful in the evaluation of PE.

11. c (Chapter 29)

Recognize the features of SBE. This patient's physical examination demonstrates peripheral manifestations of endocarditis, including digital clubbing and Janeway lesions. Other lesions that may be seen include splinter hemorrhages, Roth spots, and Osler nodes. The most common predisposing factors for SBE are structural heart diseases, including MVP. The patient's midsystolic click and apical murmur are indicative of this disorder. While pneumonia, pericarditis, and viral syndromes may cause febrile illnesses, they are not associated with the peripheral findings noted here. Although a VSD or PDA may predispose to SBE, they are not associated with the murmur of MVP. SBE should always be considered in patients presenting with a fever of unknown origin.

12. c (Chapter 38)

Recognize the clinical features and risk factors for venous thromboembolic disease. The increase in this patient's edema likely results from a DVT. Although worsening of her HF must also be considered, the asymmetric nature of the edema and the clinical scenario are much more consistent with a DVT. The diagnosis can be confirmed with a bedside lower extremity ultrasound. A number of acquired conditions are associated with venous thromboembolic disease. These conditions result in stasis of blood, vascular injury, and/or hypercoagulability and include immobilization (stroke, spinal cord injury, prolonged travel), obesity, pregnancy, advanced age, heart failure, trauma, surgery, indwelling vascular catheters, prior DVT, malignancy, oral contraceptives, smoking, and, nephrotic syndrome. Additionally, hereditary hypercoagulable states may contribute [e.g., factor V Leiden mutation, activated protein C resistance, protein C deficiency, protein S deficiency, antithrombin III deficiency, hyperhomocyst(e)inemia, antiphospholipid antibody syndrome].

13. b (Chapter 27)

Recognize the signs and symptoms of severe AS. This patient experienced the common symptoms of significant AS, including syncope, angina, and dyspnea on exertion (possible CHF). In addition, his examination is consistent with severe to critical AS with a late-peaking SEM. The diminished carotid pulse (pulsus parvus) is frequently associated with a delay in the carotid upstroke (pulsus tardus). As AS becomes more severe, the second heart sound becomes faint and may altogether disappear. Although the other choices are possible causes of syncope in this man, his clinical presentation is classic for syncope resulting from significant AS.

14. c (Chapter 25)

Recognize the indications for permanent pacemaker implantation. This patient has symptomatic bradycardia, likely a result of a tachy-brady syndrome. She is on no medications that could induce the bradycardia, and her conduction system disease is irreversible; thus, she has a clear indication for pacemaker implantation. Holter monitoring is not indicated, as the resting ECG is diagnostic. ICDs are reserved for those with life-threatening ventricular tachyarrhythmias. Simple reassurance without further therapy is inappropriate, as—without pacemaker therapy—the patient is at risk for progressive bradycardia and syncope.

15. b (Chapter 31)

Recognize the symptoms and signs of pericarditis. Pericarditis classically causes sharp, *pleuritic* chest pain and may be associated with a sensation of dyspnea. The presence of a pericardial friction rub is pathognomonic for pericarditis. This rub is often confused with a murmur but is difficult to characterize because it occurs in both systole and diastole and may have one to three components. The ECG demonstrates the classic findings of PR segment depression and diffuse STE. In this particular case, the pericarditis may relate to her SLE or may be postviral in etiology. Although an AMI may be associated with pericardial irritation, the clinical history and ECG are much more consistent with pericarditis. Mitral stenosis frequently causes exertional chest pain and dyspnea, but it is not pleuritic. Pneumonia and can cause pleuritic chest pain, but it is not associated with a pericardial friction rub or ECG changes. A PE is a distinct possibility; however, the ECG abnormality is essentially diagnostic of pericarditis.

16. c (Chapter 17)

Understand the management of decompensated HF based on hemodynamic measurements. This patient is volume-overloaded with high left and right heart filling pressure, low cardiac output, and high SVR but has an adequate systemic BP. He clearly requires diuresis; however, his markedly reduced cardiac output and elevated SVR are the predominant hemodynamic abnormalities. He requires inotropic support (dobutamine) as well as afterload reduction (nitroprusside). Although beta blockers have favorable effects on chronic HF, they are contraindicated in decompensated HF. This patient's BP is adequate; therefore he does not need a vasopressor (dopamine). Digoxin is a very weak inotrope and is unlikely to be of value in acute HF. An intraaortic balloon pump would likely help this patient significantly; however, it should be considered only after aggressive medical therapy has failed.

17. b (Chapter 19)

Recognize restrictive CMP. The clinical presentation of restrictive CMP is similar to that of severe constrictive pericarditis with exertional dyspnea and signs of biventricular HF. Additional symptoms may include orthopnea, paroxysmal nocturnal dyspnea, anorexia, and fatigue. Physical examination frequently reveals pulmonary and systemic venous congestion. The Kussmaul sign (a paradoxical rise in JVP with inspiration) may be present. Echocardiography typically reveals thickened ventricles with relatively preserved systolic function. With idiopathic dilated CMP, the heart is dilated and systolic function is usually moderately to severely depressed. With constrictive pericarditis, the LV is usually small, not thickened, and hyperdynamic. Pericardial tamponade is rarely the result of a small pericardial effusion and is not associated with the Kussmaul sign. High-output failure is usually associated with hyperdynamic ventricular function and not with biventricular thickening.

18. c (Chapter 39)

Recognize the features of pulmonary HTN. This patient's physical findings of an RV heave (prominent parasternal impulse), loud second heart sound, tricuspid regurgitant murmur, and elevated JVP all suggest elevated PA and right heart pressures. The CXR demonstrates RV enlargement and pulmonary vascular changes consistent with pulmonary HTN. CAD would be distinctly unusual in a 34-year-old woman, especially in the absence of risk factors, chest pain, or ECG abnormalities. Right HF from asthma would be unlikely in the absence of a long history of severe bronchospastic disease. Anemia may cause dyspnea but does not produce the physical findings of pulmonary HTN and right HF. Chronic PE may result in pulmonary HTN and the findings noted in this patient, but an acute PE would be unlikely given the several-month history of dyspnea.

19. c (Chapter 28)

20. a (Chapter 27)

ANSWERS

21. g (Chapter 19)

Recognize the classic features of various murmurs. The 36-year-old woman has the classic findings of MS with a loud P_2 (from pulmonary HTN), an OS in early diastole, and a diastolic rumble. Tachycardia and dyspnea are commonly seen with MS, and her palpitations likely reflect paroxysmal AF. The 75-year-old man has severe AS, as evidenced by the late-peaking systolic murmur that radiates to the carotids and the soft S_2. Diminished carotid upstrokes might also have been present. His symptoms of chest pain, dyspnea, and syncope are the cardinal symptoms of AS. The 40-year-old man has HCM. This murmur may mimic AS but does not radiate to the carotids and/or result in diminished carotid upstrokes. Additionally, the murmur of HCM is the only murmur that increases with Valsalva. The murmur of AI is a decrescendo diastolic murmur at the left sternal border. MR produces a holosystolic murmur at the cardiac apex that radiates to the axilla. An ASD results in a systolic flow murmur at the upper sternal border (owing to increased flow across the PV) and a fixed split S_2. A PDA produces a continuous (systolic and diastolic) "machine-like" murmur at the left upper sternal border that radiates to the back.

22. e (Chapter 29)

Know the appropriate tests for the evaluation of endocarditis and recognize the significance of specific causative organisms. Patients with *S. bovis* endocarditis frequently have colonic neoplasms and should be screened with colonoscopy. CT of the chest may be useful to evaluate for lung abscess in a patient with right-sided SBE and abnormal CXR, but it is unlikely to be of value in this patient. Although SBE may be associated with cerebral abscesses and intracranial aneurysms, routine scans are not indicated in the absence of CNS symptoms. Cardiac catheterization would be indicated only in the event of a complication requiring cardiac surgery (i.e., progressive valvular disease).

23. b (Chapter 13)

Recognize the ECG of a patient with an acute STEMI. This ECG demonstrates 2 to 3 mm of STEMI in leads V_1 to V_5. This is consistent with an acute infarction of the anterior wall of the LV, which most likely resulted from an acute thrombotic occlusion of the LAD. The presence of Q waves in V_1 to V_3 suggests that the infarct has been evolving for more than a few hours. Although pericarditis is also associated with chest pain and STE on ECG, the STE is usually diffuse and is concave upward in morphology. Additionally, PR-segment depression is frequently seen with pericarditis but is not present on this ECG. UA is associated with ST-segment depression on ECG, not STE. An LBBB can produce STE in the anterior precordial leads; however, it is always associated with a wide QRS complex (not present here). PE can be associated with a variety of ECG changes, most commonly tachycardia and signs of right heart strain (RBBB and T-wave inversions in the inferior and anterior leads S1Q3T3 pattern), but they rarely cause regional ST elevation.

24. c (Chapter 32)

Recognize the features and treatment of cardiac tamponade. This patient exhibits the classic signs of cardiac tamponade, including hypotension, elevated JVP, and faint heart sounds (the Beck triad). She would also likely have exaggerated respiratory variation of her SBP (pulsus paradoxus). Patients with tamponade may rapidly deteriorate unless an emergent pericardiocentesis is performed. Cardiac tamponade may be confirmed with echocardiography; however, it is a *clinical* diagnosis that requires emergent therapy. Although the patient has a small pleural effusion, it is not the cause of her deterioration; thus thoracentesis would not be helpful. Cardiac catheterization is not indicated in this setting. Heparin is contraindicated in the setting of pericarditis or tamponade. It is noteworthy that the cause of tamponade in this woman is likely recurrent lung cancer. The most common tumors that metastasize to the pericardium are lung, breast, lymphoma, and melanoma.

25. b (Chapter 12)

Recognize the difference between an ACS and chronic stable angina. This patient presents with classic crescendo exertional angina of recent onset, followed by a prolonged episode of rest angina (>20 minutes). The accelerating nature of his anginal pattern as well as rest angina are characteristic of UA. His ECG does not demonstrate ST-segment abnormalities and therefore is not consistent with a STEMI or pericarditis. Although he had a relatively prolonged episode of rest angina and may subsequently "rule-in" for a non-STEMI by serial assessment of cardiac markers (CK-MB or troponin), the ECG itself does not suggest an AMI. The presentation of an acute PE is usually that of sudden, sharp, pleuritic, chest pain associated with dyspnea.

26. d (Chapter 11)

Recognize the indications for CABG in patients with CAD. This patient's angina was easily provoked on stress testing despite multiple anti-ischemic medications, suggesting that his current medical regimen is inadequate for the control of his ischemia. Additionally, his HR and BP at rest are well controlled and unlikely to allow further uptitration of his medications without inducing bradycardia or hypotension. He has, thus, failed medical management and will require revascularization. Both percutaneous and surgical revascularization are effective in the treatment of CAD. However, patients with left main CAD, triple-vessel CAD, and double-vessel CAD (including a high-grade proximal LAD stenosis) with depressed LV systolic function, experience long-term mortality benefit from CABG when compared with multivessel PTCA or medical therapy. This is especially true for diabetic patients and patients who have depressed LV systolic function. TMR is reserved only for patients with refractory angina who are not CABG candidates (usually due to poor target vessels).

27. a (Chapter 36)

Recognize the presentation of an acute aortic dissection. Most patients with this condition present with an abrupt onset of severe pain localized to the chest or back and described as sharp, ripping, or tearing. The pain often radiates to the neck, jaw, flanks, or legs. HTN is the most common finding in patients with descending aortic dissections, whereas those with ascending aortic dissections frequently present with hypotension. Other physical findings may include pulse deficits, asymmetric extremity BPs (>30 mm Hg), short decrescendo diastolic murmur (due to acute AI), left pleural effusion (hemothorax), paraparesis or paraplegia, neurologic deficits consistent with cerebrovascular accident, abdominal pain (mesenteric ischemia), flank pain (renal infarction), acute lower extremity ischemia, cardiac tamponade (rupture into pericardial space), and Horner syndrome (compression of superior cervical sympathetic ganglion).

28. c (Chapters 24 and 25)

Understand the treatment of patients who have survived a cardiac arrest. One of the approved indications for ICDs is for the treatment of survivors of SCD. Holter monitoring and EP study in SCD survivors is unnecessary, as the possibility of recurrent cardiac arrest is sufficiently high to warrant empiric implantation of an ICD. Exercise stress testing will likely be unhelpful, as angiography did not reveal significant coronary artery stenoses. The patient has no described conduction disease that would necessitate implantation of a pacemaker.

29. d (Chapter 38)

Diagnose PE. The most common presenting symptom of PE is sudden dyspnea, which occurs in approximately 80% of patients. Additional symptoms include pleuritic chest pain, cough, hemoptysis, and syncope. Physical examination of patients with PE may be normal but often demonstrates signs of pulmonary HTN or right HF, including tachypnea, tachycardia, elevated JVP, tricuspid regurgitation murmur, accentuated pulmonic component of S_2 (P_2), and a RV heave. A pulmonary rub may be heard over the involved area of lung when pulmonary infarction has occurred. The normal CXR essentially excludes pneumonia or pneumothorax as the cause, and the absence of ECG changes makes pericarditis very unlikely. Pleurisy is a frequent cause of pleuritic chest pain but is not associated with acute shortness of breath or signs of right HF.

30. b (Chapter 39)

Understand the treatment of PPH, an incurable disease with a relatively poor prognosis. Vasodilators are the mainstay of treatment, although not all patients exhibit a significant treatment response. The oral vasodilators of choice include nifedipine and diltiazem in doses of 120–240 mg/day and 540–900 mg/day, respectively. In patients who have an inadequate response to these agents, a continuous infusion of epoprostenol, a vasodilating prostaglandin, may be beneficial. Epoprostanol acts by increasing intracellular levels of cyclic AMP and produces both acute and sustained hemodynamic improvement, symptomatic improvement, and prolonged survival in patients with PPH. It may be used either as primary treatment or as a bridge to lung transplantation. Single-lung and combined heart-lung transplantation remains the only definitive therapies for PPH and are used for patients who fail vasodilator therapy. One-year survival following lung transplantation approaches 65 to 70%. Beta blockers and ACE inhibitors do not have a role in the treatment of PPH.

31. c (Chapter 34)

Recognize and manage hypertensive emergency. This patient has marked HTN with concomitant symptoms/target-organ damage (acute pulmonary edema) and requires immediate BP reduction. Although oxygen and diuresis are clearly necessary, they are not adequate, and IV antihypertensive agents such as sodium nitroprusside, nitroglycerin, or enalaprilat should be administered expeditiously. The initial goal should be a 25% reduction in mean arterial pressure within the first 2 hours. Further reduction in BP should proceed more slowly, as rapid reductions in BP can lead to end-organ hypoperfusion. Sublingual nitroglycerin is not an effective method of controlling BP, and most oral agents are not absorbed fast enough to produce the desired effect in a short period of time. Beta blockers should be used with caution in patients with decompensated HF.

32. a (Chapter 29)

Recognize the valvular abnormalities induced by endocarditis. The course of events suggests that antibiotics have failed to eradicate the infection and progressive valvular dysfunction has occurred, resulting in HF. Acute valvular dysfunction is almost always regurgitant. The only answer that is consistent with a regurgitant lesion is the apical HSM of MR. The crescendo-decrescendo murmur is indicative of a flow murmur. The weak and delayed carotids are indicative of AS. A middiastolic murmur and an OS are features of MS, while the three-component rub indicates pericarditis.

33. a (Chapter 13)

Know the acute pharmacologic management of an AMI. Immediate therapy should include aspirin and supplemental oxygen. Morphine sulfate can help reduce the sympathetic outflow during an AMI and is the analgesic of choice. Beta blockers should be given to reduce the HR provided that the BP is >90 mm Hg and the patient is not in HF. The reduction in HR reduces MVO_2 and may limit ischemia/infarction. Anticoagulation with either unfractionated heparin or LMWH should be initiated as soon as possible if there are no contraindications. Calcium channel blockers are not routinely indicated in the setting of an AMI, although they may be useful for HR control in patients who have contraindications to beta blockers (e.g., severe bronchospasm or beta-blocker allergy). Nitrates would be reasonable for symptom control in this patient; however, diuretics are not indicated given the lack of congestion and the relatively low BP. NSAIDs are the treatment of choice for pericarditis but are contraindicated in an AMI.

34. d (Chapter 6)

Recognize the hemodynamic abnormalities associated with sepsis. The primary hemodynamic abnormality in sepsis is inappropriate vasodilation (i.e., decreased SVR), resulting in hypotension. The reduction in SVR results in an increase in CO. In general, patients with sepsis have low filling pressures unless they have associated cardiac disease (resulting in CHF) or renal disease (resulting in volume overload). Cardiogenic shock is associated with a decreased CO, increased SVR, and increased filling pressures. Hypovolemia is associated with low filling pressures, resulting in a decrease in CO and a rise in SVR. In pericardial tamponade, there is elevation and equilibration of diastolic pressures (i.e., the RA, PCW, and PA diastolic pressure are high and nearly equal). PE is associated with elevated right-sided pressures (mild to moderately increase PA and RA pressure) with low or normal PCW and CO. The SVR is usually increased in significant PE.

35. c (Chapter 33)

Recognize the symptoms and signs of constrictive pericarditis. Constrictive pericarditis results from thickening of the pericardium and inability of the ventricles to completely expand in diastole. Thus, cardiac output is reduced and RH pressures are significantly elevated. The paradoxical rise in JVP with inspiration is known as the Kussmaul sign and is commonly seen in patients with constrictive pericarditis. The "prominent" venous pulsations are the result of the rapid x and y descents that are characteristic of this disease. Right HF and hepatic congestion are common findings in these patients. TB is a common cause of this syndrome and is the likely cause in this patient. The clinical presentation is not that of acute pericarditis. Although some of the features could also be seen with pericardial tamponade, the normal cardiac size on CXR makes constrictive disease much more likely; also, the Kussmaul sign is not associated with tamponade. Although a pericardial knock may be confused with an OS, the absence of a diastolic rumble makes MS unlikely.

36. d (Chapter 21)

Identify AVNRT on ECG and recognize the treatment options. This patient's ECG demonstrates AVNRT. This is a SVT (narrow-complex tachycardia) caused by a microreentrant circuit

within the AV node. The atria and ventricles are often simultaneously activated and P waves are not usually obvious on the ECG (retrograde P waves are seen after the QRS complex in lead II and aVF on this patient's ECG). However, a "pseudo-R'" may be noted in lead V_1 that is actually a P wave superimposed on the terminal portion of the QRS complex. The tachycardia is dependent on the AV node for its perpetuation; therefore any therapy that slows or blocks AV-nodal conduction (e.g., calcium channel blockers, beta blockers, adenosine, CSM) may terminate or reduce the rate of this tachycardia. Of the listed medications, only diltiazem has effects on the AV node. Although *synchronized electrical* cardioversion is very effective at terminating this arrhythmia, it is generally reserved for hemodynamically unstable patients or patients who fail pharmacologic therapy.

37. b (Chapter 41)

Recognize the signs and symptoms of an ASD. ASDs are common congenital abnormalities in adults. In childhood, the only manifestation may be a murmur. If the ASD is large and left uncorrected, it can result in progressive RH enlargement, pulmonary HTN, and eventually right HF. As the RH pressures rise, right-to-left shunting of deoxygenated blood may occur and cyanosis develops (Eisenmenger syndrome). The physical findings of a systolic ejection murmur and fixed split S_2 are characteristic of an ASD, especially in the presence of an incomplete RBBB on ECG. The RV heave (prominent left parasternal impulse) and loud P_2 suggest associated pulmonary HTN, and the elevated JVP and hepatomegaly suggest that this patient also has right HF. Although a VSD may produce a fixed split S_2, the associated murmur is usually louder, holosystolic, and may have an associated thrill, while the murmur of an aortic coarctation is usually localized to the interscapular region, may be both systolic and diastolic, and is not associated with a split S_2 or right HF. PPH may result in right HF but is not associated with a fixed split S_2.

38. d (Chapter 26)

The patient has two of the major criteria for rheumatic fever— migratory polyarthritis and evidence of carditis—and has evidence of a recent streptococcal infection. Other major criteria include chorea, erythema marginatum, and subcutaneous nodules. Rheumatic fever follows streptococcal pharyngitis by several weeks; hence blood cultures are unlikely to be positive. However, a course of PCN should be administered to all patients with rheumatic fever to eradicate any residual infection. The risk of recurrent rheumatic fever is high in these patients, and they should receive prophylaxis against streptococcal pharyngitis for at least 15 years. A mitral middiastolic murmur and an opening snap are features of MS, which develops years to decades after acute rheumatic fever. The polyarthritis of rheumatic fever is nonerosive and is not associated with long-term deformity.

39. c (Chapter 12)

Know the appropriate management of UA. Aspirin, beta blockers, and anticoagulation with IV heparin or subcutaneous LMWH are all indicated and recommended in the initial management of UA. Patients with UA, especially those having had a prolonged episode, require admission to the hospital for telemetry monitoring and serial measurement of CK-MB and troponin levels. Patients who subsequently develop elevated cardiac enzymes are at higher risk of recurrent events and have a worse long-term prognosis. Nonemergent cardiac catheterization is often performed in this setting. Emergent cardiac catheterization in UA is indicated only when angina is refractory to medical therapy or hemodynamic instability is present. Thrombolysis is not indicated for the treatment of UA or non-STEMI; in this setting, it is associated with an increased mortality. Exercise stress testing is contraindicated in patients with *active* UA but may be performed once the patient is stabilized. TTE can identify regional wall-motion abnormalities if active ischemia or prior MI is present but would not add significant diagnostic information in this case, as the patient is currently pain-free.

40. d (Chapter 10)

Recognize the major risk factors for CAD, goal LDL levels, and the need for TLC as well as drug therapy. According to the ATP III guidelines for cholesterol management, this patient has two major risk factors: cigarette smoking and age ≥55 years. The LDL goal for this patient is <130 mg/dL. Initial recommendations should include smoking cessation and TLC (including the TLC diet, weight management, and increased physical activity). If the goal LDL cannot be achieved with these interventions after 3 months, drug therapy should be considered.

41. c (Chapter 14)

Recognize the presentation and management of papillary muscle rupture complicating an AMI. Papillary muscle rupture in AMI is rare but classically occurs 3 to 5 days after the initial infarction (earlier following thrombolysis). Its presentation is usually dramatic, with the development of acute pulmonary edema resulting from acute severe MR. The HSM at the LV apex is characteristic of MR, but can sometimes be difficult to distinguish this murmur from that of a VSD, although the latter is usually more central and not associated with pulmonary edema. Ventricular free-wall rupture is usually heralded by cardiac tamponade or SCD and is not associated with a new murmur or pulmonary edema. The diagnosis can easily be confirmed by echocardiography. Treatment of papillary muscle rupture is surgical; IABP placement preceding surgery is usually necessary to maintain hemodynamic support.

42. d (Chapter 34)

Recognize when to start antihypertensive therapy and which agent to use. This patient has stage I hypertension as defined by the JNC-7. In a patient with DM (and also in patients with chronic kidney disease), goal BP is <130/80 mm Hg. This should be achieved with agents that are also indicated for the patient's other medical conditions. In this case, an ACE inhibitor such as lisinopril is appropriate for BP control as well as for renal protection in a diabetic. If the patient had CAD, beta blockers would also be appropriate; in general, however, only one medication should be started at a time. In someone without an indication for ACE inhibition or beta blockade, HCTZ is the appropriate first line antihypertensive agent. The patient should be followed closely and medication adjusted and/or added as necessary to achieve the goal BP; many patients will require more than one drug. Of course, lifestyle modification should be emphasized with each patient, but it may not be enough to control BP in this setting. Routine stress testing is not indicated unless the patient were having symptoms suggestive of cardiac ischemia or had several cardiac risk factors.

43. b (Chapter 10)

Know the importance of risk-factor modification in the secondary prevention of CAD. This is a patient with multiple cardiac risk factors including DM, HTN, and hypercholesterolemia, all of which are modifiable. Patients with known CAD or DM should have a target LDL of <100 mg/dL. In patients at very high risk (those who have had a recent MI or have CAD combined with either DM or poorly controlled risk factors), the target LDL is <70. HMG-CoA reductase inhibitors are considered first-line therapy for LDL reduction in these patients. Tighter blood glucose control can also be achieved in this patient, although its cardiovascular benefit is not as well established as that of statins. Her BP is well controlled and there is no need for any adjustment of her antihypertensive regimen at this point. Clopidogrel is a platelet inhibitor similar to aspirin, but with a different mechanism of action. It is equivalent to aspirin in reducing mortality in CAD. However, it is unclear if it offers any additional benefit when it is added to aspirin in patients with *stable* CAD.

44. e (Chapter 42)

Recognize the cardiovascular findings of normal pregnancy. Normal pregnancy leads to an increase in plasma volume and cardiac output and may result in elevated JVP, a hyperdynamic apical impulse, and systolic murmurs. These benign murmurs are early-peaking, nonradiating, and associated with normal heart sounds. A cervical venous hum and a continuous murmur over the breasts (mammary souffle) may also be present. The expanded blood volume is normal and does not require diuretic therapy. CXR is relatively contraindicated in pregnancy. Echocardiography is safe but not necessary in this setting. Because these murmurs are related to increased flow and not due to abnormal valves, there is no need for antibiotic prophylaxis.

ANSWERS

45. b (Chapters 2 and 27)

Recognize the physical findings of AR and know the appropriate diagnostic evaluation. This patient has chronic AI, likely as a result of long-standing untreated hypertension. The most common complaint in patients with chronic AI is dyspnea. In chronic AI, the excess volume initially results in LV dilation and increased end-diastolic volume. Consequently, contractility increases via the Frank-Starling mechanism, resulting in increased stroke volume. The increased stroke volume results in the peripheral manifestations of AI and may cause a pounding sensation in the neck. The SBP is usually elevated and the pulse pressure widened. The widened pulse pressure is a consequence of peripheral vasodilation and regurgitation of blood back into the LV, thereby lowering diastolic pressure. The apical impulse is often hyperdynamic and laterally displaced as a result of LV dilation and hypertrophy. The visible pulsations in the nail beds are known as Quincke pulses and are a manifestation of the widened pulse pressure. The murmur of AI is characteristically described as a high-pitched, decrescendo, diastolic murmur at the second or third intercostal space. AS, tricuspid insufficiency, and mitral regurgitation are all systolic murmurs. Although mitral stenosis is a diastolic murmur, it is a low-pitched "rumble" at the apex.

46. b (Chapter 12)

Recognize the high-risk features of UA and how the presence of these features alters management. The ECG demonstrates 1 to 2 mm of ST-segment depression in leads V_3 to V_6 and minimal depression in leads I and aVL. This patient's prolonged rest angina and persistent ST-segment depression after resolution of his chest pain place him in a higher risk category. Other high-risk features include CHF, hemodynamic instability, and positive CK-MB or troponin. Patients with high-risk features should receive GP IIB-IIIA inhibitors and proceed to urgent cardiac catheterization. In these patients with UA for whom cardiac catheterization and percutaneous intervention are planned, clopidogrel should also be started immediately. Intermediate- to low-risk patients may undergo further risk stratification with stress testing to determine their need for catheterization and revascularization. IV NTG may be effective in preventing further ischemic episodes, but it is not a definitive treatment. NSAIDs or thrombolytic therapy is not indicated for the treatment of UA.

47. a (Chapter 29)

Know the appropriate evaluation of complicated endocarditis and recognize the indications for valve surgery in this setting. The differential diagnosis of persistent fevers in a patient with endocarditis who is on appropriate antibiotic therapy includes drug fever, an extracardiac abscess and persistent valvular infection with development of a paravalvular abscess. This patient developed a new murmur consistent with tricuspid insufficiency probably related to persistent infection with resultant valvular dysfunction. He also has developed a first-degree AV block, which suggests a paravalvular abscess with extension of the infection into the conduction system. The most useful diagnostic study when a paravalvular abscess is suspected is a TEE. Although TTE is specific when an abscess is seen, its sensitivity is ~30%, compared with the 90% sensitivity of a TEE. An electrophysiologic study is not indicated because the primary problem is infection, not conduction system disease. Neither a bronchoscopy nor cardiac catheterization would provide useful information in this patient, as his lungs and coronary arteries are not the primary problem.

48. b (Chapter 17)

Recognize the indications for PA catheterization in patients with HF. This patient has decompensated CHF and would benefit from invasive hemodynamic monitoring with a PA catheter. This would allow for the optimization of her hemodynamic status via the use of appropriate medications as guided by her hemodynamic profile—so called tailored medical therapy. Although hemodialysis to remove volume would be a consideration if she failed all medical therapy, tailored therapy should be attempted first. Coronary angiography may be a consideration later to further evaluate the etiology of her CMP; however, her hemodynamic status must first be optimized. Any type of stress testing, including dobutamine echocardiograms and exercise echocardiograms, is contraindicated in patients with this degree of decompensated HF.

49. c (Chapters 2 and 28)

Recognize the physical findings of MS. A patient with MS will have an OS, which is manifest as a crisp heart sound shortly after S_2 (i.e., early in diastole). It is heard best with the diaphragm of the stethoscope at the cardiac apex and the patient rolled to the left side. The murmur of MS is more difficult to appreciate and is a low-pitched diastolic "rumble" heard at the apex immediately following the OS. A high-pitched, descrescendo diastolic murmur at the third left intercostal space is characteristic of AI. Pulsus parvus et tardus is found in patients with severe critical AS. A midsystolic click heard at the apex is a finding of MVP. Increased pulsus paradoxus is seen in patients with cardiac tamponade or severe asthma.

50. b (Chapter 41)

All patients with PDAs are considered at high risk for endocarditis (or, more appropriately, endarteritis) and should be properly instructed on prophylaxis. The site of infection is typically in the PA opposite the site of the patent ductus. PDAs have no association with MIs, aortic dissections, tamponade, or PEs in isolation.

51. d (Chapters 22 and 25)

Recognize the indications for permanent pacemaker implantation. The patient has complete heart block (CHB) with a junctional escape rhythm, as evidenced by physical examination (cannon a waves represent atrial contraction against a closed ventricle; a variable S_1 is heard as the PR interval varies) and confirmed on ECG. There is no clear association between the p waves and QRS complexes; furthermore, the sinus rate is faster than the ventricular rate. CHB is an indication for permanent pacing, even in the absence of symptoms. The presence of symptoms makes the indication even more compelling in this patient. Emergent measures such as insertion of a temporary transvenous pacemaker are not warranted in patients with stable (narrow QRS complex) escape rhythms and stable BP. Atropine is unlikely to improve the HR, as the CHB likely reflects degenerative changes of the AV node rather than nodal suppression related to medications or high vagal tone. While an inferior MI can cause brady-arrhythmias, there is no evidence on history or ECG of ischemia or infarct as a cause of the CHB in this patient. It would be unsafe to discharge the patient home; even though she is currently stable, her conduction system disease could progress (i.e., slower escape rhythm). She should be admitted to telemetry with temporary transcutaneous pacing pads placed externally while arrangements for a dual-chamber pacemaker are made.

52. b (Chapter 37)

Recognize the symptoms of TIA and the first steps in management. The patient has several risk factors for vascular disease (smoking, HTN, DM) and likely has CAD as the cause of his neurologic symptoms, based on the presence of carotid bruits. A CT of the head is indicated, but use of IV heparin is controversial in this setting. Antiplatelet therapy with aspirin (or clopidogrel if the patient is aspirin-allergic) is appropriate, as is control of BP and assessment of potential carotid artery stenosis by ultrasound. If the patient were febrile, had a high white blood cell count, or had ongoing symptoms such as global confusion or obtundation, a lumbar puncture would be indicated to rule out meningitis. An echocardiogram to evaluate for a potential cardiac source of embolism might be indicated if other studies were unrevealing; however, it is not the best initial study in this patient. MRI of the brain and MRA of the carotid and cerebral vessels may be an appropriate adjunct test, but carotid ultrasound should be performed first.

53. a (Chapter 43)

Recognize a possible cardiac contusion. In a patient with blunt chest trauma, the RV, septum, and apical LV may be damaged. The vast majority of patients with cardiac contusions have significant chest wall trauma, and frequently have ST-T abnormalities or conduction disturbance on ECG. This patient has no physical signs of myocardial dysfunction or tamponade, but 2D echocardiography may reveal a wall-motion abnormality or pericardial effusion. Treatment consists of close observation and supportive care. Anticoagulation is contraindicated. Serial enzymes may indicate the degree of myocyte death but is not as important as an echocardiogram. Cardiac catheterization is not indicated in this setting, nor is an EPS. Any arrhythmias that will occur will probably be seen during hospitalization; an outpatient Holter monitor will not add useful information. Cardiac MRI is useful to closely evaluate cardiac structures but is not usually readily available on an emergent basis.

54. d (Chapter 28)

Identify the MVP syndrome. This clinical scenario is most consistent with MVP, a disorder characterized by redundancy of the mitral valve leaflets (usually the posterior leaflet), allowing for prolapse of the leaflets into the LA during systole and resulting in an audible sound in midsystole (a midsystolic click). Patients with MVP often report palpitations, chest pain, presyncope, and fatigue (the MVP syndrome) and frequently have atrial and ventricular premature beats. MVP is the most common cause of isolated MR and affects about 3% of the population, more commonly women. An echocardiogram is warranted to evaluate for associated MR; MVP with even mild MR warrants endocarditis prophylaxis. An event monitor is more useful than a Holter monitor in the evaluation of symptoms that occur infrequently, as the latter is worn for only 24 hours at a time. An event monitor can be worn for up to a month and is activated by the patient during symptoms. Tilt-table testing is used in the evaluation of neurocardiogenic syncope.

55. d (Chapter 40)

Understand the predictors of adverse cardiac events during noncardiac surgery and determine the appropriate preoperative evaluation. The patient has one intermediate clinical predictor (DM) and two minor clinical predictors (age and low functional capacity) of having a perioperative event such as MI, HF, or death. Because of his orthopedic limitations, he cannot achieve at least 4 METs of activity; therefore it is not clear on clinical grounds whether he has exertional cardiac symptoms. Since the surgery is elective and poses an intermediate risk (i.e., 1 to 5%) of perioperative events, further risk stratification should be considered. It is unlikely that the patient will be able to walk long enough to achieve an adequate HR and BP response, and pharmacologic nuclear testing (or dobutamine stress with echocardiographic imaging) is warranted. Further management is based upon the stress test results. BP control is indicated, and beta blockers are appropriate in patients without contraindications for their use. An echocardiogram would provide information regarding resting cardiac function and may be an adjunct test, but it is not necessary in the absence of valvular disease or HF.

ANSWERS

56. c (Chapter 14)

Recognize AIVR occurring immediately after an AMI. This patient is having an expected and not life-threatening arrhythmia within 48 hours of an STEMI. This arrhythmia is common in this setting and likely results from myocardial irritability; it often occurs after pharmacologic or mechanical reperfusion. While the rhythm is ventricular in origin, it is not fast (i.e., not VT), not sustained, and not causing hemodynamic instability; therefore cardioversion is not indicated. An ICD is not indicated for this arrhythmia. If fast ventricular rhythms (VT) occur >6 days after MI, evaluation for an ICD is warranted, especially if the LV ejection fraction is <30%. Beta blockers are indicated post-MI, but other antiarrhythmic agents such as lidocaine are not indicated for AIVR. Since this is not an ischemically mediated rhythm, repeat cardiac catheterization and IV heparin are not indicated.

57. b (Chapter 36)

Recognize the features of Marfan syndrome, an autosomal dominant disorder of the gene encoding fibrillin. The resulting abnormal protein leads to decreased integrity of connective tissue throughout the body. Clinical manifestations include tall stature, hypermobile joints, ocular lens dislocation, and cardiovascular problems. Aortic root dilation occurs in up to 80% of patients with Marfan syndrome, with resulting AR (heard in this patient as the diastolic murmur; also note wide pulse pressure of AR). These patients also have a significant risk of aortic dissection. MVP and associated MR are also common. A TTE would be useful to evaluate the aortic root, aortic valve, and mitral valve. TEE is more invasive and unlikely to yield more information unless aortic dissection is suspected. Chest CT and MRA of the chest vessels are appropriate to further evaluate aortic disease but will not be helpful in the initial valvular evaluation. Cardiac catheterization would be indicated if the patient has a thoracic aortic aneurysm that requires surgical repair.

58. d (Chapter 44)

Recognize the manifestations of carcinoid heart disease. Carcinoid tumors are rare neuroendocrine tumors that secrete serotonin and other hormones and can cause symptoms referred to as the carcinoid syndrome (flushing, diarrhea, abdominal cramping). The cells can metastasize through the venous system and affect the right-sided cardiac valves, leading to TR and right HF (as evidenced by the right-sided S$_3$, elevated neck veins, ascites, and lower extremity edema in this patient). An echocardiogram will demonstrate valvular involvement, and 24-hour urine for serotonin metabolites can confirm the diagnosis. An abdominal CT scan and urinary metanephrine level are useful in the diagnosis of a pheochromocytoma, which can also produce flushing and palpitations but is generally not associated with GI symptoms and usually produces significant HTN. Abdominal ultrasound and LFTs are adjunct tests to evaluate for other causes of hepatomegaly. Right heart catheterization would define filling pressures inside the heart and the hemodynamic profile of TR but would not demonstrate structural detail of the valves. Lower extremity ultrasound is usually performed to assess for lower extremity venous thrombosis, but in this case the edema is symmetric and is caused by right HF.

59. d (Chapter 34)

Recognize causes of secondary HTN. In a young woman with no other medical problems and no family history of high BP but with the new onset of accelerated hypertension, there is likely a secondary cause. Fibromusclar dysplasia is a rare type of hyperplasia affecting medium-sized and large arteries (including renal arteries) in younger patients, more often women. The resulting renal artery stenoses lead to relative hypoperfusion of the kidneys and a compensatory hypertensive response as the body attempts to increase perfusion. A normal body habitus makes Cushing syndrome unlikely, as it is usually associated with signs of steroid excess (e.g., moon facies, buffalo hump, truncal obesity, cutaneous striae). Equal upper and lower extremity pulses essentially rule out coarctation of the aorta. Pheochromocytoma usually presents with paroxysmal flushing and palpitations as well as labile BP. Although essential HTN can first develop in the third decade of life, it is generally gradual in onset and the majority of these patients (60 to 80%) have a family history of hypertension.

60. c (Chapter 28)

Understand the hemodynamic abnormality in MS. Patients with MS often have signs and symptoms of chronic right and left HF. Severe enlargement of the LA can compress the left recurrent laryngeal nerve, resulting in hoarseness; it can also compress the esophagus causing dysphagia. A stenotic MV impedes blood flow from the LA to the LV during diastole. This is represented on the hemodynamic tracing by a continuous pressure gradient during diastole between the PCWP and the LV pressure. AS results in a gradient between the aortic pressure tracing and the LV pressure tracing. MR produces prominent v waves on a PCWP tracing, whereas tricuspid insufficiency produces prominent v waves on the RA pressure tracing.

61. c (Chapters 17 and 25)

Recognize the indication for biventricular pacing in patients with HF. This patient has NYHA class III HF symptoms despite optimal medical management and has an LBBB on ECG. This conduction abnormality results in a delay between the contraction of the RV and LV (referred to as dysynchrony), producing discoordinated contraction of an already inefficient heart and thereby aggravating his symptoms. Biventricular pacing resynchronizes the ventricles, resulting in coordinated ventricular contraction and improved hemodynamics.

Patients treated with such therapy have demonstrated improvement in symptoms, exercise tolerance, and overall quality of life. This patient may benefit from an increase in his oral diuretics, but he has no indication for IV diuretics at this time. He also has no indication for IV nesiritide. In light of his recent cardiac catheterization, an exercise nuclear test would not provide any further information. By the same token, with no change in his symptoms or physical findings, a repeat echocardiogram would not be of benefit.

62. a (Chapter 30)

Know the appropriate type of prosthetic valve to place in a woman of childbearing age. The preferred type for this patient would be a bioprosthetic valve. Of the given choices, only the Carpenter-Edwards porcine xenograft is a bioprosthetic valve. Prosthetic valves are classified as mechanical or bioprosthetic (i.e., tissue). Mechanical prostheses are more durable than bioprostheses; however, they are thrombogenic and require lifelong anticoagulation. The main advantage of bioprostheses are that they are less thrombogenic and require only 1 to 3 months of anticoagulation after implantation; however, they are not as durable and generally need to be replaced 10 to 15 years after implantation. There are several factors to consider in selecting a valve for a patient. In this particular patient who hopes to become pregnant, a bioprosthesis is the preferred valve, as it avoids the need for long-term anticoagulation with warfarin, a known teratogen.

63. d (Chapter 42)

Know the indications for pharmacologic therapy and its safety in pregnant hypertensive patients. With repeatedly elevated BP measurements, this patient meets the criteria for antihypertensive drug therapy. She is not preeclamptic or eclamptic. Methyldopa has the best-established safety record in pregnancy and is recommended as first-line therapy. Hydralazine may also be used. Beta blockers may lead to fetal growth retardation. ACE inhibitors are associated with fetal death and renal failure in newborns and are contraindicated in pregnancy. There have also been reports of neonatal bradycardia, hyponatremia, and thrombocytopenia associated with maternal use of HCZT.

64. d (Chapter 36)

Know the initial medical management of a descending aortic dissection. In general, descending aortic dissections can be managed conservatively unless they are complicated by acute end-organ ischemia or aneurysm rupture, whereas ascending aortic dissections require emergent surgical therapy. Initial medical management is aimed at promptly lowering BP and decreasing LV contractility (dP/dT). IV beta blockers are the treatment of choice; nitroprusside may also be required. Heparin and thrombolytic therapy are absolutely contraindi-

cated in this setting. IV fluids and analgesia may be required but do not treat the underlying problem.

65. e (Chapter 38)

Recognize the appropriate test to confirm the diagnosis of PE. A V/Q lung scan remains the most frequently employed diagnostic test for PE. Although V/Q scans may yield inconclusive results, normal and near-normal tests virtually exclude the diagnosis of PE, while a high-probability test confirms the diagnosis. Arterial blood gas analysis in a patient with a PE typically demonstrates respiratory alkalosis, hypocapnea, and hypoxemia but is of low specificity. Echocardiography is an insensitive means of diagnosing PE; however, it provides a rapid assessment of RV function in patients with an established diagnosis of PE. Venous ultrasonography for the detection of DVT may be helpful in patients with an intermediate clinical probability and indeterminant V/Q scan results or clinical signs suggestive of DVT. Although venous ultrasonography has high sensitivity and specificity (both 90 to 100%) for the detection of DVT, a negative result does not exclude the diagnosis of PE, as up to 50% of patients with PE may have no sonographic evidence of DVT.

66. d (Chapter 13)

Recognize the different reperfusion strategies for AMI. Reperfusion therapy is indicated for acute STEMI presenting within 6 hours of onset of symptoms. Thrombolytic therapy and primary angioplasty are considered equivalent strategies in STEMI provided that angioplasty can be done in a timely manner (<90 minutes after presentation). Primary angioplasty is associated with a lower incidence of intracranial hemorrhage as well as a trend toward a lower mortality. Unfortunately, it is not readily available in many community hospitals. Thrombolytic therapy would usually be the preferred strategy in this setting; however, it is contraindicated in this patient because of her recent CVA. Thus, immediate transfer to a facility that has angioplasty capability is indicated. Although aortic dissections and PE may result in chest pain, the history is more consistent with myocardial ischemia, and the ECG findings are diagnostic of an acute STEMI. Further diagnostic testing to exclude aortic dissection or PE would only delay the time to myocardial reperfusion. Liberal use of analgesia is an important adjunctive therapy for AMI; however, the primary goal is to salvage the ischemic myocardium by reestablishing blood flow to the occluded coronary artery.

67. e (Chapter 33)

Identify the best test of the given choices by which to diagnose constrictive pericarditis. Cardiac catheterization allows for direct measurement of the ventricular pressures and, in the presence of constrictive pericarditis, will demonstrate *equalization* of the LV and RV diastolic pressures with a dip-and-plateau pattern. CT scan of the chest may be the best study by which to visualize the thickened pericardium, but this finding alone is not diagnostic of constrictive pericarditis without the hemodynamic confirmation. CXR may demonstrate pericardial calcification, but it is also not diagnostic. Bronchoscopy may reveal TB, but it does not prove that the patient has constrictive physiology.

68. a (Chapter 41)

Identify the most appropriate initial test to confirm the presence of an ASD. Echocardiography is an excellent method to detect an ASD. It is easily performed and noninvasive and can quantify the severity of the interatrial shunt. Cardiac MRI can also identify an ASD, but is costly and less easily accessible. CXR and ECG may be suggestive but are not diagnostic. Cardiac catheterization is useful to assess the *severity* of the shunt after initial diagnosis and concomitant CAD if surgical correction is anticipated. Exercise stress testing is not helpful for the diagnosis of an ASD.

69. e (Chapter 29)

Persistent fevers and bacteremia despite 2 weeks on antibiotic therapy are indications for valve-replacement surgery. Other indications include progressive valvular dysfunction, development of a paravalvular abscess, and recurrent embolic events. Antibiotics alone are inadequate to treat these complications.

70. a (Chapters 2 and 41)

Recognize the physical findings of a PDA. All of the given choices can result in signs and symptoms of right HF and pulmonary HTN. However, the wide pulse pressure and characteristic continuous, machinery-like murmur are classic findings of a PDA. In this patient, the chronic left-to-right shunt through the PDA (from the aorta to the PA) has caused pulmonary HTN with subsequent right-to-left shunting of poorly oxygenated blood from the PA to the descending aorta. This is apparent clinically by her differential cyanosis.

71. d (Chapter 37)

Know the appropriate management of symptomatic carotid artery disease. Carotid endarterectomy (CEA) is indicated in a symptomatic patient with carotid artery stenosis of >70%. In patients with symptoms and stenosis between 30 and 69%, CEA is more controversial, but it is probably beneficial in terms of reducing future cerebrovascular events. Risk-factor modification is always warranted but will not regress the carotid lesion sufficiently. Warfarin would be indicated in a patient with a TIA resulting from cardioembolic disease (i.e., chronic AF). Following the patient with serial ultrasounds or MRAs is not appropriate, as he has already had an event and has high-grade stenosis. Antiplatelet therapy is indicated as chronic therapy but is not as effective as carotid endarterectomy at reducing recurrent neurologic events.

72. a (Chapter 14)

Know the presentation of RV infarction. RV infarction is most commonly associated with inferior wall MI. This patient presents with an acute inferior wall MI and signs of RV infarction, including hypotension (commonly after NTG administration, owing to RV preload reduction), and elevated JVP with clear lungs. RV infarction should be suspected and excluded in all patients with acute inferior wall MI. A 12-lead ECG with right-sided precordial leads should be performed. STE of >0.5 mm in V_{4R} is diagnostic of RV infarction. PE can present similarly with chest pain, hypotension, and elevated JVP; however, ECG would not demonstrate STE characteristic of AMI. Aortic dissection characteristically presents with sharp chest pain radiating to the back. Cardiac tamponade may complicate the course of an AMI when free wall rupture is present, although its presentation tends to be more dramatic. If an ECG with right-sided precordial leads is not diagnostic and tamponade remains high on the differential diagnosis, a quick bedside echocardiogram can be performed. Papillary muscle rupture complicating AMI usually presents with dyspnea, PE, and a loud holosystolic MR murmur.

73. a (Chapters 36 and 40)

This patient has a life-threatening condition that requires emergent surgical intervention. He is at high risk of sustaining a perioperative cardiac event, given the history of CAD, recent angina, DM, and HTN; in addition, vascular surgery is a high-risk procedure, generally carrying a risk of >5% for perioperative cardiac events. However, he is already demonstrating hemodynamic compromise (likely from blood loss from the leaking aneurysm), and further evaluation of his coronary disease is contraindicated. Beta blockers are also contraindicated at this point, given his hypotension. Emergent surgery is required with close intraoperative monitoring. Beta blockers should be initiated postoperatively, when his BP is stable.

74. b (Chapter 19)

Recognize the appropriate medical therapy for HCM. This patient has the classic features of HCM, including exertional presyncope, a systolic murmur that does not radiate but worsens during Valsalva, LVH on ECG, and biventricular hypertrophy and LV outflow tract gradient on his echocardiogram. The mainstay of medical therapy is negatively inotropic agents such as beta blockers or calcium channel blockers; disopyramide is an alternative if these agents are ineffective. Diuretics should not be used in the absence of congestive symptoms and NTG is contraindicated because the reduction in preload that these agents produce make the LV cavity smaller and worsen the outflow tract obstruction. ACE inhibitors are similarly problematic, as the fall in afterload increases LV contractility and worsens the obstruction. Antiplatelet agents are not indicated in this condition.

75. e (Chapter 21)

Know the appropriate management of chronic AF. This patient reports having had an irregular heartbeat for several years and likely has been in AF during that time. However, his HR is well controlled on the metoprolol and he has not had symptoms of ischemia or HF. Recent studies suggest that management with HR control and anticoagulation is superior to that of rhythm control (i.e., electrical or chemical cardioversion), since most of these patients will have a recurrence of the arrhythmia within a year. Therefore the best option is the addition of warfarin. Since this patient's HR is already well controlled, there is no need to add digoxin. In the absence of clinical instability (e.g., angina, CHF, poorly controlled HR despite therapy), there is no need to proceed to either electrical or chemical cardioversion. In younger patients (age <60) with "lone afib," aspirin may be equivalent to warfarin in preventing thromboembolic complications. However, this patient's age and history of HTN place him in a group for whom aspirin is less effective.

Appendix A: Evidence-Based Resources

Chapter 1: The History
American Thoracic Society. **Dyspnea**: mechanisms, assessment, and management: a consensus statement. Am J Respir Crit Care Med 1999;159(1):321–340.

Lee TH, Goldman L. Evaluation of the patient with acute **chest pain**. N Engl J Med 2000;342(16):1187–1195.

Zimetbaum P, Josephson ME. Evaluation of patients with **palpitations**. N Engl J Med 1998;338(19):1369–1373.

Chapter 2: Physical Examination of the Cardiovascular System
Etchells E, Bell C, Robb K. Does this patient have an abnormal **systolic murmur**? JAMA 1997;277(7):564–571.

Lembo NJ, Dell'Italia LJ, Crawford MH, O'Rourke RA. **Bedside diagnosis** of systolic murmurs. N Engl J Med 1988;318: 1572–1578.

Chapter 4: Stress Testing
Gibbons R, Balady G, Bricker J, et al. ACC/AHA 2002 **guideline update for exercise testing**: summary article: a report of the American College of Cardiology/American Heart Association Task Force on Practice Guidelines. Circulation 2002;106: 1883–1892.

Tavel ME. **Stress testing** in cardiac evaluation: current concepts with emphasis on the ECG. Chest 2001;119(3):907–925.

Chapter 5: Echocardiography
Melvin D, Cheitlin M, Alpert J, et al. ACC/AHA **guidelines** for the clinical application of **echocardiography**. Circulation 1997;95: 1686–1744.

Peterson GE, Brickner ME, Reimold SC. **Transesophageal echocardiography**: clinical indications and applications. Circulation 2003;107(19):2398–2402.

Chapter 6: Cardiac Catheterization
Arjomand H, Turi ZG, McCormick D, Goldberg S. **Percutaneous coronary intervention**: historical perspectives, current status, and future directions. Am Heart J 2003;146(5):787–796.

Chapter 7: Diagnostic Modalities for Arrhythmias
Sutton R, Bloomfield DM. Indications, methodology, and classification of results of **tilt-table testing**. Am J Cardiol 1999; 84(8A):10Q–19Q.

Zimetbaum PJ, Josephson ME. The evolving role of **ambulatory arrhythmia monitoring** in general clinical practice. Ann Intern Med 1999;130(10):848–856.

Chapter 8: Other Imaging Modalities
Cerqueira MD, Lawrence A. **Nuclear cardiology** update. Radiol Clin North Am 2001;39(5):931–946.

Constantine G, Shan K, Flamm SD, Sivananthan MU. Role of **MRI** in clinical cardiology. Lancet 2004;363(9427):2162–2171.

Lipton MJ, Boxt LM. How to approach cardiac diagnosis from the **chest radiograph**. Radiol Clin North Am 2004;42(3): 487–495.

Nasir K, Budoff MJ, Post WS, et al. **Electron beam CT** versus helical CT scans for assessing coronary calcification: current utility and future directions. Am Heart J 2003;146(6): 969–977.

Chapter 9: Coronary Artery Disease Pathophysiology
Casscells W, Naghavi M, Willerson JT. Vulnerable **atherosclerotic plaque**: a multifocal disease. Circulation 2003;107(16): 2072–2075.

Fruchart JC, Nierman MC, Stroes ES, et al. New **risk factors** for atherosclerosis and patient risk assessment. Circulation 2004; 109(23 suppl 1):III15–III19.

Libby P. **Vascular biology** of atherosclerosis: overview and state of the art. Am J Cardiol 2003;91(3A):3A–6A.

Chapter 10: Dyslipidemia
Executive Summary of the Third Report of the National Cholesterol Education Program (NCEP) Expert Panel on Detection, Evaluation, and Treatment of **High Blood Cholesterol** in Adults (Adult Treatment Panel III). JAMA 2001; 285:2486–2497.

Grundy SM, Cleeman JI, Merz CNB, et al. Implications of recent clinical trials for the National Cholesterol Education Program Adult Treatment Panel III Guidelines. Circulation 2004;110: 227–239.

Chapter 11: Chronic Stable Angina

CAPRIE Steering Committee. A randomized, blinded, trial of **clopidogrel** versus **aspirin** in patients at risk of ischaemic events (CAPRIE). Lancet 1996;348:1329–1339.

Gibbons RJ, Abrams J, Chatterjee K, et al. ACC/AHA 2002 **guideline** update for the management of patients with **chronic stable angina**: a report of the ACC/AHA Task Force on Practice Guidelines. J Am Coll Cardiol 2003;41:159–168.

The BARI Investigators. Seven-year outcome in the Bypass Angioplasty **Revascularization** Investigation (BARI) by treatment and diabetic status. J Am Coll Cardiol 2000;35:1122–1129.

Chapter 12: Unstable Angina and Non-ST-Elevation Myocardial Infarction

Antman EM, Cohen M, Bernink PJ, et al. The **TIMI risk score** for unstable angina/non-ST elevation MI: a method for prognostication and therapeutic decision making. JAMA 2000;284: 835–842.

Braunwald E, Antman EM, Beasley JW, et al. ACC/AHA 2002 **guideline update** for the management of patients with unstable angina and non ST-segment elevation MI: a report of the ACC/AHA Task Force on Practice Guidelines. J Am Coll Cardiol 2002;40:1366–1374.

Cannon CP, Weintraub WS, Demopoulos LA, et al. (TIMI-TACTICS 18 investigators) Comparison **of Early Invasive and Conservative Strategies** in Patients with Unstable Coronary Syndromes treated with the Glycoprotein IIb/IIIa Inhibitor Tirofiban. N Engl J Med 2001; 344:1879–1887.

The Clopidogrel in Unstable Angina to Prevent Recurrent Events Trial Investigators. Effects of **clopidogrel in addition to aspirin** in patients with acute coronary syndromes without ST-segment elevation. N Engl J Med 2001;345:494–502.

Yeghiazarians Y, Braunstein JB, Askari A, Stone P. **Unstable angina pectoris**. N Engl J Med 2000;342:101–114.

Chapter 13: ST-Elevation Myocardial Infarction

Antman E, Anbe D, Armstrong P, et al. ACC/AHA **guidelines** for the management of patients with ST-elevation myocardial infarction—executive summary [ACC/AHA practice guidelines]. J Am Coll Cardiol 2004;44(3):e1–e211.

Keeley EC, Boura JA, Grines CL. **Primary angioplasty versus intravenous thrombolytic therapy** for acute myocardial infarction: a quantitative review of 23 randomised trials. Lancet 2003;361(9351):13–20.

Chapter 14: Complications of Myocardial Infarction

Birnbaum Y, Fishbein M, Blanche C, Siegel R. **Ventricular septal rupture** after acute myocardial infarction. N Engl J Med 2002; 347:1426–1432.

Reeder GS. Identification and treatment of **complications of myocardial infarction**. Mayo Clin Proc 1995;70(9):880–884.

Chapter 15: Cardiovascular Hemodynamics

Amin DK, Shah PK, Swan HJC. Deciding when **hemodynamic monitoring** is appropriate. J Crit Illness 1993;8:1053–1061.

Amin DK, Shah PK, Swan HJC. The **technique** of inserting a Swan-Ganz catheter. J Crit Illness 1993;8:1147–1156.

Assessment of normal and abnormal cardiac function. In: Braunwald E, ed. Heart Disease: A Textbook of Cardiovascular Medicine, 5th ed. Philadelphia: Saunders, 1997;479–502.

Chapter 16: Mechanisms of Heart Failure

Jessup M, Brozena S. **Heart failure**. N Engl J Med 2003;348: 2007–1018.

Zile MR, Brutsaert DL. New concepts in diastolic dysfunction and **diastolic heart failure**. Part I: diagnosis, prognosis, and measurements of diastolic function. Circulation 2002;105(11): 1387–1393.

Chapter 17: Clinical Manifestations and Treatment of Heart Failure

Cazeau S, Leclercq C, Lavergne T, et al. Effects of multisite **biventricular pacing** in patients with heart failure and intraventricular conduction delay. N Engl J Med 2001;344: 873–880.

Foody JM, Farrell MH, Krumholz HM. **Beta-blocker therapy in heart failure**: scientific review. JAMA 2002;287:883–889.

Hunt SA, Baker DW, Chin MH, et al. ACC/AHA **guidelines** for the evaluation and management of chronic heart failure in the adult: executive summary: a report of the ACC/AHA Task Force on Practice Guidelines. J Am Coll Cardiol 2001;38: 2101–2113.

Zile MR, Brutsaert DL. New concepts in diastolic dysfunction and **diastolic heart failure**: Part II: causal mechanisms and treatment. Circulation. 2002;105(12):1503–1508.

Chapter 18: Myocarditis

Feldman AM, McNamara D. Medical progress: **myocarditis**. N Engl J Med 2000;343:1388–1398.

McCarthy RE 3rd, Boehmer JP, Hruban RH, et al. Long-term outcome of fulminant myocarditis as compared with acute (nonfulminant) myocarditis. N Engl J Med 2000;342: 690–695.

Chapter 19: Cardiomyopathies
Kushwaha SS, Fallon JT, Fuster V. Medical progress: **restrictive cardiomyopathy.** N Engl J Med 1997;336:267–276.

Maron BJ, McKenna WJ, Danielson GK, et al. AC/European Society of Cardiology Clinical Expert Consensus Document on **Hypertrophic Cardiomyopathy:** a report of the ACC Task Force on Clinical Expert Consensus Documents and the European Society of Cardiology Committee for Practice Guidelines. J Am Coll Cardiol 2003:42:1687–1713.

Chapter 20: Mechanisms of Arrhythmogenesis
Chiang CE, Roden DM. The **long QT syndromes:** genetic basis and clinical implications. J Am Coll Cardiol 2000;36(1):1–12.

Mazgalev TN, Ho SY, Anderson RH. **Anatomic-electrophysiological correlations** concerning the pathways for atrioventricular conduction. Circulation 2001;103(22):2660–2667.

Chapter 21: Tachyarrhythmias
ACC/AHA/ESC **guidelines** for the management of patients with **supraventricular arrhythmias**—executive summary. A report of the American College of Cardiology/American Heart Association Task Force on Practice Guidelines and the European Society of Cardiology Committee for Practice Guidelines (writing committee to develop guidelines for the management of patients with supraventricular arrhythmias) developed in collaboration with NASPE–Heart Rhythm Society. J Am Coll Cardiol 2003;42(8):1493–1531.

Ganz L, Friedman P. Supraventricular **tachycardia.** N Engl J Med 1995;332(3):162–173.

Saliba WI, Natale A. **Ventricular tachycardia** syndromes. Med Clin North Am 2001;85:267–304.

Chapter 22: Bradyarrhythmias
Mangrum M, diMarco J. The evaluation and management of **bradycardia.** N Engl J Med 2000;342(10):703–709.

Chapter 23: Syncope
Kapoor W. **Syncope.** N Engl J Med 2000;343:25:1856–1862.

Chapter 24: Sudden Cardiac Death
Huikuri H, Castellano A, Myerburg R. **Sudden death** due to cardiac arrhythmias. N Engl J Med 2001;345:20:1473–1481.

Josephson M, Wellens HJ. **Implantable defibrillators** and sudden cardiac death. Circulation 2004;109(22):2685–2691.

Chapter 25: Pacemakers and Implantable Cardioverter Defibrillators
Gregoratos G, Abrams J, Epstein A, et al. ACC/AHA/NASPE 2002 **guideline update** for implantation of cardiac pacemakers and antiarrhythmia devices: summary article. A report of the American College of Cardiology/American Heart Association Task Force on Practice Guidelines. Circulation 2002;106: 2145–2161.

Leclercq C, Kass DA. Retiming the failing heart: principles and current clinical status of **cardiac resynchronization.** J Am Coll Cardiol 2002;39(2):194–201.

Moss AJ, Zareba W, Hall WJ, et al. **Prophylactic implantation of a defibrillator** in patients with myocardial infarction and reduced ejection fraction. N Engl J Med 2002;346:12:877–883.

Trohman RG, Kim MH, Pinski SL. **Cardiac pacing:** the state of the art. Lancet 2004;364(9446):1701–1719.

Chapter 26: Rheumatic Fever
Stollerman GH. **Rheumatic fever.** Lancet 1997;349(9056): 935–942.

Chapters 27 and 28: Aortic Valve and Mitral Valve Disorders
Bonow RO, Carabello B, de Leon AC Jr, et al. ACC/AHA **guidelines** for the management of patients with valvular heart disease: a report of the American College of Cardiology/American Heart Association Task Force on Practice Guidelines (Committee on Management of Patients With Valvular Heart Disease). J Am Coll Cardiol 1998;32:1486–1588.

Borer JS, Bonow RO. Contemporary approach to aortic and **mitral regurgitation.** Circulation 2003;108(20):2432–2438.

Carabello BA. **Aortic stenosis.** N Engl J Med 2002;346: 677–682.

Carabello BA, Crawford FA. **Valvular heart** disease. N Engl J Med 1997;337:32–41.

Enriquez-Sarano M, Tajik AJ. **Aortic regurgitation.** N Engl J Med 2004;351:1539–1546.

Pellerin D, Brecker S, Veyrat C. Degenerative mitral valve disease with emphasis on **mitral valve prolapse.** Heart 2002; 88(suppl 4):iv,20–28.

Zile MR, Gaasch WH. Heart failure in **aortic stenosis:** improving diagnosis and treatment. N Engl J Med 2003;348:1735–1736.

Chapter 29: Infective Endocarditis
Bayer AS, Bolger AF, Taubert KA, et al. AHA Scientific Statement: **diagnosis and management of infective endocarditis** and its

complications. From an ad hoc writing group of the Committee on Rheumatic Fever, Endocarditis, and Kawasaki Disease, American Heart Association. Circulation 1998;98:2936–2948.

Dajani AS, Taubert KA, Wilson W, et al. **Prevention of bacterial endocarditis**: recommendations by the American Heart Association. From an ad hoc writing group of the Committee on Rheumatic Fever, Endocarditis, and Kawasaki Disease, American Heart Association. JAMA 1997;277:1794–1801.

Mylonakis E, Calderwood SB. Medical progress: **infective endocarditis in adults.** N Engl J Med 2001;345:1318–1330.

Wilson WR, Karchmer AW, Dajani AS et al. **Antibiotic treatment** of adults with infective endocarditis due to streptococci, enterococci, staphylococci, and HACEK microorganisms. From an ad hoc writing group of the Committee on Rheumatic Fever, Endocarditis, and Kawasaki Disease, American Heart Association. JAMA 1995;274:1706–1713.

Chapter 30: Prosthetic Heart Valves
Seiler C. Management and follow up of **prosthetic heart valves.** Heart 2004;90(7):818–824.

Vongpatanasin W, Hillis LD, Lange RA. **Prosthetic heart valves**. N Engl J Med 1996;335(6):407–416.

Chapter 31: Pericarditis
Lange RA, Hillis LD. Acute pericarditis. N Engl J Med 2004; 351:2195–2202.

Chapter 32: Cardiac Tamponade
Spodick DH. Current concepts: **acute cardiac tamponade.** N Engl J Med 2003;349:684–690.

Spodick DH. **Pathophysiology** of cardiac tamponade. Chest 1998;113(5):1372–1378.

Chapter 33: Constrictive Pericarditis
Myers RB, Spodick DH. **Constrictive pericarditis**: clinical and pathophysiologic characteristics. Am Heart J 1999;138: 219–232.

Nishimura RA. **Constrictive pericarditis** in the modern era: a diagnostic dilemma. Heart 2001;86(6):619–623.

Sagrista-Sauleda J, Angel J, Sanchez A, et al. **Effusive-constrictive pericarditis.** N Engl J Med 2004;350:469–475.

Chapter 34: Hypertension
Garg J, Messerli AW, Bakris GL. Evaluation and treatment of patients with **systemic hypertension.** Circulation 2002;105 (21):2458–2461.

National Heart, Lung, and Blood Institute. Seventh Report of the **Joint National Committee** on Prevention, Detection, Evaluation, and Treatment of High Blood Pressure (JNC 7). Available at: http://www.nhlbi.nih.gov/guidelines/hypertension/jnc7full.htm/, accessed 2003.

Chapter 35: Peripheral Arterial Disorders
Hiatt W. Medical treatment of peripheral arterial disease and claudication. N Engl J Med 2001;344(21):1608–1621.

Chapter 36: Diseases of the Aorta
Hallet J. Management of abdominal **aortic aneurysms.** Mayo Clin Proc 2000;75:395–399.

Nienaber C, Ealge K. **Aortic dissection**: new frontiers in diagnosis and management. Circulation 2003;108:628–635 (Part 1); Circulation 2003;108:772–778 (Part 2).

Chapter 37: Carotid Arterial Disease
Barnett H, Taylor W, Eliasziw M, et al. Benefit of carotid **endarterectomy** in patients with symptomatic moderate or severe stenosis. N Engl J Med 1998;339(20):1415–1425.

MRC Asymptomatic Carotid Surgery Trial (ACST) Collaborative Group. Prevention of disabling and fatal strokes by successful carotid **endarterectomy** in patients without recent neurological symptoms: randomised controlled trial. Lancet 2004; (363):1491–1502.

Sacco R. Extracranial **carotid stenosis**. N Engl J Med 2001; 345:15:113–118.

Chapter 38: Deep Venous Thrombosis and Pulmonary Embolic Disease
Goldhaber S. **Pulmonary embolism.** Lancet 2004;363: 1295–1305.

McRae SJ, Ginsberg JS. Initial treatment of **venous thromboembolism.** Circulation 2004;110(9 supp I1):I3–I9.

Chapter 39: Pulmonary Hypertension
Farber H, Loscalzo J. **Mechanisms** of disease: pulmonary arterial hypertension. N Engl J Med 2004;351:1655–1665.

Humbert M, Sitbon O, Simonneau G. **Treatment** of pulmonary arterial hypertension. N Engl J Med 2004;351:1425–1436.

Chapter 40: Preoperative Evaluation of the Cardiac Patient
Eagle K, Berger P, Calckins H, et al. ACC/AHA **guideline** update for perioperative cardiovascular evaluation for noncardiac surgery—executive summary. J Am Coll Cardiol 2002;39(3): 542–553.

Fleisher LA, Eagle KA. Clinical practice. Lowering cardiac **risk in noncardiac surgery.** N Engl J Med 2001;345(23):1677–1682.

Chapter 41: Congenital Heart Disease
Hoffman JI, Kaplan S. The incidence of congenital heart disease. J Am Coll Cardiol 2002;39:1890–1900.

Therrien J, Webb G. Clinical update on **adults with congenital heart disease.** Lancet 2003;362:1305–1313.

Chapter 42: Pregnancy and Cardiovascular Disease
James P, Nelson-Piercy C. Management of **hypertension** before, during, and after pregnancy. Heart 2004;90:12: 1499–1504.

Reimold S, Rutherford J. Clinical practice: **Valvular heart disease** in pregnancy. N Engl J Med 2003;349:52–59.

Thorne SA. **Pregnancy in heart disease.** Heart 2004;90(4): 450–456.

Chapter 43: Traumatic Heart Disease
Asensio JA, Stewart BM, Murray J, et al. Penetrating cardiac injuries. Surg Clin North Am 1996;76:685–724.

Prêtre R, Chilcott M. Blunt trauma to the heart and great vessels. N Engl J Med 1997;336:626–632.

Sybrandy KC, Cramer MJ, Burgersdijk C. Diagnosing cardiac contusion: old wisdom and new insights. Heart 2003;89: 485–489.

Chapter 44: Cardiac Tumors
al-Mohammad A, Pambakian H, Young C. **Fibroelastoma:** case report and review of the literature. Heart 1998;79:301–304.

Reynen K. Cardiac **myxomas.** N Engl J Med 1995;333: 1610–1617.

Appendix B: Electrocardiograms

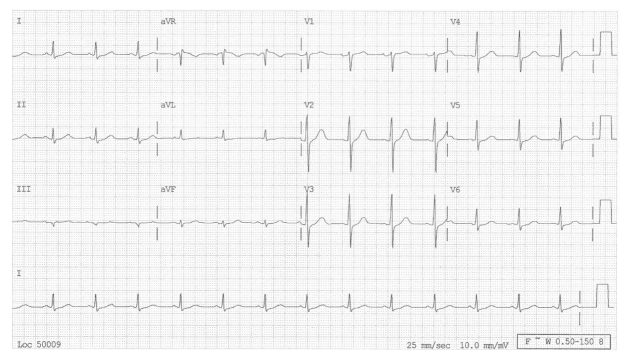

I   aVR   V1   V4

II   aVL   V2   V5

III   aVF   V3   V6

I

Loc 50009   25 mm/sec 10.0 mm/mV   F ~ W 0.50~150 8

1. Normal ECG.

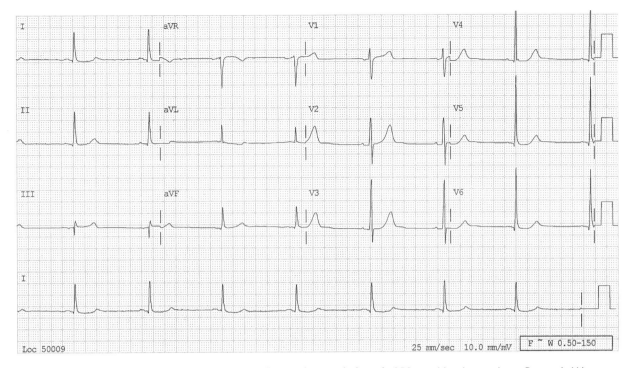

2. Sinus bradycardia at a heart rate of 46 bpm. Other abnormalities include early QRS transition (a prominent R wave in V$_2$).

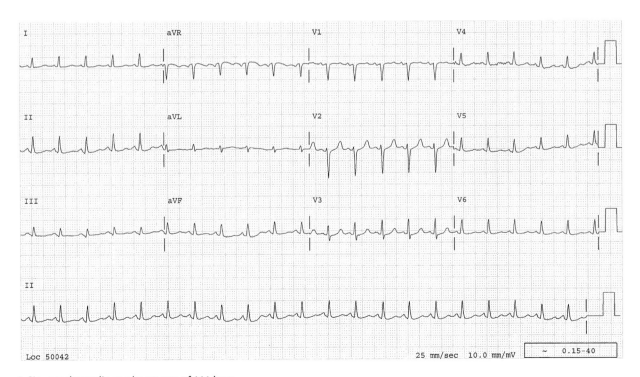

3. Sinus tachycardia at a heart rate of 111 bpm.

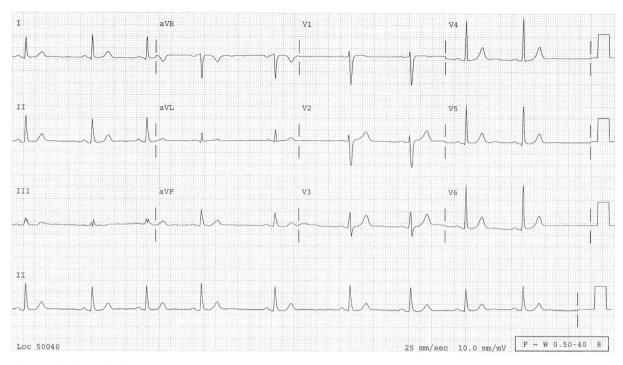

4. Sinus arrhythmia. The heart rate varies from 45 to 62 bpm. The variability in rate is secondary to changes in autonomic tone during the respiratory cycle.

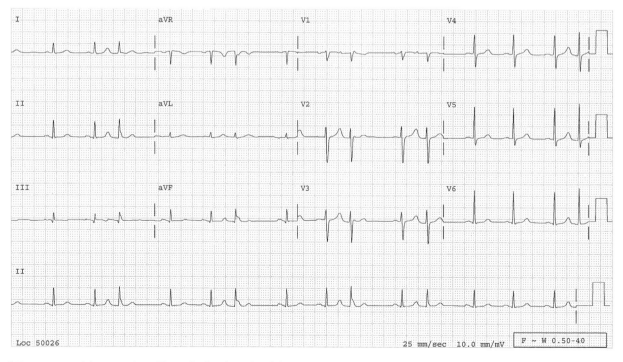

5. Premature atrial contractions. The 3rd, 6th, 9th, and 11th beats are premature, have a narrow QRS complex, and are of similar morphology as the normal beats. Each premature complex is preceded by a P wave. This is best seen in lead V_1. In other leads the premature P wave is buried in (and distorting) the preceding T wave.

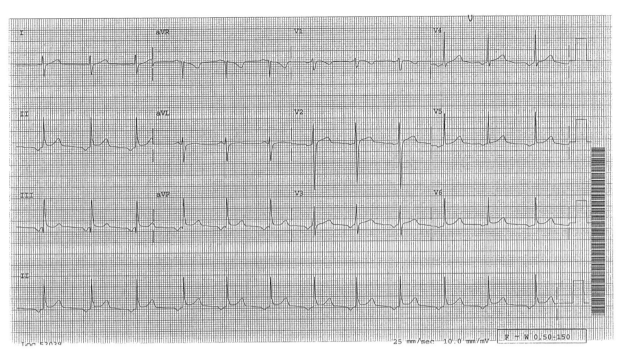

6. Ectopic atrial rhythm. The atrial impulse originates low in the atrium instead of high in the atrium at the SA node. This produces an inverted P wave in the inferior leads (II, III, F) and a relatively short PR interval.

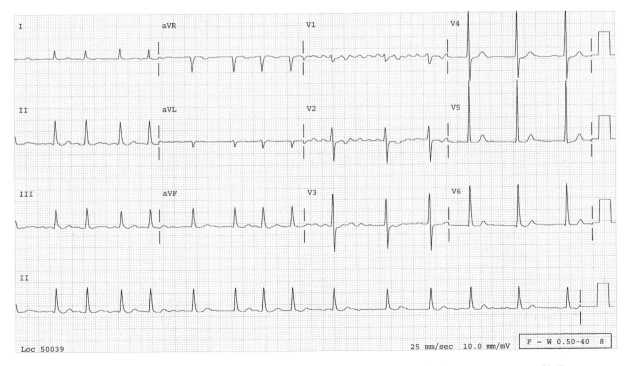

7. AF. The rhythm is irregularly irregular without definable P waves. The irregular baseline in lead V₁ represents coarse fibrillatory waves.

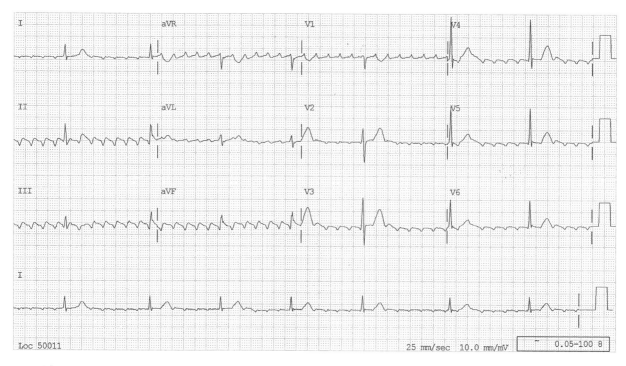

8. Atrial flutter. Notice the well-defined flutter waves, inverted in the inferior leads, resulting in the classic "sawtooth" pattern. The atrial rate is ~300 bpm. There is a 6:1 AV conduction, resulting in a ventricular rate of ~50 bpm.

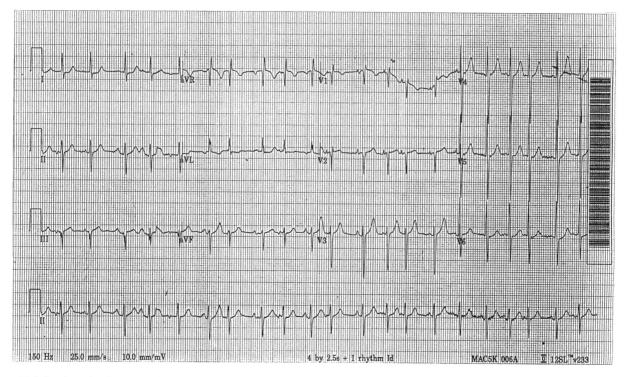

9. Multifocal atrial tachycardia. The rhythm is irregularly irregular with an overall rate of 128 bpm. Each QRS complex is preceded by a well-defined P wave; however, there are more than three different P-wave morphologies without a predominant underlying sinus rhythm.

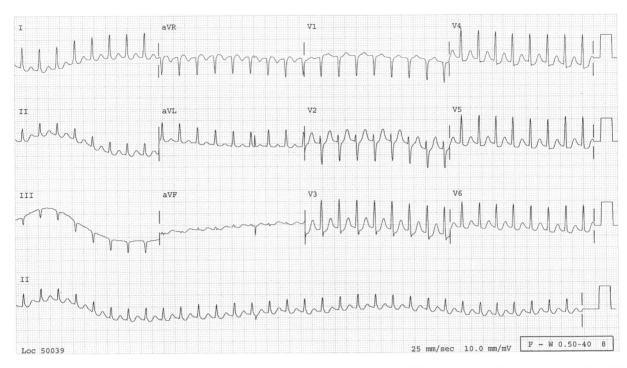

10. AV-nodal reentrant tachycardia. There is a narrow-complex tachycardia at a rate of 195 bpm without P waves preceding the QRS complexes. The narrow QRS indicates a supraventricular origin of the arrhythmia. The small S waves in V_3 and V_4 were not present when the patient was in normal sinus rhythm and likely reflect retrograde atrial activation ("pseudo-S waves").

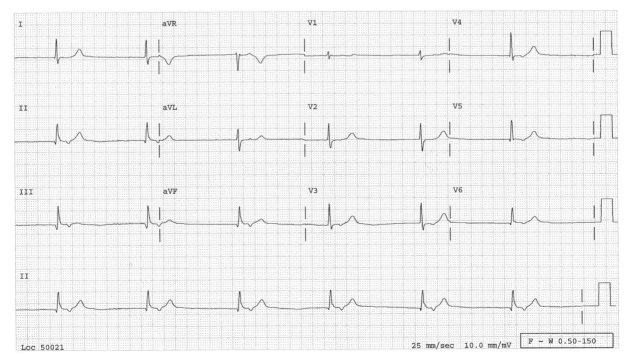

11. Junctional rhythm. There is a slow, narrow-complex, regular rhythm with QRS complexes that are not preceded by P waves. P waves are seen following each QRS complex (seen best in the lead II rhythm strip), representing retrograde conduction from the AV node to the atria.

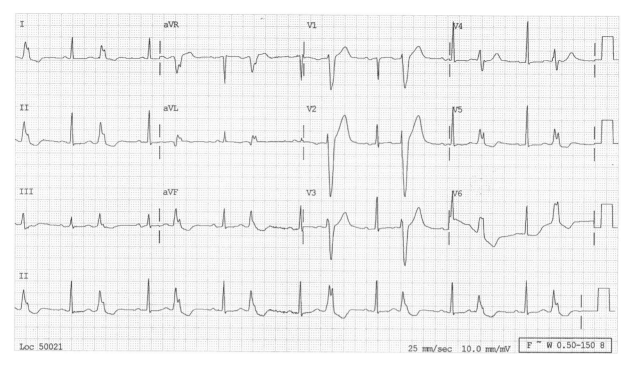

12. VPCs. The underlying rhythm is sinus (notice the P waves preceding each narrow QRS complex). There are frequent, premature, wide QRS complexes. The wide QRS reflects origin of the complexes in the ventricles with slow conduction through the ventricular myocardium. The morphology and axis of these complexes are much different than those of the underlying rhythm. In this tracing, every other complex is a VPC, a pattern known as ventricular bigeminy.

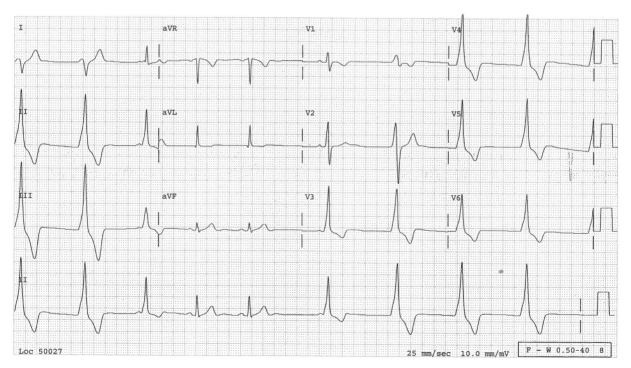

13. AIVR. The 4th and 5th QRS complexes represent the underlying normal sinus rhythm (NSR). The 1st, 2nd, and 7th to 9th complexes are wide and regular and reflect a ventricular rhythm at a rate of 54 bpm. The usual escape rate of the ventricle is 30 to 40 bpm; thus the rhythm is accelerated. This rhythm is competing with the underlying sinus rhythm. The 3rd and 6th complexes are fusion complexes, resulting from the simultaneous depolarization of the ventricles from the NSR and AIVR.

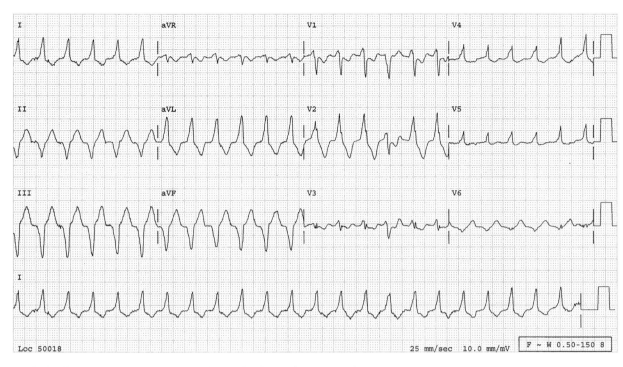

14. VT. The rhythm is rapid (140 bpm), regular, and with a wide QRS complex.

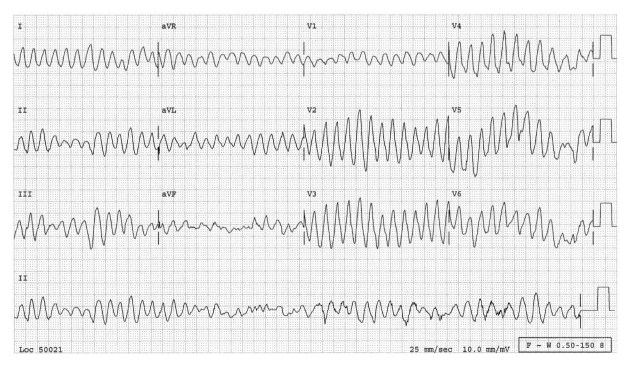

15. Polymorphic VT (torsades de pointes). Notice the rapid wide-complex rhythm with a cyclically changing axis, giving the appearance that the complexes are rotating around the isoelectric line.

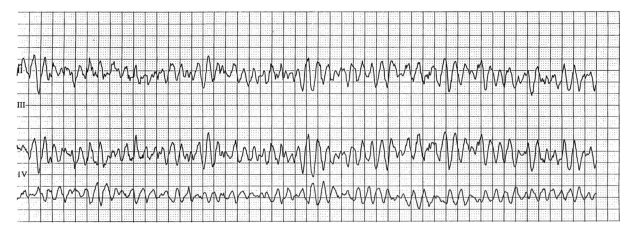

16. VF. There is coarse electrical activity without a definable underlying rhythm.

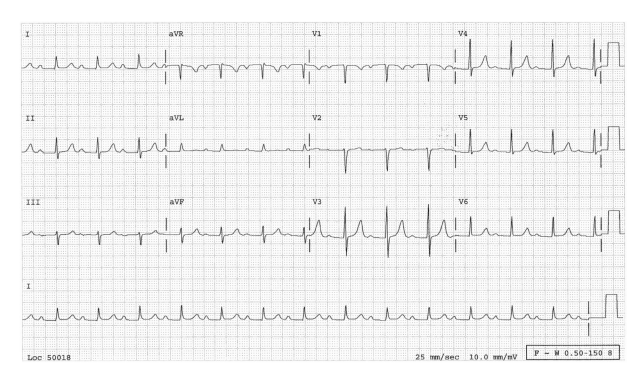

Loc 50018

25 mm/sec   10.0 mm/mV   F ~ W 0.50-150 8

17. First-degree AV block. The PR interval is prolonged (~310 milliseconds), reflecting a delay in conduction from the atria to the ventricles.

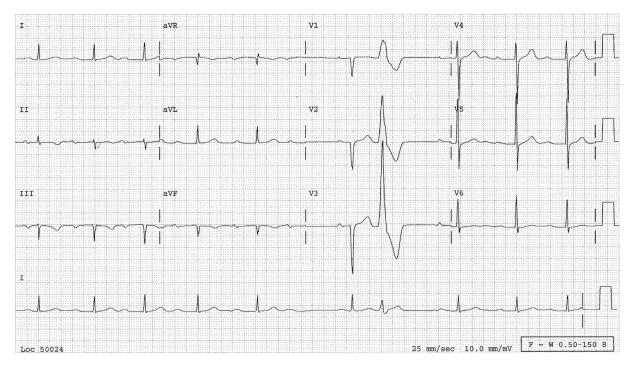

18. Mobitz type I second-degree AV block (Wenckebach). The underlying rhythm is sinus. Notice the gradual prolongation of the PR interval from the first to the fifth complex. The sixth P wave is blocked and does not conduct to the ventricles (best seen in lead aVF). The cycle starts again on the sixth QRS complex and is interrupted by a premature ventricular complex (seventh complex). Other abnormalities include left axis deviation, probable old anteroseptal MI (Q waves in V_1 to V_2), and a possible old inferior MI (Q-wave lead in aVF, T-wave inversion leads II, III, and aVF).

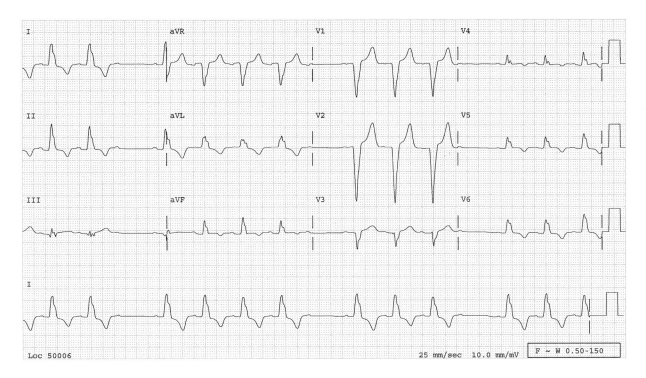

19. Mobitz type II second-degree AV block. The underlying rhythm is sinus. Notice the frequent nonconducted P waves (3rd, 8th, and 12th P waves), which are not premature and are not preceded by a gradual prolongation of the PR interval. An LBBB is also present.

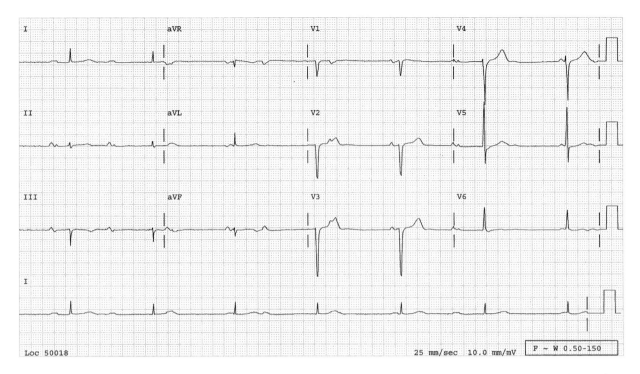

20. Complete HB. The atrial rate (P waves) is ~60 bpm. However, there is AV dissociation present (the atria and ventricles are functioning independently), with a narrow-complex escape rhythm at a rate of 41 bpm. The QRS complexes are narrow because the depolarization originates in the AV node (junctional escape rhythm) and propagates to the ventricles through the normal conduction system. An old anteroseptal MI is also present (minimal R waves V_1 to V_3).

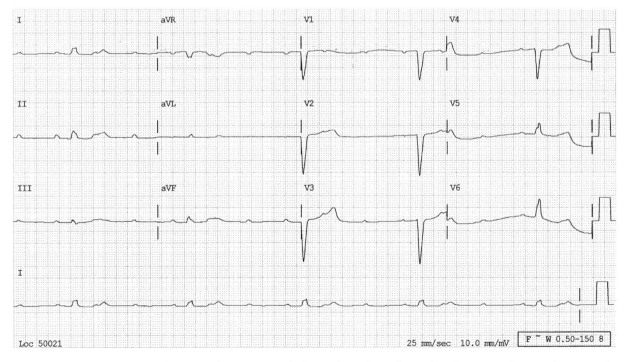

21. Complete HB. As in ECG 20, there is AV dissociation, with the atrial rate being faster than the ventricular rate. The ventricular depolarizations originate in the ventricular myocardium, resulting in a wide and slow rhythm at a rate of ~28 bpm (ventricular escape rhythm).

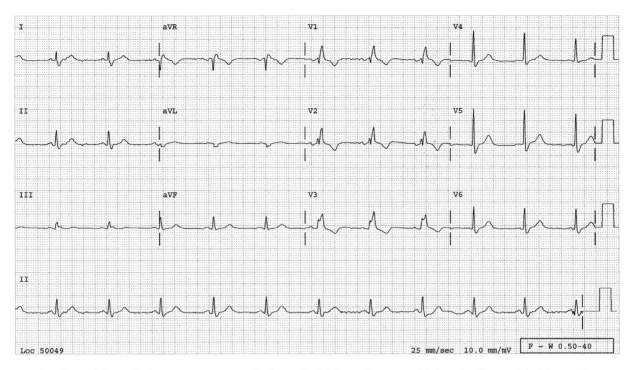

22. RBBB. The underlying rhythm is sinus at a rate of 66 bpm. The QRS complexes are wide (>120 milliseconds) with an rsR' pattern in V_1 and a wide, deep, "terminal S wave" in the lateral leads (V_6, I, and aVL). Secondary repolarization changes are seen with downsloping ST segments and T-wave inversions in leads V_1 to V_3.

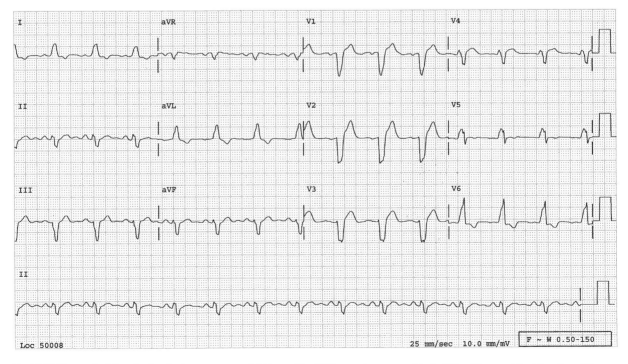

23. LBBB. The underlying rhythm is sinus at a rate of 84 bpm. The QRS complexes are wide (>120 milliseconds) with a deep QS complex in V_1, prominent R complexes in the lateral leads (V_6, I, and aVL), and absence of the normal "septal Q waves" in V_6. There are secondary repolarization changes with ST-T abnormalities opposite the major deflection of the QRS complex in most leads. Left atrial enlargement is also present (the P wave is more than one box deep and wide in lead V_1 and more than three boxes wide in lead II).

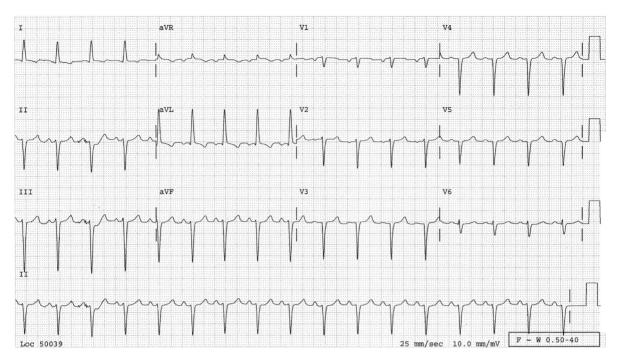

24. Left anterior fascicular block. The axis is more negative than –45 degrees (QRS is positive in lead I and negative in leads II, III, and aVF); there is a small Q wave and tall R wave in lead I and a small R wave and deep S wave in lead III. Other abnormalities include LA enlargement, an old anterior MI (Q waves V_3 to V_5), and LV hypertrophy (R wave more than 11 boxes high in lead aVL).

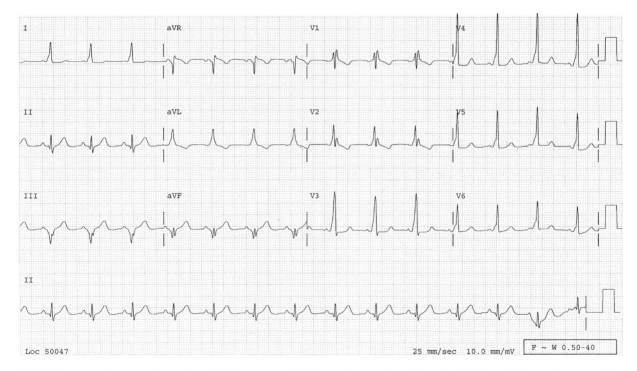

25. WPW syndrome (normal sinus rhythm). Notice the short PR interval (accelerated AV conduction). The QRS complexes are fusion complexes. The initial portion of the QRS complex is slurred (a delta wave), reflecting conduction through the bypass tract with early ventricular depolarization (ventricular preexcitation). The latter portion of the QRS is narrow complex and represents more rapid depolarization through the normal conduction system.

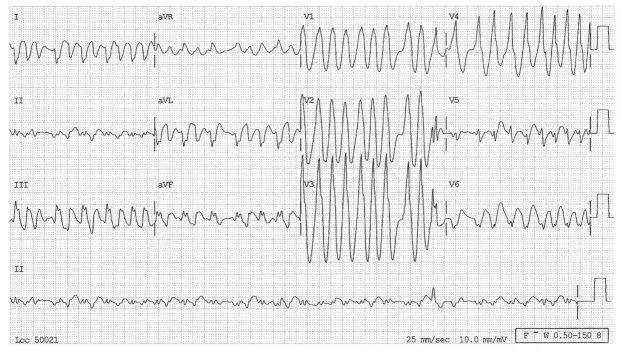

26. WPW syndrome (AF). Notice that the rhythm is irregularly irregular, tachycardic, and without P waves (i.e., AF). There is marked variation in the QRS morphology reflecting varying conduction down the bypass tract. The narrow complex seen in the rhythm strip reflects conduction through the AV node. The very wide complexes reflect conduction through the bypass tract. Intermediate width complexes reflect varying degrees of fusion between these two pathways.

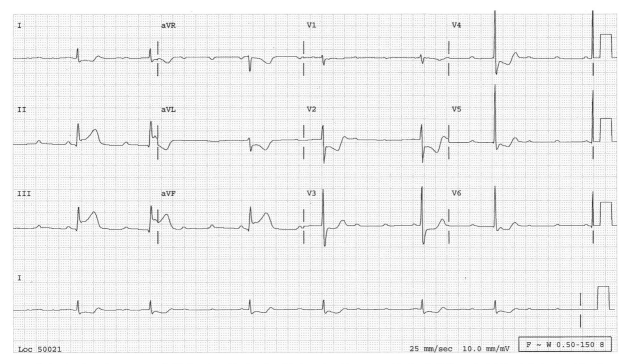

27. Inferior ST elevation myocardial infarction. Notice the ST elevation (3 to 4 mm) in leads II, III, and aVF (the inferior leads) reflecting acute occlusion of the RCA. The ST depression in the anterior leads likely reflects posterior wall infarction, whereas the ST depression in the lateral leads reflects lateral wall ischemia. Sinus tachycardia is present (atrial rate ~110 bpm) with high degree AV block (the P waves are only intermittently conducted to the ventricles). Inferior MIs are often associate with transient HB, usually as a result of high vagal tone or AV nodal ischemia.

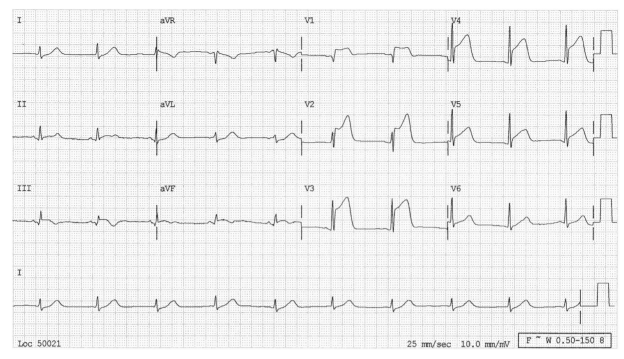

28. Anterior ST elevation MI. The underlying rhythm is sinus at a rate of 56 bpm. There is marked concave-downward ST elevation ("tombstones") in the anterior leads (V_1 to V_5) consistent with acute occlusion of the proximal LAD coronary artery. There is also mild ST elevation in the inferior leads (III, aVF), indicative of acute inferior infarction, likely reflecting a region of the distal inferior wall that is subserved by the large occluded LAD.

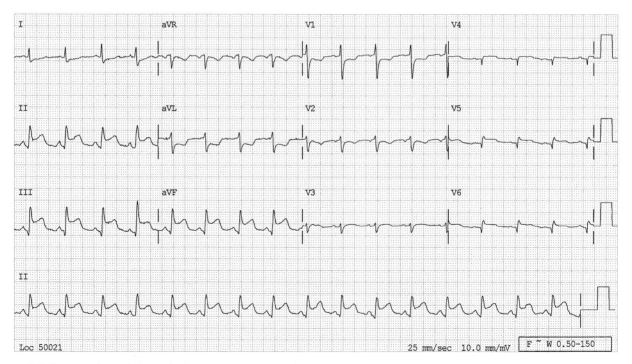

29. RV infarction. The underlying rhythm is a sinus at a rate of 98 bpm. There is ST elevation in the inferior leads, reflecting an acute inferior infarction. The precordial leads have been placed on the right side of the chest, resulting in diminutive R waves in the precordial leads. There is >1 mm of ST elevation in the right precordial leads (RV_4 to RV_6), consistent with an acute RV infarction. The right ventricle is supplied by proximal branches of the RCA; thus inferior infarctions are often associated with RV infarctions. RV leads should be checked in all patients with acute inferior STEMI.

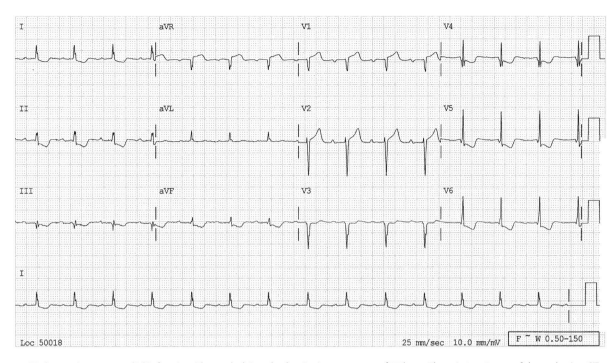

30. ST-depression myocardial infarction. The underlying rhythm is sinus at a rate of 87 bpm. There is 1 to 2 mm of downsloping ST-segment depression in leads V_4 to V_6, I, II, III, and aVF, indicating widespread ischemia. Additionally, there is evidence of an old anterior MI (Q wave in V_3 to V_4) and a first-degree AV block (PR interval >200 milliseconds). At cardiac catheterization, the patient had severe CAD.

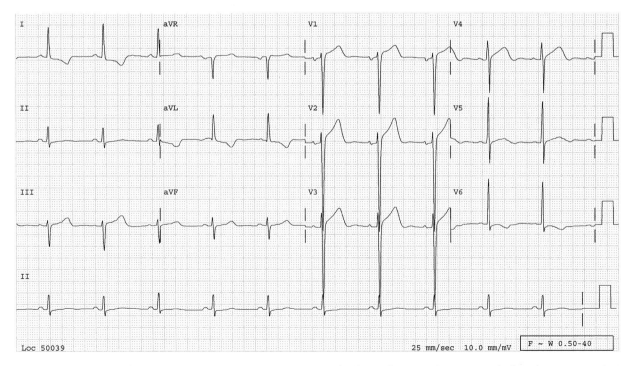

31. LVH with "strain" pattern. The underlying rhythm is sinus at a rate of 62 bpm. The QRS voltage is quite high and meets several criteria for LVH: depth of S wave in V_1 +height of R wave in V_5 or V_6 >35 mm, depth of S wave in V_2 +height of R wave in V_5 or V_6 >45 mm, R wave height >11 mm in aVL. Additionally, there are secondary repolarization changes with ST-elevation in leads with a predominant S wave and ST depression and T-wave inversion in leads with a predominant R wave (a "strain" pattern). LA enlargement is also present (common with LVH).

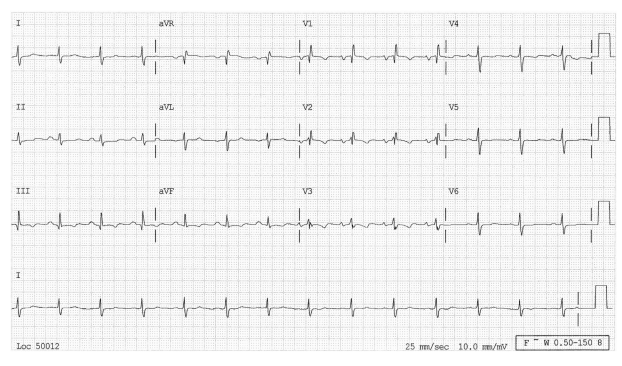

32. RVH. The underlying rhythm is sinus at a rate of 82 bpm. There is right axis deviation, and the R/S ratio is >1 in V_1 and <1 in V_5 and V_6.

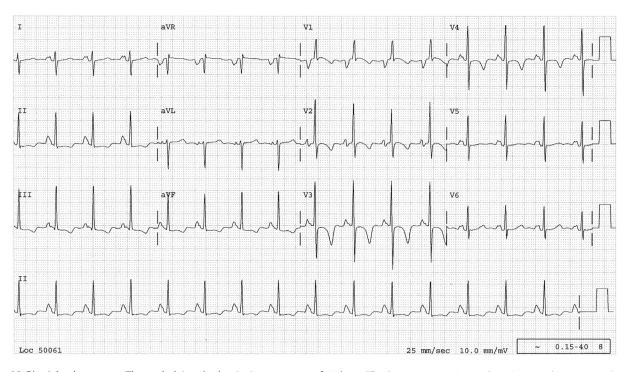

33. Biatrial enlargement. The underlying rhythm is sinus at a rate of 91 bpm. The P waves are >1 mm deep in V_1 and >3 mm wide in lead II, consistent with LA enlargement. Additionally the P wave in lead II is >2.5 mm tall, consistent with RA enlargement. Additional findings include right axis deviation (QRS is negative in lead I and positive in aVF) and RV hypertrophy (R >S in V_1, R wave in V_1 >7 mm). The T-wave inversions in V_1 to V_4 result from RVH (a "strain" pattern). This patient had severe MS.

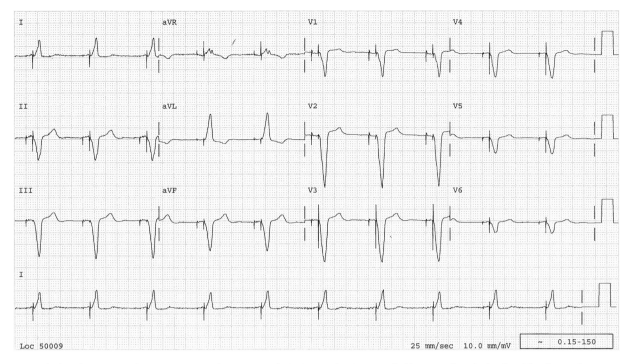

Loc 50009   25 mm/sec   10.0 mm/mV   ~   0.15-150

34. Dual-chamber pacemaker: AV sequential pacing. Each QRS complex is preceded by two electrical spikes. The first spike represents discharge of the atrial pacing lead; the subsequent P wave is best seen in lead II. The second spike represents discharge of the ventricular pacing lead; the subsequent QRS complex is wide and in an LBBB pattern because the RV is the site of initial depolarization. The time between the atrial and ventricular pacing spikes is set by the pacemaker and is referred to as the AV delay. Note that the pacemaker is set at a rate of 60 bpm. If the patient's own HR exceeds this rate, the pacemaker will be inhibited.

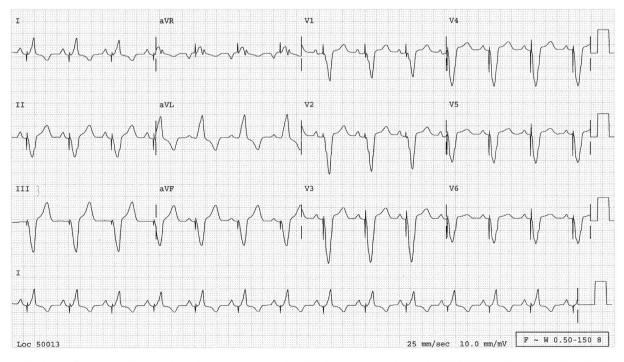

Loc 50013   25 mm/sec   10.0 mm/mV   F ~ W 0.50-150 8

35. Dual-chamber pacemaker: atrial sensing, ventricular pacing. This is the same patient as in ECG 35. The patient's own sinus rhythm has return at a rate of 81 bpm. This suppresses the atrial pacemaker. The ventricles are subsequently paced because the native impulse did not reach the ventricles in the set period of time (the AV delay).

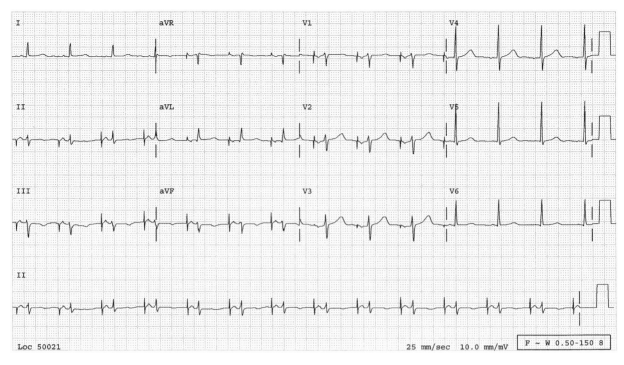

36. Atrial paced rhythm. Atrial pacing spikes are seen prior to each P wave and occurring at a rate of 80 bpm. The P waves all conduct to the ventricles with a PR interval of ~200 msec. The native QRS complexes are essentially normal albeit with left axis deviation and are not preceded by pacing spikes.

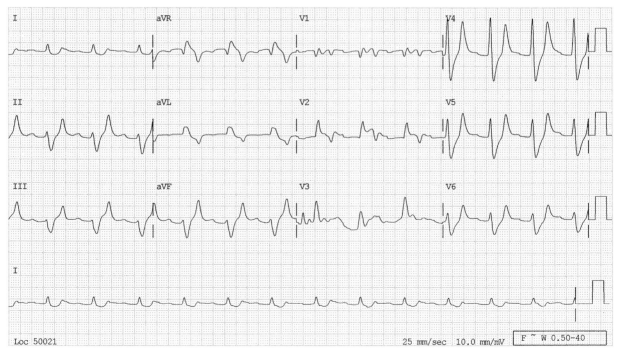

37. Hyperkalemia. The underlying rhythm is sinus at a rate of 78 bpm. There is a first-degree AV block (PR interval >200 msec). The QRS complexes are wide and extend almost to the T wave. The T waves are narrow and peaked. The patient's potassium level was >7.

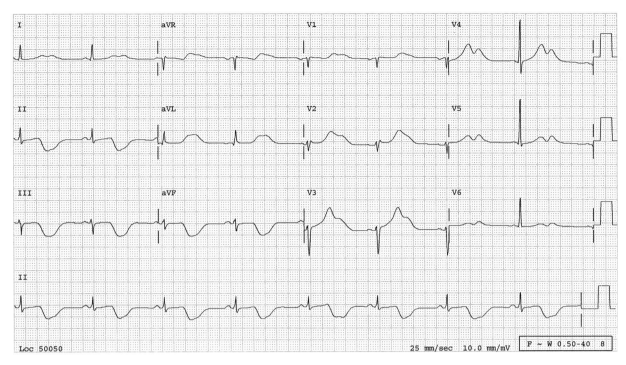

38. Long-QT syndrome. The underlying rhythm is sinus bradycardia at a rate of 48 bpm. The QT interval is exceedingly long (almost 700 msec), and there is a double-peaked T wave in the precordial leads. The long QT interval predisposes to the development of polymorphic VT.

Appendix C: Commonly Used Cardiovascular Medications

Class	Examples	Usual Dosage Range	Indications	Side Effects
ACE inhibitors	Captopril	6.25–100 mg tid		Hypotension
	Enalapril	5–20 mg bid		Hyperkalemia
	Fosinopril	10–80 mg qd	HTN	Renal dysfunction
	Lisinopril	10–80 mg qd	CHF	Rash
	Quinapril	10–80 mg qd	S/p MI	Cough
	Ramipril	2.5–20 mg qd		Angioedema
Angiotensin receptor–blocking agents	Candesartan	16–32 mg qd	HTN	Hypotension
	Irbesartan	150–300 mg qd	CHF	Hyperkalemia
	Losartan	50–100 mg qd	S/p MI	Renal dysfunction
	Valsartan	80–320 mg qd		Angioedema (rare)
Alpha-adrenergic blocking agents	Clonidine	Tablets: 0.1–1.2 mg bid Patch: 0.1–0.6 mg/24 h		Hypotension
	Doxazosin	1–16 mg qhs	HTN	
	Prazosin	1–20 mg bid		
	Terazosin	1–20 mg qd		
Antiarrhythmic agents	Adenosine	6–12 mg IV bolus	SVT	Hypotension, bronchospasm
	Amiodarone	Load: 1 g IV over 24 h or 400 mg bid/tid for 10 g Maintenance: 200–400 mg qd	VT/VF AF	Hypo- or hyperthyroidism, LFT abnormalities, pulmonary fibrosis, photosensitivity
	Atropine	0.5–1.0 mg IV q 3–5 min	Symptomatic bradycardia	Acute glaucoma
	Digoxin	0.125 qd–0.25 mg qd	Control of SVT; CHF	Bradycardia, nausea
	Lidocaine	Bolus: 1 mg/kg IV, then 1–4 mg/min infusion	Life-threatening ventricular arrhythmias	Confusion
	Procainamide	Bolus: 1 g IV at 20 mg/min then 2–6 mg/min infusion	Ventricular and supraventricular arrhythmias	Lupus-like syndrome, torsades de pointes, hypotension
Anticoagulants	Unfractionated heparin	Weight-based	Acute need for anticoagulation	Bleeding, thrombocytopenia
	Low-molecular-weight heparin	1 mg/kg bid (treatment) 30 mg SC q12 h (prophylaxis)	Treatment: ACS, DVT, PE Prophylaxis: DVT	Bleeding, thrombocytopenia (rare)
	Warfarin	Varies depending on INR goal	Chronic need for anticoagulation	Bleeding, birth defects
Antiplatelet agents	Aspirin	81–325 mg qd		
	Clopidogrel	75 mg qd		
	Eptifibatide	Bolus: 180 μg/kg IV, then 2 μg/kg/min for up to 72 h	ACS	Bleeding, thrombocytopenia
	Tirofiban	0.4 μg/kg/min infusion × 30 min, then 0.1 μg/kg/min infusion × 48 h	ACS	Bleeding, thrombocytopenia

Class	Examples	Usual Dosage Range	Indications	Side Effects
Beta-adrenergic blocking agents	Atenolol	25–100 mg qd	Treatment of HTN, angina	
	Carvedilol	3.125–25 mg bid	Rate control of SVT	
	Labetalol	100–1,200 mg bid	Secondary prevention post-MI	
	Metoprolol	25–100 mg qd	CHF (metoprolol XL, carvedilol)	
	Propranolol	80–640 mg qd		
Calcium channel blockers	Amlodipine	2.5–10 mg qd	HTN, angina, CHF	Hypotension, edema
	Diltiazem	120–360 mg qd	HTN, angina, SVT	Hypotension, bradycardia
	Nifedipine	30–90 mg qd	HTN	Hypotension, bradycardia
	Verapamil	120–480 mg qd	HTN, angina, SVT	Hypotension, edema
Diuretics	Amiloride	5–20 mg qd	HTN, edema	Hyperkalemia
	Furosemide	20–300 mg daily	HTN, CHF, edema	Hypokalemia
	Hydrochlorothiazide	12.5–25mg qd	HTN, CHF, edema	Hypokalemia, hyponatremia
	Metolazone	2.5–10 mg qd	HTN, CHF, edema	Hypokalemia, hypomagnesemia
	Spironolactone	25 mg qd	Class III–IV CHF	Hyperkalemia, gynecomastia
Lipid-lowering therapy	Atorvastatin	10–80 mg qd	Treatment of elevated LDL in patient with (or at risk for) CHD	LFT abnormalities Myalgias/myositis
	Lovastatin	10–80 mg qd		
	Pravastatin	10–80 mg qd		
	Rosuvastatin	10–40 mg qd		
	Simvastatin	10–80 mg qd		
	Ezetimibe	10 qd	Treatment of elevated LDL	None significant
	Fenofibrate	54–160 mg qd	Treatment of elevated triglycerides	LFT abnormalities
	Gemfibrozil	600 bid		
	Niacin (extended release)	500–2,000 mg qhs		
Nitrates	Isosorbide dinitrate	10–40 mg tid	Chronic stable angina, CHF	Headache, hypotension
	Isosobide mononitrate	30–120 mg qd	Chronic stable angina, CHF	
	Nitroglycerine IV	10–400 μg/min infusion	ACS, acute CHF	
Other vasodilators	Hydralazine	10–100 mg tid or qid	HTN, chronic CHF	Tachycardia, lupus-like syndrome
	Nitroprusside	0.3–10 μg/kg/min infusion	Hypertensive crisis, acute CHF	Hypotension, cyanide toxicity
Vasopressors/ inotropes	Dobutamine	2–20 μg/kg/min infusion	HTN	Tachycardia
	Dopamine	2–20 μg/kg/min infusion	CHF	Arrhythmias
	Milrinone	Load: 50 μg/kg IV over 10 min, then 0.375–0.75 μg/kg/min	Shock	Ischemia
	Norepinephrine	2–12 μg/min infusion		
	Phenylephrine	40–180 μg/min infusion		

qd, once daily; bid, twice daily; tid, thrice daily; qid: four times daily; qhs, at bedtime.

Index

Index note: page references with a *b*, *f*, or *t* indicate a box, figure or table on the designated page; references in **bold** indicate discussion of the subject in the Questions and Answers sections.

Abdominal aneurysm, **190, 205–206**

Ablation, 35–36, 94, 96

Accelerated idioventricular rhythm (AIVR), 67*t*, **200, 201***f,* **214,** 230*f*

Action potential (AP), 90–91, 91*f*

Activities of daily living (ADLs), metabolic equivalent (METs) levels of, 23, 23*t*

Acute arterial occlusion, 151–152

Acute bacterial endocarditis (ABE), 126

Acute coronary syndrome (ACS), 55–56, 56*f*, 57, 57*b*, 58

Acute heart failure, 73–74, 74*t*

Acute inferior MI with RV infarction, **203, 216**

Acute marginal branch, 42, 43*f*

Acute myocardial infarction (AMI)
 criteria for thrombolysis in, 60–61, 61*b*
 as differential dx for myocarditis, 84
 mechanical complications of, 66, 66*f/t*, 68
 pharmacologic management of, 59–61, **195, 202, 209–210, 215**
 See also ST-elevation myocardial infarction

Acute rheumatic fever (RF), 114–115, 115*b*, 116

Adenovirus
 as cause of myocarditis, 83
 as cause of pericarditis, 137*t*

Afterload, 70, 72*f*

Airway obstruction, as differential dx for dyspnea, 5, 5*t*

Alpha-adrenergic blocking agents, 244

Ambulatory ECG monitoring, 34

Amphetamines, as differential dx for palpitations, 7*t*

Amyloidosis, as cause of pericarditis, 137*t*

Anemia, as differential dx
 for dyspnea, 5, 5*t*
 for palpitations, 7*t*

Anemia, heart sounds associated with, 10*t*

Aneurysms
 abdominal, **190, 205–206**
 focal or diffuse, 154
 saccular vs. fusiform, 154
 true or pseudoaneurysms, 68, 154
 ventricular, 68

Angina, 2
 as differential dx for left-sided HF, 77
 pharmacologic agents for, 52–53, 53*t*
 Prinzmetal variant of, 53–54
 revascularization therapies, 53, 53*t*
 variant angina in, 53–54

Angina, chronic stable, 51–52, 52*t*, 53, 53*t*, 54

Angina pectoris, 51

Angioplasty, 61, 62*f*

Angiotensin-converting enzyme (ACE) inhibitors, 57, 244

Angiotensin receptor-blocking agents, 244

Ankle-brachial index (ABI), 151

Ankylosing spondylitis, aortic aneurysms associated with, 154*t*

Antiarrhythmic agents, 244

Anticoagulants, 244

Antidromic AVRT, 97

Antiplatelet agents, 244

Anxiety, as differential dx
 for chest pain, 4*t*
 for palpitations, 7*t*
 for PE, 164
 for syncope, 103, 103*b*

Aorta, diseases of, 154, 154*t*, 155–156, 156*f*, 157, 157*f*, 158, 158*f/t*, 159

Aortic aneurysms
 diseases associated with, 154, 154*t*, 155
 indications for surgery of, 156
 radiographic findings of, 38*t*

Aortic dissection
 classification of, 156, 156*f*
 diagnostic evaluation of, 38*t*, 157, 157*f*, 158, 158*f/t*, **194, 209**
 as differential dx for chest pain, 3, 4*t*, 56
 dissecting aortic aneurysm, as cause of pericarditis, 173*t*
 pathogenesis of, 156–157, 157*f*
 treatment of, 158–159, **190, 194, 202, 206, 209, 215**

Aortic insufficiency (AI), 118–119, 119*t*, 120, **197–198, 212**
 epidemiology and etiology of, 118
 murmur associated with, 11*t*
 peripheral signs of, 119*t*

Aortic regurgitation (AR), 115, **197–198, 200, 212, 214**

Aortic sclerosis, murmur associated with, 11*t*

Aortic stenosis (AS), 11*t*, 12, 117, 117*f*, 118, **191, 192, 193, 207**

Aortic stenosis (AS), as differential dx for chest pain, 3, 4*t*
 heart sounds associated with, 10*t*, 11
 for syncope, 103, 103*b*

Aortic valve disorders, 117, 117*f*, 118–119, 119*t*, 120

Aortitis, 159

Aortography, 31–32

Apolipoprotein C-II (apo C-II), 46, 47*f*

Arrhythmias
 action potential (AP) in, 90–91, 91*f*
 associated with prosthetic heart valves, 132
 bradyarrhythmias in, 90*t*, 92
 as complication of acute MI, 67*t*, 68
 delayed afterdepolarization as, 91, 92, 92*f*
 diagnostic modalities for, 34–35, 35*f*, 36
 mechanisms of, 90, 90*t*, 91, 91*f*, 92, 92*f*
 reentrant mechanism in, 91–92, 92*f*
 tachyarrhythmias in, 90*t*, 91–92, 92*f*

Arterial embolus, as complication of acute MI, 68

Arterial occlusion, acute, 151–152

Arthritis, associated with rheumatic fever, 114, 115

Aschoff body, 114

Asthma, as differential dx for dyspnea, 5, 5t

Asymmetric septal hypertrophy (ASH), 86

Atherosclerosis
    aortic aneurysms associated with, 154, 154t
    foam cells and fatty streaks in, 44
    pathogenesis of, 43–44, 44b/f, 45
    risk factors for, 44b, 45

Atherosclerotic plaque, 44, 44f, 45

Atrial fibrillation (AF)
    as complication of acute MI, 67t
    heart sounds associated with, 10t
    as tachyarrhythmia, 95, 95f, 96, **204, 217,** 227f

Atrial flutter, 96, 96f, 228f
    as complication of acute MI, 67t
    RF ablation therapy for, 36

Atrial septal defects (ASDs)
    characteristic findings with, 177, 177t, 178, **196, 203, 210, 216**
    heart sounds associated with, 10, 10t
    indications for surgical closure of, 178
    ostium primum defects, 176, 176f, 177, 177t
    ostium secundum defects, 176, 176f, 177, 177t
    radiographic findings of, 38t
    sinus venosus defect, 176, 176f, 177, 177t

Atrioventricular (AV) block
    as complication of acute MI, 67t
    See also Heart block (HB)

Atrioventricular (AV) node, 16, 16f

Atypical chest pain, 2

Atypical Mycobacteria, as cause of IE, 126b

Austin-Flint murmur, 119

Autograft tissue heart valve, 130

Autoimmune disease, as cause of myocarditis, 83

Automaticity, 91, 92

Autoregulation, 42

AV dissociation, 10t, 97, 102

AV fistula, murmur associated with, 11t

AV-nodal block, as differential dx for syncope, 103, 103b

AV-nodal reentrant tachycardia (AVNRT), 96, 96f, 97, **196, 196f, 210,** 229f

as differential dx for palpitations, 7
    RF ablation therapy of, 35, 36

AV node conduction disorders (Heart block), 99t, 101, 101f, 102, 102f

Bacilli, gram-negative, as cause of IE, 126b

Baker cyst, ruptured, as differential dx for DVT, 164

Ball-in-cage mechanical valves, 130, 130f, 132

Barlow syndrome, 123

Bartonella spp., as cause of IE, 127

Bayes theorem, 24

Beats per minute (BPM), 17, 18f

Beck triad, 139

Benign flow murmur, 11t

Beta blockers, 53, 53t, 245

Biatrial enlargement, 240f

Bicuspid aortic valve, heart sounds associated with, 7t

Bile-acid sequestrants, 49t, 50

Bileaflet tilting disc heart valves, 130, 130f

Bioprosthetic valves (BPVs), 130, 130f

Bisferiens pulse, 9

Biventricular pacing, 80, 111–112, **201–202, 214–215**

Blalock-Taussig shunt, 179

Blunt trauma cardiac injuries, 154t, 184, 184b, 185, **200, 213**

Borrelia burgdorferi, as cause of myocarditis, 83

Brachytherapy, 33

Bradyarrhythmias
    differential dx of, 100, 100f, 101, 101f, 102, 102f
    escape rhythms in, 92
    functional and structural causes of, 99, 99t
    heart blocks (HB) with, 92
    mechanisms of, 90t, 92
    See also Heart block (HB)

Bradyarrhythmias, as differential dx
    for palpitations, 7, 7t
    for syncope, 103, 103b

Brain natriuretic peptide (BNP), 6

Breast cancer, as cause of pericarditis, 137t

Breath sounds, diminished, 12

Bronchospasm, 12

Brucella abortus, as cause of IE, 127

Bruce protocol, 21–22

B-type natriuretic peptide (BNP), 77

Buerger disease, 152–153

Bundle of HIS, 16f

Bypass tract, 18

Caffeine, as differential dx for palpitations, 7t

Calcium channel blockers, 53, 53t, 245

Candida, as cause of IE, 126b

Carcinoid heart disease, 188, **200–201, 214**

Cardiac asthma, 12

Cardiac catheterization
    complications associated with, 33
    contraindications to, 33
    hemodynamic profiles with, 31, 31t
    left heart catheterization (LHC), 29f, 31–32, 32f
    percutaneous coronary intervention (PCI) in, 32–33
    right heart catheterization (RHC) in, 29, 29f, 30, 30f, 31
    techniques of, 29, 29f

Cardiac contusion, as cause of pericarditis, 137t

Cardiac electrophysiology, 16, 16f, 17, 17b/f, 18, 18f, 19, 19t, 20

Cardiac enzymes, 56, 56f, 59, 84

Cardiac evaluation, preoperative, 172, 172t, 173, 173t, 174, 174f, 175, **200, 213**

Cardiac imaging, 37, 37f, 38, 38t, 39, 39f, 40, 40f

Cardiac index, 70, 70t

Cardiac injury/trauma, nonpenetrating and penetrating, 184, 184b, 185, 186, **200, 213**

Cardiac MRI, 39–40, 40f

Cardiac output (CO), 6, 70–71

Cardiac rupture, 184, 184b

Cardiac tamponade
    causes of, 137t, 139
    as differential dx for syncope, 103, 103b
    echocardiogram and ECG changes with, 140, 140f
    features of, 139–140, 140f, **193–194, 208**

Cardiac transplantation, 81

Cardiac tumors, 187, 187b, 188, 188f

Cardiogenic shock, 31t, 65

Cardioinhibitor response, as differential dx for syncope, 103, 103b

Cardiomyopathy, 73, 85–88, 88f
    as differential dx for palpitations, 7t
    dilated, 85–86
    hypertrophic, 85, 86–87
    restrictive, 85, 87–88, 88f, **191–192, 207**

Cardiopulmonary exercise testing (CPET), 25

Cardiovascular hemodynamics
afterload, 70, 72, 72f
alterations with heart failure, 72
cardiac index, 70, 70t
cardiac output (CO), 70–71
changes with pericardial diseases, 142, 142f, 143
contractility, 70, 71, 71f, 72
of critical aortic stenosis (AS), 117f
ejection fraction (EF), 70t, 71–72
filling pressure of, 70
intracardiac pressures, 70, 70t
of mitral regurgitation (MR), 124f
of pericardial diseases, 143t
during pregnancy, 181, 181t, 182
preload, 71, 71f, 72f
problems associated with prosthetic heart valves, 132

Cardiovascular system, physical exam of, 9–10, 10f/t, 11, 11f/t, 12, 12t, 13

Cardioversion, 94

Carditis, with acute rheumatic fever, 114–115

Carotid arterial disease
clinical syndromes of, 160, **200, 213**
treatment of, 161, 161t, 162, **203, 216**

Carotid bruit, 160

Carotid endarterectomy, 161, 161t, 162, **203, 216**

Carotid sinus hypersensitivity, as differential dx for syncope, 103, 103b

Carotid sinus massage (CSM), 94

Carotid stenosis, 160

Catheterization, cardiac, 29, 29f, 30, 30f, 31, 31t, 32, 32f, 33

Cellulitis, as differential dx for DVT, 164

Central cyanosis, 12

Cerebrovascular accident (CVA), 160

Cerebrovascular disease (CVD), 160

Chagas disease, as cause of myocarditis, 83

Chest
auscultation of, 10, 10t, 11, 11f/t, 12, 12t
inspection and palpation of, 9

Chest leads, 16, 17f

Chest pain, 2–3, 4t

Chest radiography (CXR), 37, 37f, 38, 38t

Chlamydia pneumoniae, as cause of IE, 127

Cholelithiasis, as differential dx for chest pain, 56

Cholesterol, calculating total serum level of, 46–47

Chorea, associated with rheumatic fever, 114, 115

Chronic heart failure, 74, 74t

Chronic obstructive pulmonary disease (COPD), as differential dx
for dyspnea, 5, 5t
for left-sided HF, 77

Chronic stable angina, 51–52, 52t, 53, 53t, 54
pharmacologic agents for, 52–53, 53t
revascularization therapies, 53, 53t

Chylomicrons, 46, 47f/t

Cine CT, 39, 39f

Cirrhosis, as differential dx for right-sided HF, 77

Clicks, 7t

Cocaine use
as cause of myocarditis, 83
as differential dx for palpitations, 7t

Codominant circulation, 42

Collagen vascular disease, as cause of myocarditis, 83

Color Doppler echocardiography technique, 27

Complete heart block, 102, 102f, 234f

Complicated endocarditis, 125

Congenital cardiac shunts, 176, 176f, 177, 177t, 178

Congenital heart disease, 176, 176f, 177, 177t, 178–180
See also Atrial septal defect; Congenital cardiac shunts; Corrected transpositions; Cyanotic heart disease; Eisenmenger syndrome; Patent ductus arteriosus; Tetralogy of Fallot; Ventricular septal defect

Congenital long-QT syndrome, 98

Congestive heart failure (CHF)
developing after an MI, 64
radiographic findings of, 38t

Congestive heart failure (CHF), as differential dx
for dyspnea, 5t
for PE, 164

Conservative therapy, for UA or NSTEMI, 58

Constrictive pericarditis
causes of, 142, 142t
diagnostic modalities for, 143–144, 144t, **195, 202–203, 210, 215–216**
as differential dx for restrictive cardiomyopathy, 87, 88f

radiographic findings of, 38t
ventricular pressures associated with, 142, 142f

Continuous murmur, 11t

Contractility, 70, 71, 71f, 72

Contrast echocardiography, 27

Coronary angiography, 31, 32f

Coronary arteries
autoregulation of, 42
coronary flow reserve of, 42–43
endothelial walls of, 42–43
injury/trauma to, 184b
normal anatomy of, 42, 43f
physiology of, 42–43, 43f

Coronary artery bypass graft (CABG), 53, **194, 208–209**

Coronary artery disease (CAD)
angina of, 2
indications for CABG, 53, **194, 208–209**
modifiable risk factors for, 52, 52t, **197, 211**
pathophysiology of, 42–43, 43f, 44, 44b/f, 45
risk factors for, 44b, 45, **197, 211**

Coronary flow reserve, 42, 42f

Coronary stents, 61

Cor pulmonale, hemodynamic profiles of, 31t

Corrected transpositions, 179

Corrigan pulse, associated with aortic insufficiency (AI), 119t

Coxiella burnetti, as cause of IE, 127

Coxsackie A virus, as cause of pericarditis, 137t

Coxsackie B virus
as cause of myocarditis, 83
as cause of pericarditis, 137t

Crackles, 12

Cyanotic heart disease, 178–180

Cystic medial necrosis, aortic aneurysms associated with, 154t, 155

DeBakey class of aortic dissection, 156f

Decompensated heart failure, 78, 78f, 79, 79f/t, 80, **191, 198–199, 207, 212**

Decrescendo diastolic murmur, 11t

Deep venous thrombosis (DVT)
causes of, 163, 164b
diagnostic algorithm for, 164, 164f, 165, **190–191, 206–207**
as differential dx for right-sided HF, 77
indications for inferior vena cava filter placement, 166, 166b
prophylaxis against, 166

DeMusset sign, associated with aortic insufficiency (AI), 119t

Dependent rubor, 150

Depression, as differential dx for palpitations, 7t

Diabetes mellitus (DM), atypical chest pain of, 2

Diagonal branch, 42, 43f

Diaphragmatic paralysis, as differential dx for dyspnea, 5, 5t

Diastolic heart failure, 73–74, 74t, 82

Diastolic rumble, 11t

Digital clubbing, 12, 126

Dilated cardiomyopathy (DCM), 85–86

Dilated cardiomyopathy (DCM), as differential dx for palpitations, 7t

Diphtheroids, as cause of IE, 126b

Diuretics, 245

Doppler echocardiography, 27

Dressler syndrome, 68, 137t

Drug abuse, endocarditis associated with IV drug use, 125, **198, 212**

Drugs/medications
    as cause of pericarditis, 137t
    commonly used cardiovascular medications, 244–245

Drugs/medications, as differential dx
    for chest pain, 3
    for palpitations, 7t
    for syncope, 103, 103b

Dual-chamber pacemakers, 241f

Duroziez sign, associated with aortic insufficiency (AI), 119t

Dyslipidemia, 46–47, 47f/t, 48, 48t, 49, 49b/t, 50
    goals in treatment of, 48, 48t, 49, 49t, 50
    primary dyslipidemias in, 46, 48t
    Dyspnea, 5, 5t, 6–7

Early invasive strategy, for UA or NSTEMI, 58

Early-peaking systolic ejection murmur, 11t

Echocardiography, 26, 26f, 27, 27b, 28
    color Doppler echocardiography technique of, 27
    contrast, 27
    Doppler technique of, 27
    intravascular (IVUS), 27
    three-dimensional (3D) echocardiography, 27
    transesophageal echocardiography (TEE) technique of, 26, 27

transthoracic echocardiography (TTE) technique of, 26, 27
    two-dimensional (2D) technique of, 26, 26f, 27
    uses and limitations of, 27b

Ectopic atrial tachycardia, 95

Einthoven, Willem, 16

Eisenmenger syndrome, 178

Ejection fraction (EF), 70t, 71–72

Electrocardiogram (ECG)
    ambulatory, 34
    cardiac physiology, 16, 16f
    diagnostic criteria for abnormalities 19t, 20
    features of normal ECG, 17–18, 18f, 19–20, 224f
    lead system of, 16, 17f
    limb leads of, 16, 17f
    mechanism and generation of, 16
    precordial leads of, 16, 17f
    PR interval, 18, 18f
    P wave, 17–18, 18f
    QRS complex, 18, 18f, 19
    QT interval, 18f, 20
    steps in analyzing, 16, 17b
    with stress testing, 24, 24f, 25
    strips of normal and abnormal, 224f–243f
    ST segment, 18f, 19
    T wave, 18f, 19–20

Electron-beam computed tomography (EBCT), 39, 39f

Electrophysiologic study (EPS), 35, 35f, 36

Emotional stress, as differential dx for palpitations, 7t

Endocardial structural injury/trauma, 184b

Endocarditis, infective (IE), 125–126, 126b, 127, 127f/t, 128, 128b, 129t, **193, 208**

Endothelial dysfunction, 43–44

Enterococcus, as cause of IE, 126b

Epstein-Barr virus (EBV), as cause of pericarditis, 137t

Erythema marginatum, associated with rheumatic fever, 114, 115

Escape rhythm, 92, 102

Esophageal rupture, as differential dx for chest pain, 4t

Esophageal spasm, as differential dx for chest pain, 3, 4t

Exercise stress testing, 21–22, **189–190, 205**

Exercise tolerance testing (ETT), 58

Ezetimibe, 49t, 50

Fatty streaks, 44

Fenofibrate, 49t, 50

Fever, as differential dx
    for IE, 126
    for palpitations, 7t

Fever, heart sounds associated with, 10t

Fibric-acid derivatives, 49t, 50

Filling pressure, 70

First-degree AV block, 101, 101f, 102, 232f

Fixed splitting, 10, 10t

Flip-flops, 7

Flow-mediated vasodilation, 42

Frank-Starling curve, 71f, 119

Gallavardin phenomenon, 118

Gallbladder disease, as differential dx for chest pain, 3

Gastroesophageal reflux disease (GERD), as differential dx for chest pain, 3, 4t, 56

Giant-cell arteritis
    aortic aneurysms associated with, 154t
    as cause of aortitis, 159

Glycoprotein (GP) IIb-IIIa inhibitors, 57

Granulomatous disease, as cause of myocarditis, 83

HACEK (*Haemophilus parainfluenzae, Haemophilus aphrophilus, Actinobacillus actinomycetemcomitans, Eikenella corrodens*, and *Kingella kingae*), 126

Heart block (HB), 92, 99t, 101, 101f, 102, 102f
    first-degree AV block in, 101, 101f, 102, 232f
    Mobitz I (Wenckebach) second-degree, 101, 101f, 102, 233f
    Mobitz II second degree in, 101, 101f, 102, 233f
    second-degree AV block in, 101, 101f, 102, 102f, 233f
    third-degree (complete) AV block in, 102, 102f, 234f

Heart failure (HF)
    acute or chronic, 73–74, 74t
    classifications of, 73–74, 74t
    clinical manifestations of, 72, 76–77
    common causes of, 74t
    compensatory responses to, 74, 74t, 75
    as complication of MI, 64
    decompensated, 78, 78f, 79, 79f/t, 80, **191, 198–199, 207, 212**
    device therapies for, 80
    etiologies of, 76, 76t

functional status of patients with, 77, 77b

high-output or low output, 73–74, 74t

mechanisms of, 73–74, 74t, 75

outpatient management of, 81f

pharmacologic therapies for, 78, 78f, 79, 79f/t, 80, 80t, 81f, 82

right-sided or left-sided, 73–74, 74t

surgical therapies for, 80–81

systolic or diastolic, 73–74, 74t, 78, 78f, 79, 79f/t, 80, 80t, 81, 81f, 82

Heart rate, calculation of, 17, 18f

Heart sounds, auscultation of, 10, 10t, 11

Hemodialysis, as cause of pericarditis, 137t

Hemodynamics, cardiovascular, 70, 70t, 71, 71f, 72, 72f

Herpes zoster, as differential dx for chest pain, 4t

Heterograft tissue heart valves, 130, 130f

High-density lipoproteins (HDL), 46, 47f/t

High-output heart failure, 73–74, 74t

Hill sign, associated with aortic insufficiency (AI), 119t

His-Purkinje system, 16f, 90, 99

History and physical, 2

HMG-CoA reductase inhibitors, 49t, 50, **189, 205**

Holosystolic murmur, 11t

Holter monitors, 34

Homograft tissue heart valves, 130

Human immunodeficiency virus (HIV)
as cause of myocarditis, 83
as cause of pericarditis, 137, 137t

Hypercholesterolemia, treatment of, 49, 49t, 50

Hyperkalemia
as differential dx for palpitations, 7t
ECG changes with, 242f
Hyperlipidemia
goals in treatment of, 48, 48t, 49, 49t, 50
primary, 46, 48t
secondary causes of, 46, 49b

Hypersensitivity reactions, as cause of myocarditis, 83

Hypertension (HTN)
classification of, 146, 146t
heart sounds associated with, 10t
pharmacologic therapies for, 148, 148t, 149, **197, 211**
pregnancy and, 182, **202, 215**
target organ damage associated with, 147, 147t
treatment recommendations for, 147–148, 148t, **197, 211**

Hypertensive crisis, 149, 149t, **195, 209**

Hypertensive heart disease, as differential dx for cardiomyopathy, 88

Hyperthyroidism, as differential dx for dyspnea, 5, 5t

Hypertriglyceridemia, 49, 49t, 50

Hypertrophic cardiomyopathy (HCM), 10t, 11t, 85, 86–87, **203–204, 216–217**

Hypertrophic cardiomyopathy (HCM), as differential dx for palpitations, 7t

Hypertrophic obstructive cardiomyopathy (HOCM), 12t, 86, **192, 193, 208**

Hypertrophic obstructive cardiomyopathy (HOCM), as differential dx for syncope, 103, 103b

Hypoglycemia, as differential dx
for palpitations, 7t
for syncope, 103, 103b

Hypokalemia
as differential dx for palpitations, 7t
hemodynamic profiles of, 31t

Hypomagnesemia, as differential dx for palpitations, 7t

Idiopathic hypertrophic subaortic stenosis (IHSS), 86

Idiopathic restrictive cardiomyopathy, 87

Implantable cardioverter-defibrillator (ICD), 95, 111, 111b, 112, **194, 209**

Infected indwelling vascular catheters, as differential dx for IE, 126

Infective endocarditis (IE), 125–126, 126b, 127, 127f/t, 128, 128b, 129t, **193, 195, 208, 209**
antibiotic prophylaxis for patients at risk, 129, 129t
associated with prosthetic heart valves, 133, **203, 216**
complicated endocarditis of IV drug users, 125, **198, 212**
criteria for diagnosis of, 127, 128b
cutaneous manifestations of, 127, 127t
differential diagnosis of, 126
indication for surgery in, 128, 128b
microorganisms causing, 125–126, 126b, **193, 195, 208, 209**
native valve endocarditis (NVE) as, 125, 128b
prosthetic valve endocarditis (PVE) as, 125, 128b

Inferior vena cava filter, indications for, 166

Infiltrative cardiomyopathy, as differential dx for dyspnea, 5t

Influenza, as cause of myocarditis, 83

Inotropes, 245

Inotropy, 71, 71f

Inspiratory crackles, 12

Intermediate-density lipoproteins (IDL), 46, 47f/t

Intraaortic balloon pump (IABP), 65, 81

Intracardiac pressures, 70, 70t

Intravascular ultrasound (IVUS), 27

Intraventricular block, as complication of acute MI, 67t

Irregularly irregular pulse, 9

Ischemia, as differential dx for dyspnea, 5t

Ischemic heart disease, as differential dx for cardiomyopathy, 88

Ischemic/nonischemic cardiomyopathy, as differential dx for dyspnea, 5t

Janeway lesions, associated with IE, 127b

J♥NES (joints, carditis, subcutaneous nodules, erythema marginatum, Sydenham chorea), 114

Jones criteria for rheumatic fever, 115, 115b

Jugular venous pressure (JVP), 6, 9, 10f, 143t

Junctional rhythm, 229f

Knocks, 7t, 143

Kussmaul sign, 65, 143t

Late-peaking systolic ejection murmur, 11t

Lead system of ECG, 16, 17f

Left anterior descending (LAD) artery, 42, 43f

Left anterior fascicle, 16f

Left anterior fascicular block, abnormal ECG associated with, 19t, 236f

Left atrium (LA) enlargement
abnormal ECG associated with, 19t
radiographic findings of, 38t

Left-axis deviation, abnormal ECG associated with, 19t

Left bundle branch, 16f

Left bundle branch block (LBBB), 67t
abnormal ECG associated with, 19t, 235f
heart sounds associated with, 10, 10t

Left circumflex (LCx) artery, 42, 43f

Left-dominant circulation, 42

Left heart catheterization (LHC), 29f, 31–32, 32f

Left main coronary artery, 42, 43f

Left posterior block, abnormal ECG associated with, 19t

Left-sided heart failure, 73–74, 74t

Left ventricular end-diastolic pressure (LVEDP), 70, 70t, 72

Left ventricular enlargement, 38t

Left ventricular hypertrophy (LVH), 19t, 38t, 239f

Leriche syndrome, 150

Levine's sign, 2

Lifestyle changes, therapeutic (TLC), 50

Limb leads, 16, 17f

Lipid-lowering therapy, 49t, 50, 245

Lipids, normal metabolism of, 46, 47f

Lipoprotein a [Lp(a)], 46, 47f/t

Lipoprotein lipase (LPL), 46, 47f

Lipoproteins, 46, 47f

Lone atrial-fibrillation, 96

Long-QT syndrome, 98, 243f

Low-density lipoprotein (LDL), 43, 46, 47f/t

Low-molecular-weight heparin (LMWH), 57, 165–166

Low-output heart failure, 73–74, 74t

Lung cancer, as cause of pericarditis, 137t

Lungs, assessment of, 12

LV dysfunction, following an MI, 64

LV end-diastolic volume, 71

Lyme disease, as cause of myocarditis, 83

Lymphedema, as differential dx for DVT, 164

Lymphoma, as cause of pericarditis, 137t

"Machinery" murmur, 11t, 203

Marfan syndrome, 200, 214

Medications. See Drugs/medications

Melanoma, as cause of pericarditis, 137t

Metabolic equivalents (METs), 23, 23t

Missed beats, 7

Mitral regurgitation (MR)
    associated with rheumatic fever, 115
    etiology and epidemiology of, 123, 123b
    hemodynamic tracing of, 124f
    murmur associated with, 11t, 12t

Mitral stenosis (MS), 121, 121f, 122, 122f, 123, 240f
    as differential dx for syncope, 103, 103b
    dyspnea associated with, 6, 192, 201, 207, 210f, 214
    heart sounds associated with, 10t, 192–193, 199, 207, 212
    hemodynamic changes associated with, 121f
    murmur associated with, 11t, 199, 212

Mitral valve disorders, 121, 121f, 122, 122f, 123, 123b, 124, 124f

Mitral valve prolapse (MVP), 7t, 123, 200, 213

Mitral valve prolapse (MVP), as differential dx for palpitations, 7t

Mitral valve prolapse (MVP) with mitral regurgitation (MR), 11t, 12t

Mnemonics
    J♥NES (joints, carditis, subcutaneous nodules, erythema marginatum, Sydenham chorea), 114
    "six Ps" of arterial occlusion, 152

Mobitz I (Wenckebach) second-degree heart block, 101, 101f, 102, 233f

Mobitz II second-degree heart block, 101, 101f, 102, 233f

Muller sign, associated with aortic insufficiency (AI), 119t

Multifocal atrial tachycardia (MAT), 95, 95f, 228f

Multiple gated acquisition (MUGA), 38–39

Murmurs
    with aortic stenosis (AS), 11t, 118, 192, 193, 207
    assessment of, 11, 11f/t, 12, 12t
    Carey-Coombs, 114
    maximal intensity of, 11, 11f, 12
    origins of, 11, 11t

Musculoskeletal pain, as differential dx
    for chest pain, 4t
    for DVT, 164

Mycoplasma spp., as cause of IE, 126b

Myocardial contusion, 184, 184b

Myocardial infarction (MI)
    complications of, 64–66, 66f/t, 67t, 68
    ECG changes with, 19, 239f

Myocardial infarction (MI), as differential dx
    for chest pain, 2, 3, 4t
    for PE, 164

Myocardial ischemia, ST-segment depression with, 19

Myocardial perfusion imaging, 22, 22f, 23–24, 24t

Myocarditis, 83–84, 114–115

Myoxmas, 187, 187b, 188, 188f

National Cholesterol Education Program (NCEP), 48

Native valve endocarditis (NVE), 125, 128b

Neisseria spp., as cause of pericarditis, 137t

Nephrotic syndrome, as differential dx for right-sided HF, 77

Neurocardiogenic syncope, as differential dx for syncope, 103, 103b

New York Heart Association (NYHA), classification of functional status of HF patients, 77b

Nicotine, as a precipitant of palpitations, 7t

Nicotinic acid, 49t, 50

Nitrates, 52, 53t, 245

Nodules, subcutaneous, associated with rheumatic fever, 114, 115

Nonpenetrating cardiac injury/trauma, 184–185, 200, 213

Non-Q-wave MI. See Non-ST-elevation myocardial infarction (NSTEMI)

Non-ST-elevation myocardial infarction (NSTEMI), 55–56, 56f, 57, 57b, 58

Obesity, as differential dx for dyspnea, 5, 5t

Obtuse marginal (OM) branch, 42, 43f

Opening snap (OS), 6, 7t

Orthodromic AVRT, 97

Orthostatic hypotension, as differential dx for syncope, 103, 103b

Osler nodes, associated with IE, 127b

Ostium primum defects, 176, 176f, 177, 177t

Ostium secundum defects, 176, 176f, 177, 177t

Pacemaker, as differential dx for palpitations, 7t

Pacemakers
    biventricular pacing with, 80, 111–112, 201–202, 214–215
    choosing modes of, 111
    dual-chamber, 241f
    ECG manifestations of, 110f, 241f, 242f
    indications for, 110–111, 111b, 191, 199, 199f, 207, 213
    placement of, 110, 110f

Palpitations, 7, 7t, 8, 8f

Pancreatitis, as differential dx for chest pain, 3, 56

Panic attacks, as differential dx for palpitations, 7t

Papillary muscle rupture, 66, 66f/t, 184b, 197, 211

Paradoxical splitting, 10, 10t

Patent ductus arteriosus (PDA)
    heart sounds associated with, 10, 10t, 11
    murmur associated with, 11t, 203, 216
    risks associated with, 199, 212

Pathologic Q wave, ECG associated with, 19*t*

Patient history, 2

Peaked T wave, abnormal ECG associated with, 19*t*

Penetrating cardiac injury/trauma, 185, 186

Peptic ulcer disease (PUD), as differential dx for chest pain, 3

Percutaneous coronary intervention (PCI), 32–33, 61

Percutaneous transluminal angioplasty (PTA), 151

Percutaneous transluminal coronary angioplasty (PTCA), 53

Pericardial constriction, as differential dx for dyspnea, 5, 5*t*

Pericardial disease, as differential dx for right-sided HF, 77

Pericardial diseases, 135–144
　　See also Cardiac tamponade; Constrictive pericarditis; Pericarditis

Pericardial effusion, 38*t*

Pericardial friction rub, 11*t*, 12

Pericardial injury/trauma, 184*b*

Pericardial knock, 7*t*, 143

Pericardial tamponade
　　diagnosis of, **190, 206**
　　as differential dx for dyspnea, 5, 5*t*
　　hemodynamic profiles of, 31*t*

Pericardial window, 141

Pericarditis
　　with acute rheumatic fever, 115
　　as complication of acute MI, 68
　　ECG abnormalities with, 137, 137*f*, 138*t*, **191, 192f, 207**
　　etiology of, 136, 137*t*, **189, 190, 191, 192f, 205, 206, 207**
　　murmur associated with, 11*t*

Pericarditis, as differential dx
　　for chest pain, 3, 4*t*, 56
　　for PE, 164

Perioperative risk, assessment for
　　postoperative surveillance and, 175
　　predictors of, 172, 172*t*, 173, 173*t*, 174, **203, 216**
　　revascularization and, 175

Peripartum cardiomyopathy, 182–183

Peripheral arterial disease (PAD), 150–151

Petechiae, associated with IE, 127*b*

Pharmacologic stress testing, 21–22

Pheochromocytoma, as differential dx for palpitations, 7*t*

Pleural effusion, as differential dx for dyspnea, 5, 5*t*

Pleurisy, as differential dx for PE, 164

Pneumococcus spp., as cause of pericarditis, 137*t*

Pneumonia, as differential dx
　　for chest pain, 3, 4*t*, 56
　　for dyspnea, 5, 5*t*
　　for left-sided HF, 77
　　for PE, 164

Pneumothorax, as differential dx
　　for chest pain, 56
　　for dyspnea, 5, 5*t*
　　for PE, 164

Point of maximal impulse (PMI), 9

Polygenic hypercholesterolemia, 46, 48*t*

Polymorphic ventricular tachycardia, 97–98, 98*f*, 231*f*

Posterior descending artery (PDA), 42, 43*f*

Pott shunt, 179

Precordial leads, 16, 17*f*

Preeclampsia, 182

Pregnancy
　　cardiac testing during, 182
　　cardiovascular disorders related to, 182–183, **202, 215**
　　cardiovascular physiology during, 181, 181*t*, 182–183, 183*t*, **197, 211**
　　as differential dx for palpitations, 7*t*
　　preexisting cardiac disease and, 182
　　risks associated with prosthetic heart valves, 133

Preload, 70, 71, 71*f*, 72*f*

Premature atrial contractions (PACs), 226*f*

Premature atrial contractions (PACs), as differential dx for palpitations, 7

Premature pulmonary valve (PV) closure, associated with PDA, 11

Premature ventricular contractions (PVCs), as differential dx for palpitations, 7

Preoperative cardiac evaluation
　　algorithmic approach to, 173, 174*f*
　　diagnostic evaluation for, 173
　　managing other cardiac conditions, 174–175
　　predictors of perioperative cardiac risk, 172, 172*t*, 173, 173*t*, 174, **200, 203, 213, 216**

Presyncope, 103

Primary dyslipidemias, 46, 48*t*

Primary hypertension, 146

Primary pulmonary hypertension (PPH), 167–168, 168*f*, 169, **194–195, 209**

Primary restrictive cardiomyopathy, 87–88

PR interval, 18, 18*f*

Prinzmetal's angina, 53–54

Probucol, 49*t*, 50

Prosthetic heart valves
　　autograft tissue type in, 130
　　Ball-in-cage mechanical, 130, 130*f*, 132
　　bileaflet tilting disc valves in, 130, 130*f*
　　bioprosthetic valves (BPVs) in, 130, 130*f*
　　factors affecting choice of, 131, 131*t*, 132
　　heterograft (xenograft) tissue valves, 130, 130*f*, **202, 215**
　　homograft tissue type, 130
　　lifetime anticoagulation with, 132
　　mechanical prosthetic valves (MPVs) in, 130, 130*f*
　　problems associated with, 132–133, **203, 216**
　　Single tilting disc valves in, 130, 130*f*, 132
　　sounds of, 131
　　tissue valves in, 130, 130*f*, **202, 215**
　　types of, 130, 130*f*, **202, 215**

Prosthetic valve endocarditis (PVE), 125, 128*b*

Pseudoaneurysms, 68

Pseudoclaudication, 150–151

Pseudoseizure, as differential dx for syncope, 103, 103*b*

Pulmonary capillary wedge pressure (PCWP), 70, 70*t*, 72

Pulmonary embolus (PE)
　　causes of, 163, 164*b*
　　diagnostic algorithm for, 164, 164*f*, 165, **194, 202, 209, 215**
　　differential dx of, 164
　　indications for inferior vena cava filter placement, 166, 166*b*

Pulmonary embolus (PE), as differential dx
　　for chest pain, 3, 4*t*, 56
　　for dyspnea, 5*t*
　　for left-sided HF, 77

Pulmonary fibrosis, as differential dx for dyspnea, 5, 5*t*

Pulmonary hypertension
　　differential dx of, 168
　　ECG changes with, 168
　　heart sounds associated with, 10*t*, **192, 207**
　　hemodynamic profiles of, 31*t*
　　primary (PPH) and secondary (SPH) forms of, 167–168, 168*f*, 169, **194–195, 201, 209, 214**
　　radiographic findings of, 38*t*

Pulmonary hypertension, as differential dx
  for chest pain, 4t
  for dyspnea, 5, 5t
  for syncope, 103, 103b
Pulmonic insufficiency, murmur
  associated with, 11t
Pulmonic stenosis (PS), 7t, 11t, 12t
Pulse, assessment of, 9
Pulsus alternans, 9
Pulsus paradoxus, 9, 139, 143t
Pulsus parvus et tardus, 9, 118
P wave, 17–18, 18f

QRS complex, 17, 18, 18f, 19
QT interval, 18f, 20
Quincke pulses, associated with aortic
  insufficiency (AI), 119t
Q wave, pathologic, 19t
Q-wave MI. See ST-elevation MI
(STEMI)

Radiation, as cause of pericarditis, 137t
Radiofrequency ablation (RFA), 35–36,
  94, 96
Radionuclide ventriculography (RVG),
  38–39
Rales, 12
Raynaud phenomenon, 152
Reentrant arrhythmias, mechanisms,
  91–92, 92f
Reflex-mediated syncope, as differential
  dx for syncope, 103, 103b
Reiter syndrome, aortic aneurysms
  associated with, 154t
Restrictive cardiomyopathy (RCM), 85,
  87–88, 88f, 191–192, 207
Restrictive heart disease, as differential
  dx for dyspnea, 5t
Revascularization, 151
Reversible ischemic neurologic deficit
  (RIND), 160
Rheumatic carditis, 114–115
Rheumatic endocarditis, 114
Rheumatic fever (RF), 114–115, 115b,
  116, 196, 210–211
  as cause of myocarditis, 83
  criteria for diagnosis of, 115, 115b,
    116
  organs involved in, 114
  prevention of, 116
Rheumatoid arthritis
  aortic aneurysms associated with,
    154t
  as cause of pericarditis, 137t
Right anterior fascicle, 16f

Right atrium (RA) enlargement, 19t, 38t
Right-axis deviation, abnormal ECG
  associated with, 19t
Right bundle branch, 16f
Right bundle branch block (RBBB)
  abnormal ECG associated with, 19t,
    235f
  as complication of acute MI, 67t
  heart sounds associated with, 7
Right coronary artery (RCA), 42, 43f
Right-dominant circulation, 42
Right heart catheterization (RHC), 29,
  29f, 30, 30f, 31
Right-sided heart failure, 73–74, 74t
Right ventricular enlargement, 38t
Right ventricular hypertrophy (RVH),
  19t, 240f
Right ventricular infarction (RVI),
  65–66, 203, 216, 238f
Ross procedure, 132
Roth spots, associated with IE, 127b
RPA/reteplase, 61

Saddle embolus, 163
Sarcoidosis, as cause of pericarditis, 137t
Scleroderma, as cause of pericarditis,
  137t
Secondary hyperlipidemia, 46, 49b
Secondary hypertension, 146
Secondary pulmonary hypertension
  (SPH), 167–168, 168f, 169, 201, 214
Seizure, as differential dx for syncope,
  103, 103b
Sepsis, hemodynamic profiles of, 31t,
  195, 210
Septal myomectomy, 87
Septic thromboembolism, as differential
  dx for IE, 126
Serum markers of myocardial injury, 56f
Shear stress, 43
Sick sinus syndrome (SSS), 100–101
Sick sinus syndrome (SSS), as differential
  dx for syncope, 103, 103b
Single tilting disc heart valves, 130, 130f,
  132
Sinoatrial (SA) node, 16, 16f, 90
Sinus arrhythmia, 226f
Sinus bradycardia, 67t, 100, 225f
Sinus node dysfunction (SND), 100,
  100f, 101
Sinus tachycardia, 67t, 95, 225f
Sinus venosus defects, 176, 176f, 177, 177t
Situational syncope, as differential dx for
  syncope, 103, 103b

Smoking, TAO associated with, 152–153,
  190, 206
Splenomegaly, associated with IE, 126
Splinter hemorrhages, associated with IE,
  127b
Spondyloarthropathy, aortic aneurysms
  associated with, 154t
Spontaneous pneumothorax, as
  differential dx for chest pain, 3, 4t
St. Vitus dance, associated with
  rheumatic fever, 115
Stable angina, 2
Stanford class of aortic dissection, 156f
Staphylococcus aureus, as cause of IE,
  126b, 198
Staphylococcus epidermis, as cause of IE,
  126b
"Statins," 49t, 50, 245
ST-elevation myocardial infarction
  (STEMI), 55, 59–60, 60f, 61, 61b, 62f,
  63, 202, 215, 238f
  acute and post-MI treatment of,
    59–61, 62f, 63
  ECG changes with, 59, 60f, 193,
    193f, 200, 201f, 208, 214, 238f
Streptococcus, rheumatic strains of, 114
Streptococcus bovis, as cause of IE, 126,
  193, 208
Streptococcus spp.
  as cause of IE, 126b
  as cause of pericarditis, 137t
Streptococcus viridans, as cause of IE,
  126b, 195, 209
Streptokinase, 61
Stress testing
  indications/contraindications for, 21,
    21t
  interpreting exercise ECG testing,
    24, 24f, 25
  METs attained during, 23, 23t
  monitoring modalities of, 22, 22f,
    23–24, 24t
  testing modalities of, 21–23, 23f,
    24t, 189–190, 205
  in women, 25
Stroke, 160
Stroke volume (SV), 71, 71f
ST segment, 18f, 19, 24, 24f
Subacute bacterial endocarditis (SBE),
  126, 190, 206
Substance use/abuse, as differential dx
  for palpitations, 7t
Sudden cardiac death (SCD), 68, 95, 97,
  107–108, 108f, 109
  cardiac causes of, 107, 108t
  managing survivors of, 108–109

Sudden infant death syndrome (SIDS), 107

Supraventricular tachycardia (SVT), as complication of acute MI, 67t

Supraventricular tachycardia (SVT), as differential dx
    for palpitations, 7, 7t
    for syncope, 103, 103b

Sydenham chorea, associated with rheumatic fever, 114, 115

Sympathomimetic agents, as differential dx for palpitations, 7t

Syncope, 103–104, 104b/t, 105, 105t, 106, **189, 205**
    diagnostic modalities for, 105, 105t
    differential dx of, 103, 104b
    historic features and causes of, 104, 104t
    treatment of specific causes of, 105t, 106

Syphilis, aortic aneurysms associated with, 154t

Systemic lupus erythematosus (SLE), as cause of pericarditis, 137t, **191, 207**

Systemic vascular resistance (SVR), 70t, 71, 71f, 72

Systolic blood pressure (SBP), 71

Systolic dysfunction, 72

Systolic heart failure, 73–74, 74t, 78, 78f, 79, 79f/t, 80, 80t, 81, 81f

Systolic murmurs, differential dx for, 12t

Tachyarrhythmias
    atrial fibrillation (AF), 95, 95f, 96, **204, 217**
    atrial flutter, 96, 96f
    atrioventricular reentrant tachycardia (AVRT), 97, 97f
    AV-nodal reentrant tachycardia (AVNRT), 96, 96f, 97, **196, 196f, 210**, 229f
    as differential dx for palpitations, 7, 7t
    differential dx of, 93–94, 94t
    differentiating wide-complex tachycardias in, 98
    ectopic atrial tachycardia in, 95
    mechanisms of, 90t, 91–92, 92f
    multifocal atrial tachycardia (MAT), 95, 95f, 228f
    QRS morphology (narrow vs. wide complex) of, 94t, 98
    sinus tachycardia, 95
    treatment of, 94–95
    ventricular tachycardia (VT), 97, 97f, 98, 98f, 231f

Tachy-brady syndrome, 100f, 101

Takayasu arteritis
    aortic aneurysms associated with, 154t
    as cause of aortitis, 159

"Tet fits," 179

Tetralogy of Fallot (TOF), 176f, 178–179

Therapeutic lifestyle changes (TLC), 50

Three-dimensional (3D) echocardiography, 27

Thromboangiitis obliterans (TAO), 152–153, **190, 206**

Thrombolytic therapy, 60
    agents for, 60–61
    criteria for, 60–61, 61b

Thrombophlebitis, 163

Thyrotoxicosis, as differential dx for palpitations, 7t, 8

Tilt-table testing, 34–35, 35f

Tissue plasminogen activator (TPA), 43

TNK-TPA/tentecteplase, 61

Torsades de pointes, 97–98, 98f, 108, 231f

Toxins, as cause of myocarditis, 83

Transesophageal echocardiography (TEE), 26, 27

Transient ischemic attack (TIA), 160, **200, 213**

Transmural myocardial infarction. See ST-elevation myocardial infarction (STEMI)

Transplantation. See Cardiac transplantation

Transthoracic echocardiography (TTE), 26, 27, **190, 206**

Trauma
    as cause of pericarditis, 137t
    nonpenetrating and penetrating cardiac injuries, 184, 184b, 185, 186

Tricuspid regurgitation (TR), murmur associated with, 11t, 12t

Tricuspid valve, disease associated with rheumatic fever, 115

Triglycerides (TG), 46, 47f/t

True aneurysms, 68

Trypanosoma cruzi, as cause of myocarditis, 83

Tuberculosis (TB)
    aortic aneurysms associated with, 154t
    as cause of constrictive pericarditis, 142, 142t
    as cause of pericarditis, 137, 137t

Tumors of the heart, 187, 187b, 188, 188f

T wave, 18f, 19–20

Two-dimensional (2D) echocardiography, 26, 26f, 27

Ultrafast CT, 39, 39f

Unstable angina (UA), 55–56, 56f, 57, 57b, 58, **190, 194, 196–197, 198, 198f, 206, 208, 211, 212**
    as differential dx for chest pain, 2, 3, 4t
    ECG changes with, 56f, 198, 198f, **212**
    risk categories of, 57b

Uremia, as cause of pericarditis, 137t

Vagal maneuvers, 94

Valsalva maneuver, 94

Valve degeneration, 132

Valve thrombosis, 132

Valvular heart disease
    pregnancy and, 182
    See also Aortic valve disorders; Infective endocarditis; Mitral valve disorders; Prosthetic heart valves; Rheumatic fever

Valvular heart disease, as differential dx
    for cardiomyopathy, 88
    for dyspnea, 5, 5t
    for palpitations, 7, 7t

Valvular stenosis, associated with rheumatic fever, 115

Valvulitis, 114

Variant angina, 53–54

Vascular diseases, 145–169
    See also Aorta, diseases of; Carotid arterial disease; Deep venous thrombosis (DVT); Hypertension (HTN); Peripheral arterial disorders; Pulmonary embolic disease; Pulmonary hypertension

Vascular endothelium
    dysfunction of, 43–44

Vasculitis, aortic aneurysms associated with, 154t

Vasodepressor response, as differential dx for syncope, 103, 103b

Vasodilation, as differential dx for syncope, 103, 103b

Vasodilators, 245

Vasodilators, as differential dx for palpitations, 7t

Vasopressors, 245

Vasovagal syncope, 34–35, 35f, **189, 205**

Vasovagal syncope, as differential dx for syncope, 103, 103b, **189, 205**

Venous embolus, as complication of acute MI, 68

Venous insufficiency, as differential dx for DVT, 164

Venous stasis, as differential dx for right-sided HF, 77

Venous thromboembolism (VTE), 163–164, 164*b/f*, 165–166, 166*b*

Ventricular aneurysms, as complication of acute MI, 68

Ventricular assist devices (VADs), 81

Ventricular dysfunction, heart sounds associated with, 10*t*

Ventricular fibrillation (VF), 67*t*, 232*f*

Ventricular free-wall rupture, as complication of MI, 66, 66*f/t*

Ventricular premature beats, as complication of acute MI, 67*t*

Ventricular premature complex (VPC), 230*f*

Ventricular septal defect (VSD), 38*t*
  as complication of MI, 66, 66*f/t*
  membranous or muscular VSDs, 176
  murmur associated with, 11*t*, 12*t*

Ventricular tachycardia (VT), 97, 97*f*, 98, 98*f*, 231*f*
  as complication of acute MI, 67*t*
  RF ablation therapy of, 36

Ventricular tachycardia (VT), as differential dx
  for palpitations, 7, 7*t*
  for syncope, 103, 103*b*

Ventriculography, 31–32

Vertebrobasilar insufficiency, as differential dx for syncope, 103, 103*b*

Very low density lipoproteins (VLDL), 46, 47*f/t*

Viral pericarditis, 136, 137*t*, **189, 205**

Virchow triad, 163

Volume overload, heart sounds associated with, 10*t*

Water-hammer pulse, 9

Watterson shunt, 179

Wegener granulomatosis, as cause of pericarditis, 137*t*

Wenckebach type heart block, 101, 101*f*, 102

Wheezing, 12

Wolff-Parkinson-White (WPW) syndrome, 35, 97, 97*f*, 236*f*

Xenograft heart valves, 130, 130*f*, **202, 215**

NOTES

Additional praise for Blueprints *Cardiology*, 2nd edition

"I read the original edition cover to cover during my cardiology rotation as a med student, and definitely would recommend this book to others on cardiology or internal medicine."

—Vivian Yu, MD, Resident, University of Minnesota—Minneapolis

"The overall strength of the Blueprints texts is the simplistic and basic style that the books have. I found using Blueprints really gave me a good solid foundation during my third year that I was able to build upon later. The material covered by Blueprints is also consistent with what is seen on board and shelf exams."

—Sarah Davis, 4th year student, Drexel University College of Medicine

"These chapters provide an excellent introduction to the topics they cover. The use of imaging such as echos, chest x-rays, and CT scans make the chapters more interesting and help in understanding what will be encountered on the wards. The management and treatment sections are generally very strong. They really help lay out all the options and when they are appropriate for each disease. . . . I would recommend this book to third year and especially fourth year students. Students on internal medicine rotations would definitely benefit from this book if they use it as a quick reference."

—Simin Bahrami, 4th year student, David Geffen School of Medicine at UCLA

"I found that the Q&A section is right on target for Step 2 prep. The questions are the appropriate length and the appropriate level. These questions were much better than Qbank, which I just used before taking Step 2. The answer sets were also terrific and extraordinarily useful for reinforcing the material learned in the book as well as prep for Step 2 or a medicine shelf exam."

—Larissa Lee, 4th year student, Harvard Medical School

"I like the Key Points sections the best. They always pull out the most important 3 or 4 points and present them again, in case the student missed them. This is essential for wards reading."

—Jaspal Singh Ahluwalia, 3rd year student, Ohio State University